Seminars in Practical
Forensic Psychiatry

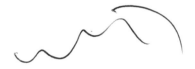

College Seminars Series

Series Editors

Professor Hugh Freeman, Honorary Professor, University of Salford, and Honorary Consultant Psychiatrist, Salford Health Authority

Dr Ian Pullen, Consultant Psychiatrist, Dingleton Hospital, Melrose, Roxburghshire

Dr George Stein, Consultant Psychiatrist, Farnborough Hospital, and King's College Hospital

Professor Greg Wilkinson, Editor, *British Journal of Psychiatry*, and Professor of Liaison Psychiatry, University of Liverpool

Other books in the series

Seminars in Alcohol and Drug Misuse. Edited by Jonathan Chick & Roch Cantwell

Seminars in Basic Neurosciences. Edited by Gethin Morgan & Stuart Butler

Seminars in Child and Adolescent Psychiatry. Edited by Dora Black & David Cottrell

Seminars in Clinical Psychopharmacology. Edited by David King

Seminars in General Adult Psychiatry. Edited by George Stein & Greg Wilkinson

Seminars in Liaison Psychiatry. Edited by Elspeth Guthrie & Francis Creed

Seminars in Psychiatric Genetics. By Peter McGuffin, Michael J. Owen, Michael C. O'Donovan, Anita Thapar & Irving Gottesman

Seminars in the Psychiatry of Learning Disabilities. Edited by Oliver Russell

Seminars in Psychology and the Social Sciences. Edited by Digby Tantam & Max Birchwood

Seminars in Psychosexual Disorders. Series editors: Hugh Freeman, Ian Pullen, George Stein & Greg Wilkinson

Seminars in Old Age Psychiatry. Edited by: Rob Butler & Brice Pitt

Forthcoming titles

Seminars in Psychotherapy. Edited by Sandra Grant & Jane Naismith

Seminars in Practical Forensic Psychiatry

Edited by
Derek Chiswick & Rosemarie Cope

GASKELL

British Library Cataloguing-in-Publication Data
A catalogue record for this book is available from the British Library.

ISBN 0-902241-78-8

Distributed in North America
by American Psychiatric Press, Inc.
ISBN 0-88048-637-6

TC00841

Gaskell is an imprint of the Royal College of Psychiatrists,
17 Belgrave Square, London SW1X 8PG
The Royal College of Psychiatrists is a registered charity, number 228636

Printed by Bell & Bain Ltd, Thornliebank, Glasgow

Contents

Contributors

Professor Robert Bluglass, Professor of Forensic Psychiatry, University of Birmingham; Clinical Director and Consultant, Reaside Clinic, Bristol Road South, Rubery, Rednal, Birmingham B45 9BE

Dr Paul Bowden, Consultant Forensic Psychiatrist at Bethlem and Maudsley NHS Trust, Denmark Hill, London SE5 8AZ, and to the Home Office at HM Prison, Brixton

Dr Fred Browne, Consultant Forensic Psychiatrist, Knockbracken Healthcare Park, Belfast

Dr Derek Chiswick, Consultant Forensic Psychiatrist, Affleck Centre, Royal Edinburgh Hospital, Morningside Place, Edinburgh EH10 5HF; Honorary Senior Lecturer in Psychiatry, University of Edinburgh

Dr Rosemarie Cope, Consultant Forensic Psychiatrist, Reaside Clinic, Bristol Road South, Rubery, Rednal, Birmingham B45 9DE; Senior Clinical Lecturer in Forensic Psychiatry, University of Birmingham

Dr Christopher Cordess, Consultant Forensic Psychiatrist, North West Thames Forensic Psychiatry Service, 304 Westbourne Grove, London W11 2PS

Dr Enda Dooley, Director of Prison Medical Services, Department of Justice, Dublin, Ireland

Dr Adrian Grounds, University Lecturer in Forensic Psychiatry, Institute of Criminology, 7 West Road, Cambridge CB3 9DT, and Department of Psychiatry, University of Cambridge; Honorary Consultant Forensic Psychiatrist, Addenbrooke's NHS Trust, Cambridge

Dr James Higgins, Consultant Forensic Psychiatrist, Scott Clinic, Rainhill Hospital, Prescott, Liverpool L35 4PQ

Dr Martin Humphreys, Lecturer in Forensic Psychiatry, University of Edinburgh

Dr Peter Snowden, Consultant Forensic Psychiatrist, Edenfield Centre, Prestwich Hospital, Bury New Road, Prestwich, Manchester M25 7BL; Honorary Clinical Lecturer in Forensic Psychiatry, University of Manchester

Foreword

Every psychiatrist should be competent to deal with those patients who are referred by the police, courts, prisons or secure hospitals. Such work forms a significant part of the general psychiatrist's working week. All psychiatrists therefore need to acquire theoretical knowledge and practical skills in forensic psychiatry. The subject, in theory and practice, draws on a number of disciplines. It is firmly rooted in the medical science of psychiatry, but also requires some knowledge of criminology, the law, criminal justice, public policy, institutional dynamics, ethics, and the organisation of services for mentally disordered offenders. Psychiatrists have difficulty in locating information on these diverse topics at a level appropriate to their needs. We hope that in the 12 chapters that follow they will find the information they require.

Forensic psychiatry is a clinical speciality and our contributors have written from a practical perspective. Learning in forensic psychiatry requires wide clinical experience and *Practical Forensic Psychiatry* should supplement that experience. Clinical aspects of forensic psychiatry are similar throughout the UK and Ireland, but the law and forensic psychiatry services have geographical differences. Therefore we have included addenda, and made reference where appropriate, concerning the distinctive features of the law and services in Scotland, Northern Ireland and the Republic of Ireland. Fred Browne, Enda Dooley and one of us (DC) have provided all these "international" contributions.

We are very grateful to our contributors for their chapters. The staff of the Publications department of the Royal College of Psychiatrists have been extremely helpful, and we particularly thank their anonymous assessors for their valuable comments. Finally, our thanks to Michelle Casamassa, Charlotte Cope and Joyce Mackay who typed the script with skill and forbearance.

Derek Chiswick
Rosemarie Cope

1 Introduction
Derek Chiswick

*Evolution of forensic psychiatry • What do forensic psychiatrists do? •
Personal attributes • Training • Career opportunities*

Most trainees enjoy forensic psychiatry: and so they should. The patients,
the circumstances of their referral and the clinical settings in which the
subject is practised cannot fail to stimulate intellectual, clinical and
emotional curiosity. The scope of the subject is broad. All shades and
degrees of psychopathology are seen, although in institutional settings
patients with gross forms of mental illness or personality deviation are
overrepresented. Men outnumber women in any forensic psychiatrist's
case-load but, this apart, the specialty is no respecter of class, race or
creed.

For many, the particular fascination of the subject comes from two main
sources. Firstly, in the fabric of individual psychopathology are woven
complex social, environmental, cultural and familial threads which make
each patient, and the manner of his presentation, unique. Secondly, there
is nearly always a legal context to the examination and treatment of the
patient which provides an additional, sometimes daunting, dimension to
clinical practice. Mentally ill patients commonly present to the forensic
psychiatrist in the most dire and tragic circumstances. It is a challenging
but immensely satisfying task to make a sound assessment of such patients,
provide proper treatment and steer them through the ramifications of the
criminal justice system.

There is no official definition of forensic psychiatry. The Latin word
forensis was the forum or public place in ancient Rome for conducting
judicial business. In general terms the subject is concerned with the area
where psychiatry and the law meet. In practice, the meat of forensic
psychiatry is the clinical assessment and treatment of mentally disordered
offenders in a variety of settings and under a range of circumstances. Non-
offender patients suffering from severe mental disorder in association with
significant behavioural disturbance are also likely to be referred to forensic
psychiatry services for both advice and treatment. Within the range of
psychiatric populations, these latter patients, often with multiple
psychopathology, are among the most disturbed and difficult to manage.
In addition, forensic psychiatrists should be knowledgable in the
application of the law to clinical practice; they should be skilled in
presenting relevant psychiatric information and conclusions to various
legal and statutory agencies. Forensic psychiatry is a developing specialty;

some appreciation of its evolution is necessary for a full understanding of current practice.

Evolution of forensic psychiatry

The last decade has seen major expansion in the field of forensic psychiatry in England and Wales. The specialty barely existed before the 1970s, although certain practitioners had already made important contributions to the subject. Historically, 'forensic psychiatrist' was the title given to those doctors who regularly gave expert psychiatric evidence in the criminal courts; many acquired fame by their involvement in the dramatic hanging trials of the pre- and post-war years. At the same time, there were calls to provide treatment for juvenile delinquents, either within prisons or in the community.

The only designated facilities then for treatment outside ordinary psychiatric hospitals were the three special hospitals in England (Broadmoor, Moss Side and Rampton), and the State Hospital at Carstairs in Scotland. These institutions, all with their administrative origins closer to the prison service than the health service, were chronically overcrowded and generally uncongenial. With some notable exceptions they often had difficulty in attracting staff of high calibre.

The 1960s saw the establishment of two out-patient forensic clinics. The first, the Douglas Inch Centre in Glasgow, was initially developed for delinquents and sex offenders. The Midland Centre for Forensic Psychiatry in Birmingham provided assessment and treatment for a wider range of offenders. By the early 1970s, apart from the special hospital consultants, there were a handful of forensic psychiatrists in Britain; most held joint appointments between psychiatric hospitals (within the National Health Service) and prisons (the responsibility of the Home Office). These posts were not entirely successful; indeed, their failure was one facet of the general problem of securing appropriate psychiatric care for mentally disordered patients in the criminal justice system. Not for the first time in forensic psychiatry, crisis and scandal were to prove decisive factors in precipitating change.

Through the 1960s and 1970s, periodic complaints about conditions for mentally disordered offenders became a persistent clamour that touched political nerves. In the public's mind, unlocking the mental hospital doors had become associated with an increase in disturbed and violent psychiatric patients on the streets. Simultaneously, the prison service drew attention to the increasing numbers of inmates with mental disorders, for whom prison medical staff were unable to obtain psychiatric hospital treatment. Meanwhile, overcrowding in Broadmoor Hospital, although of little interest to the public, had reached intolerable and dangerous proportions. In 1974 the Glancy Report (Department of Health and Social

Security, 1974) recommended that each regional health authority should develop secure hospital facilities for psychiatric patients who could not be managed in open conditions, but who did not require treatment in special hospitals. Glancy suggested 1000 beds would be necessary in England and Wales.

Butler Report

If a final event was needed to spur the government to action, it was provided by a young man named Graham Young. In 1962, Young (then aged 14) had been committed to Broadmoor Hospital after conviction for the attempted poisoning of three victims. He was conditionally discharged after nine years, only to obtain a job in a laboratory. Within months of his discharge he murdered two workmates by poisoning. His court appearance and conviction provoked intense public reaction, and once again placed mentally disordered offenders in the public and political domain. The government appointed a committee under the chairmanship of the late Lord Butler of Saffron Walden to look at the problems of mentally abnormal offenders.

Lord Butler and his distinguished committee produced a report (Home Office & Department of Health and Social Security, 1975) which was to prove decisive in the development of forensic psychiatry in England and Wales (it had no remit and therefore no effect in Scotland or Northern Ireland). The report covered all aspects of the legal provisions, facilities for assessment and treatment, and court disposals relating to mentally abnormal offenders. Sadly, much of the report has not been implemented by successive governments, but one major aspect has. Butler recommended the establishment of a secure unit in each of the regional health authorities of England and Wales. This would function as the hub of a comprehensive regional forensic psychiatric service linking with the special hospitals, ordinary psychiatric facilities, the prison medical service and the probation service. The development of the secure unit programme has been slow (see Chapter 7) but now each health authority in England and Wales has a regional secure unit and a forensic psychiatry service in varying degrees of sophistication and development. More than half of the 90 consultant forensic psychiatrists in Britain are based in regional secure units and their services.

Reed Report and *Health of the Nation*

The development of regional secure units and the expansion of services in forensic psychiatry have been insufficient to deal with current problems in relation to mentally disordered offenders. Difficulties have been identified in the community, in prisons, in general psychiatry services, in the newly established regional secure units, and in the special hospitals.

During a period of reorganisation and severe cash limiting in local authorities and in health services, the needs of mentally disordered offenders have been neglected. Failure to provide adequate services for the chronically mentally ill results in such patients coming to the attention of the police and entering the criminal justice system. Usually this is by virtue of a minor offence, such as a breach of the peace or damage to property, but sometimes the offence may be more serious.

In practice, inadequacy of services reveal themselves in many ways. At the point of arrest, police are required to deal with offenders whose presentation results from illness and who should more properly be dealt with by health and social services. Lack of alternatives, particularly for homeless mentally disordered offenders, results in the remand of defendants into prison for preparation of a psychiatric report. Facilities in prisons for managing both remanded and sentenced prisoners with a mental disorder are inadequate; those who are disturbed or suicidal are often locked up for long periods in bare, insanitary strip cells. There may be difficulties and long delays in obtaining a bed in a local psychiatric service for an offender patient. Waiting lists for entry to regional secure units have become common, and such units do not provide long-term care for chronically ill patients who require continuing care in secure conditions. Patients in special hospitals awaiting transfer to regional secure units may be similarly trapped in a queue for beds.

In the light of these and other problems, a joint committee of the Department of Health and the Home Office, under the chairmanship of Dr John Reed, was established in 1990. Its deliberations, known as the Reed Report (Department of Health & Home Office, 1992), have been published and are considered in Chapter 7. Reed emphasises the principle that the needs of mentally disordered offenders should be met by health and social services and not by the criminal justice system. Initiatives and developments have been recommended across a range of services. Early indications are that the government recognises the importance of extra services and the requirement for new funding.

The seriousness of the government's intentions on services for mentally disordered offenders is also revealed in its important document, *Health of the Nation* (Department of Health, 1992a; Jenkins, 1994). Mental illness is recognised as one of five priority areas for improvement, and the document emphasises the need "to ensure that mentally disordered offenders who need specialist health and social care are diverted from the criminal justice system as early as possible".

In Scotland, Northern Ireland and the Republic of Ireland, services in forensic psychiatry have not developed as they have in England and Wales (see Chapter 7). They have no regional secure units; in-patient services are provided by local intensive psychiatric care units, and by the State Hospital, Carstairs (for Scotland and Northern Ireland), and the Central Mental Hospital, Dundrum (for the Republic of Ireland).

What do forensic psychiatrists do?

Forensic psychiatrists assess and treat a wide range of patients in various clinical settings. Sometimes they function essentially on their own, at other times as part of a clinical team with colleagues of other disciplines. It is convenient, although the distinction is often blurred, to consider separately the work carried out in an in-patient setting from that done elsewhere.

In-patients

This takes place in a special hospital, regional secure unit, intensive psychiatric care unit, or in a conventional psychiatric ward or hospital. In addition, there are approximately 600 beds in secure provision within the private sector. Almost invariably the patients are detained under civil or criminal compulsory measures. The forensic psychiatrist may care for these patients at the initial stage of their presentation to the psychiatric services (e.g. while remanded in hospital after being arrested and charged with a crime), or while detained under a hospital order, or at any other stage during the patient's psychiatric career (e.g. in the course of a difficult-to-treat chronic psychosis).

A clinical team with multidisciplinary staffing will exist at varying degrees of sophistication and depth in forensic psychiatry in-patient units. Its description on paper is not a guarantee that it functions in practice. In theory, the multidisciplinary team should be well developed in special hospitals and regional secure units, since these are likely to have more staff from a wider range of professions than is found in ordinary psychiatric units. Sometimes, however, institutional factors can disrupt effective interdisciplinary working. This has been a particular problem in the special hospitals (NHS Health Advisory Service & DHSS Social Services Inspectorate, 1988; Department of Health, 1992*b*).

Is the work of a forensic psychiatrist with in-patients any different from the conventional work of a general psychiatrist? In essence the work is similar. Proper diagnosis is followed by appropriate treatment during which clinical progress is carefully monitored. As elsewhere, diagnosis depends on history-taking, mental state examination and obtaining information from other sources. As for treatments, these are similar to those used in general psychiatry. What is different is the invariable need to give careful thought to any dangerous implications of the patient's mental condition and to provide safeguards for the patient, fellow patients, staff and general public. Thus there is concern in forensic units with matters that can loosely be called 'security'; how these concerns are practically implemented is a finely balanced art. There must be careful consideration of the degree of supervision incorporated into a patient's care, but also for other matters. Crucially, there must be due regard for formulating the conditions under which a patient may or may not leave the hospital, unit, or even a ward.

Of course, these issues are familiar in general psychiatry, but in forensic psychiatry they are of daily and constant importance (see Chapter 7).

Other settings

Patients are seen in out-patient clinics, prisons or in other settings for a variety of reasons. Most have had previous contact with psychiatric services; the most common disorders seen are schizophrenia, personality disorder and substance abuse (Mendelson, 1992). The majority are seen for a psychiatric report to a court, solicitor or to the probation service. Other patients will be referred with a view to admission. These may be patients with their first episode of illness, or those for whom a change in the location of treatment is under consideration (e.g. from ordinary psychiatric ward to regional secure unit, or from special hospital to regional secure unit). Finally, some patients are referred from general practitioners, consultant colleagues or other agencies for advice or treatment. Forensic psychiatrists provide treatment in the community for a range of patients including those for whom in-patient care is not necessary, and others who are being followed up after a period of in-patient care. High standards of care for patients after discharge are crucial in preventing dangerous behaviour.

Some forensic psychiatrists provide a consultative service to probation officers, whereby the latter can obtain psychiatric advice in respect of clients who appear to have mental health problems. Out-patient psycho-therapeutic groups, usually for sex offenders, run jointly by psychiatrists and probation officers have also been described.

Work in prisons

Most prisons use the services of visiting psychiatrists, although these are not always forensic psychiatrists. The work of psychiatrists in prison is of three main types (see Chapter 9). Firstly, there is the assessment of prisoners at the request of the prison medical officer; these may be remanded or sentenced prisoners. The remanded prison population is likely to contain a significant number of mentally ill prisoners. Work with convicted prisoners may involve longer-term treatment of mentally ill and personality disordered prisoners, depending on the nature of the mental condition and the type of prison. Secondly, there may be requests from the prison governor to examine sentenced prisoners who present particular problems in manage-ment. Thirdly, there is the provision of statutory reports on prisoners eligible for early release on parole. In summary, in addition to the provision of court and statutory reports, the forensic psychiatrist in prison is likely to carry out short-term crisis work and medium or longer-term support of prisoners with chronic illness and personality disorders. Some may undertake psychotherapeutic work with selected offenders.

Other clinical work

The work outlined above indicates the principal tasks of forensic psychiatrists. Some develop other skills and pursue special interests.

Violence clinics

The presentation to medical agencies of patients with problems of violence has led to the development of so-called violence clinics. These are usually run in conjunction with clinical psychologists and require an eclectic approach, sometimes using techniques of anger management.

Analytically-based forensic psychiatry

A small number of psychoanalysts take a particular interest in forensic patients with problems of sexual deviance. The Portman Clinic in London has established expertise in this subject.

Therapeutic work with victims

The psychiatric sequelae for victims of violent and sexual crime are well recognised, and some forensic psychiatrists have special skills in the treatment of such patients.

Civil litigation

Some forensic psychiatrists acquire distinguished reputations as expert witnesses in civil litigation where there is a mental element in the case. These may include actions for compensation after injury, claims for medical negligence, disputes concerning custody of (and access to) children in divorce cases, and disputed wills. The consultant must guard against this work swamping his clinical practice. Much is carried out by general psychiatrists.

Personal attributes

Not every psychiatrist will want to be a forensic psychiatrist. Some psychiatrists have misguided notions of what forensic psychiatrists do, imagining, for example, that most time is spent in court or in examination of serial killers. Others may understand the tasks, but are simply not cut out to be forensic psychiatrists; perhaps they do not enjoy the work or they find prison or court work unpleasant. Certain attributes are necessary for a successful and satisfying career in forensic psychiatry (see Box 1.1).

Box 1.1 Eight personal attributes for a forensic psychiatrist

Good clinical skills
Natural curiosity
Tolerance for difficult patients
Balanced attitudes towards offenders
Clear thinking and clear speaking
Attention to detail
Capacity to lead a clinical team
Good self-organisation and energy

---

(1) *Good clinical skills* are a prerequisite. Sound experience in general psychiatry and good diagnostic skills across the whole range of psychiatric disorders are essential. Mistaken diagnoses, or previously unrecognised features of serious psychiatric illness, are commonly found in patients who present to a forensic psychiatry service. The capacity to take a fresh look at a patient with a chronic disorder, and an ability to recognise where previous treatment may have been inadequate or inappropriate, are frequently required.

(2) *A natural curiosity* about unusual behaviour and a willingness to examine it in a multidimensional manner is important. In addition to clinical knowledge and acumen, an understanding of dynamic, social, criminological and institutional factors is required. One or more of these will nearly always be relevant in any assessment.

(3) It is important to develop *tolerance* for difficult patients. Many patients do not (at least initially) accept the need for treatment. Even more have chronic or recurrent disorders. The forensic psychiatrist must learn to accept the short-term problems in treating patients with long-term disorders.

(4) *Appropriate attitudes* are needed to avoid compromising clinical appraisal. The forensic psychiatrist must free himself of moralistic judgements, and always seek to be balanced in approach. A capacity to accept, without condoning, antisocial behaviour is a virtue. It is vital not to allow emotional attitudes to interfere with clinical judgement. It is equally important to avoid dismissive attitudes in relation to violent acts carried out by patients. The forensic psychiatrist, in carrying out assessments and in report-writing, must maintain a professional, balanced and sensible approach. Anything short of this is immediately apparent and diminishes the status of the assessment or report.

(5) *Clarity of thought*, together with *clarity of expression* (written and oral) are essential. Sorting the tangled issues in a forensic case requires clear

thinking. Making oneself understood to non-medical personnel is a skill. It is particularly important in the preparation of court reports (see Chapter 6) where muddled reports usually result from muddled thinking.

(6) *Thoroughness and attention to detail* must be cultivated. Careful reading of additional information (e.g. old case notes) is often essential. Sometimes it requires an effort of will to obtain such documents, but persistence in this task will invariably produce a more thorough and sound assessment. The statements of witnesses and reports from other professionals require detailed perusal in the assessment of a forensic patient. Allocating sufficient time, usually at home in the evenings, for this task is important.

(7) *Willingness to adopt a leadership role* in a clinical team is necessary. Coupled with this is the capacity to cope with unpopularity among psychiatric colleagues. Forensic psychiatrists will find themselves, on occasions, having to say "no" to colleagues perhaps with regard to the transfer of a patient. Courteous determination is necessary, while short-term unpopularity must be tolerated.

(8) Forensic psychiatrists need to be *well organised and energetic*. The working week is full of deadlines (e.g. for delivery of reports) which must be respected. Sometimes patients must be seen at short notice, and a willingness to respond to emergencies is vital. Frequently the forensic psychiatrist will need to travel many miles to see a patient. It can be an exhausting exercise and not all psychiatrists cope with, for example, a 300-mile round trip and a careful clinical examination all in the same day. A tolerance for driving, a reliable car (preferably with a good radio!) and a preparedness to "get up and go" are all important.

Training

Arrangements for specialist training will be modified in light of the Calman Report (Department of Health, 1993; Caldicott, 1993); in psychiatry, a single training grade post to replace those of senior house officer and registrar seems likely. Specialist training over six years will be possible, rather than seven years. The description below is based on current training requirements.

The apprenticeship experience provided by general professional training in psychiatry is essential. There is no placement within a rotational training scheme that does not have relevance for the trainee aspiring to a specialist career in forensic psychiatry. A thorough grounding in general psychiatry, including the continuing management of patients with chronic disorders, is essential. Few trainees can gain experience of the complete range of psychiatric services during their training, but placements in learning disability, child and adolescent psychiatry, substance misuse and the psychotherapies are likely to pay dividends.

Most trainees in psychiatry will deal with patients from a forensic source during their general professional training. Indeed, such experiences may stimulate interest in the subject. It is important to seize any opportunity to accompany a consultant on a visit to a prison, special hospital or regional secure unit. There may also be opportunities to attend court and hear psychiatrists giving evidence – it can be a chastening experience for those who give the evidence.

Some rotational training schemes include a formal placement in forensic psychiatry. This may provide clinical experience in an in-patient setting such as a special hospital, regional secure unit, or general psychiatry service with a special interest in offender and disturbed patients. It is ideal for a trainee to gain early experience of a forensic psychiatry service, rather than simply the management of in-patients (see Chapter 7). In this way a trainee is more likely to appreciate the range of clinical components and their interrelationships.

Higher professional training

After completing general professional training and obtaining membership of the Royal College of Psychiatrists, the trainee will be eligible to pursue higher professional training by obtaining a post at senior registrar grade. Full higher professional training currently extends over four years, and the Royal College of Psychiatrists recommends that appointments at consultant grade should not be made until a minimum of three years of higher training has been completed. The length of higher training required for consultant posts in forensic psychiatry is as follows:

Consultant in forensic psychiatry. Minimum three years of higher training in an approved forensic psychiatry training scheme.

Consultant with a special responsibility in forensic psychiatry. Minimum two years of higher training in forensic psychiatry and two years in general psychiatry. A consultant with a special responsibility is likely to have some involvement in the organisation of a sub-regional service in forensic psychiatry.

Consultant with a special interest in forensic psychiatry. One year of full-time higher training in forensic psychiatry and three years in general psychiatry. A consultant with a special interest is likely to have involvement in a district-based service.

There are separate requirements for consultant posts in child and adolescent forensic psychiatry.

Approximately 20 centres in the UK provide higher training in forensic psychiatry. They range from single-trainee posts to large schemes providing training for six or more senior registrars. All must satisfy the educational standards laid down by the Joint Committee on Higher Psychiatric Training; the latter body is jointly established by the Royal College of Psychiatrists and the Association of University Teachers of Psychiatry.

The Joint Committee on Higher Psychiatric Training (1995) identifies the basic knowledge and skills in forensic psychiatry which the properly trained senior registrar should possess. These are:

(1) Assessment
    (a) Assessment of behavioural abnormalities
    (b) Assessment of risk and dangerousness
    (c) Writing reports for courts and mental health review tribunals
(2) Knowledge
    (a) Mental health legislation and relevant criminal and civil law
    (b) The range of services for mentally disordered offenders and how to use them
    (c) Ability to give evidence in court
(3) Therapeutic skills
    (a) Understanding and using security as a means of control and treatment
    (b) The treatment of chronic disorders, especially where behavioural problems are exhibited, such as severe psychoses and personality disorders
    (c) Skills in psychological treatments for behaviour disorder (particularly psychotherapy)

A good training programme for the senior registrar in forensic psychiatry should provide experience in a range of settings for the assessment and treatment of mentally disordered offenders. These include hospitals (special security, medium security, intensive care and open ward), prisons (of the various types described in Chapter 9), and in the community (out-patient clinics, hostels, supported accommodation and probation services).

All general psychiatrists who have responsibility for a defined catchment area will be required to see mentally disordered offenders in the course of their work; indeed, the majority of mentally disordered offenders are treated by general, rather than by forensic, psychiatrists. Therefore all senior registrars in general psychiatry benefit from a placement in forensic psychiatry during their higher training.

Career opportunities

Taking into account retirement and anticipated expansion, there are expected to be 7.5 consultant opportunities per year in forensic psychiatry

(Allen, 1993) The Joint Planning Advisory Committee (JPAC) of the Department of Health announced in 1994 an increase in the national target figure from 40 to 60 for senior registrar posts in forensic psychiatry. In addition, full implementation of the Reed Report would require a significant expansion of posts in forensic (and general) psychiatry.

Reorganisation of the National Health Service, changes in the provision of health care within prisons and the Reed Report will provide new challenges for forensic psychiatry. Morale within the profession has been boosted by these developments and by governmental declarations of interest in, and concern for, mentally disordered offenders. Within the Royal College of Psychiatrists the forensic psychiatry section is active in overseeing the professional implications of the changes. In recent years, two major textbooks (Bluglass & Bowden, 1990; Gunn & Taylor, 1993) have appeared, and two journals have also been launched (*Journal of Forensic Psychiatry* and *Criminal Behaviour and Mental Health*). The chapters that follow are intended to provide an outline of essential knowledge in forensic psychiatry.

References

Allen, P. (1993) Medical and dental staffing prospects in the NHS in England and Wales 1991. *Health Trends*, **25**, 4–12.

Bluglass, R. & Bowden, P. (eds)(1990) *Principles and Practice of Forensic Psychiatry*. Edinburgh: Churchill Livingstone.

Caldicott, F. (1993) Response to the Chief Medical Officer's report on specialist training. *Bulletin of the Royal College of Psychiatrists*, **17**, 577–579.

Department of Health (1992*a*) *Health of the Nation*. Cm 1986. London: HMSO.

—— (1992*b*) *Report of the Committee of Inquiry into Complaints about Ashworth Hospital*. Vols I-II. Cm 2028-I-II. London: HMSO.

—— (1993) *Hospital Doctors: Training for the Future. Report of the Working Group on Specialist Medical Training* (Calman Report). London: DoH.

—— & Home Office (1992) *Review of Health and Social Services for Mentally Disordered Offenders and others requiring Similar Services* (Reed Report) Cm 2088. London: HMSO.

Department of Health and Social Security (1974) *Revised Report of the Working Party on Security in NHS Psychiatric Hospitals* (Glancy Report). London: DHSS.

Gunn, J. & Taylor, P. J. (eds)(1993) *Forensic Psychiatry: Clinical, Legal and Ethical Issues*. Oxford: Butterworth-Heinemann.

Home Office & Department of Health and Social Security (1975) *Report of the Committee on Mentally Abnormal Offenders* (Butler Report) Cmnd. 6244. London: HMSO.

Jenkins, R. (1994) The Health of the Nation: recent government policy and legislation. *Psychiatric Bulletin*, **18**, 324–327.

Joint Committee on Higher Psychiatric Training (1995) *Handbook* (7th edn). London: Royal College of Psychiatrists & Association of University Teachers of Psychiatry (in press).

Mendelson, E. F. (1992) A survey of practice at a regional forensic service: what do forensic psychiatrists do? I. Characteristics of cases and distribution of work. *British Journal of Psychiatry*, **160**, 769–772.

NHS Health Advisory Service & DHSS Social Services Inspectorate (1988) *Report of Services provided by Broadmoor Hospital*. London: DHSS.

2 Crime and mental disorder
I. Criminal behaviour
Christopher Cordess

Nature and classification of crime • Homicide • Other assaultive crimes • Sexual offences • Offences against property • Victimology

This chapter is about crime in general and the ways in which psychiatric pathology may be associated with specific crimes such as murder, sex offences and arson. The interrelationship between crime and mental disorder is complex. Most psychotic patients are neither criminal nor violent, most criminals are not mentally ill, and there is dispute about the association between psychiatric disorder and crime. Indeed, the proven association of crime is not with psychiatric disorder but with youth. Young males between 10 and 20 years of age account for approximately half of all recorded crime; the peak age for offending is in the age group 14–17 years. Such figures understate the actual level of juvenile crime because of the current policy of informal action (e.g. unrecorded cautioning of some offending juveniles). Few juvenile offenders will yet have attracted a psychiatric diagnosis. They will generally be a dispossessed group in emotional, social, economic and educational terms. A sizeable minority will go on to careers of recidivism (i.e. repeated offending) and some may develop psychiatric disorders. For others, juvenile offending may be a prodromal manifestation of later more obvious personality difficulties.

Nature and classification of crime

Crime is a man-made concept. It may be defined as an "act that is capable of being followed by criminal proceedings". The rules of the state define which acts are criminal, and at what age and in what situations people may be considered to have committed a crime. Currently in England and Wales, children under the age of 10 years are held not to be responsible. In Scotland, the age of criminal responsibility is 8 years. Some acts have been regarded as criminal at one time in history but not at another; for example, attempted suicide and suicide were decriminalised in the Suicide Act of 1961.

Measurement of crime

Criminal activity is measured in various ways, and an accurate assessment of the prevalence of crime is beset by methodological problems. The term 'notifiable offence' is used for recording crime for statistical purposes. Information about crime rates is recorded by official criminal statistics and self-report surveys.

Official criminal statistics

The Home Office publishes annual *Criminal Statistics* which consist of all notifiable crimes committed in England and Wales. Similar statistics are published in Scotland (Scottish Office, 1994), in the Republic of Ireland (Commissioner Garda Siochana, 1993) and in Northern Ireland (Northern Ireland Office, 1993).

However, they are not a measure of the true rate of criminal activity because of the extent of "hidden" crime (i.e. discretionary decisions by the police not to record crimes) and the amount of unreported and undetected crime. The *Criminal Statistics, England and Wales* (Home Office, 1993) recorded that there were 0.5 million indictable offences per year in the 1950s, rising to 1 million in the 1960s, 2 million in the 1970s, and over 5.6 million notifiable offences recorded in 1992; the numbers continue to rise. Although the prison population reached a peak of some 51 000 in 1988, there was a reduction over the years to 1991, when a rise in numbers began again.

Figure 2.1 shows notifiable offences recorded by the police by type of offence in 1992. The most common type of offence is acquisitive (property) offences, particularly those involving motor vehicles. Violent crime (including violence against the person, sexual offences and robbery) accounts for only 5% of the total. There has been a real increase in the number of recorded violent offences, rising from 63 000 in 1974 to 114 000 in 1984, and 284 000 in 1992. The increase is mainly in the various categories of assault rather than in homicide, which has increased at a slow but steady rate of some 10% each decade. Figure 2.2 shows crimes of violence recorded by the police in 1992.

In Scotland there has been a near three-fold increase in drugs offences between 1982 and 1992. In Ireland there has been a substantial rise in the number of sex offences reported and prosecuted. In Northern Ireland, as a consequence of "the Troubles", the homicide rate over the last ten years has been four to eight times that in England and Wales (Browne, 1992).

Self-report studies and population surveys

West & Farrington (1977) carried out a longitudinal self-report study in which they estimated the number of offences committed by Camberwell

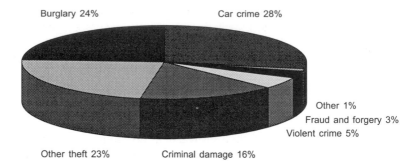

Burglary 24%   Car crime 28%

Other 1%
Fraud and forgery 3%
Violent crime 5%

Other theft 23%   Criminal damage 16%

Fig. 2.1 Notifiable offences recorded by the police in England and Wales in 1992 (Home Office, 1993) by type of offence (total no. 5 592 000).

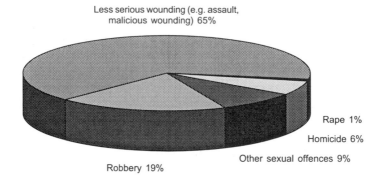

Less serious wounding (e.g. assault,
malicious wounding) 65%

Rape 1%

Homicide 6%

Other sexual offences 9%

Robbery 19%

Fig. 2.2 Violent crimes recorded by the police in England and Wales in 1992 (Home Office, 1993) by type of offence (total no. 284 000).

boys. They found that the real rate of offending was much higher than the official statistics suggest. For example, 80% of the boys in their study had committed an act which could have resulted in a court appearance by age 17, but only 20% had been caught. Females have traditionally been said to be much less criminal than males (see below).

The British Crime Surveys (Home Office Research Sudy, 1988, 1992) reported information from 11 000 households about their experiences of being victims of crime. They confirmed that the majority of offences were against property, particularly against vehicles. Violence and assault accounted for some 17% of incidents. Sexual offending emerged as less common than expected (1 rape among 6000 women) but this may have reflected reticence on the part of the subjects, or the effects of sampling.

Other recent surveys have found rape, for example, to be far more common (Koss *et al,* 1988). A large proportion of the crimes in these surveys had not been reported to the police. Reporting generally occurred because of a sense of the perceived seriousness of the offence or, for example, in the case of property offences, for insurance purposes. It was also confirmed that the police only record a proportion of crimes reported to them (e.g. 30% of property offences). The survey did confirm an overall rise in the crime rate (50% between 1981 and 1991) but a lesser rise than appears in the Home Office statistics, which show a near doubling of recorded crime over the same period. It seems likely, therefore, that there has been a real increase in the reporting of offences to the police and also the recording of offences by the police.

Female offenders

Women account for a relatively small proportion of recorded crime. In 1990, only 17% of those found guilty or convicted for indictable offences were women. Overall, the male to female ratio for recorded crime is approximately 5:1, but this ratio varies for different types of offences. Some crimes, for example, soliciting for prostitution, are committed mainly by women. Other offences, especially sexual crimes, but also burglary and violent crimes, are committed predominantly by men. Women are more likely to commit offences of theft (especially shoplifting) and fraud. Of the female population, 7% will have had a conviction for a serious offence by the age of 31, compared with 33% of males (Home Office, 1992). The age distribution of female offenders is similar to that of males, but with a secondary peak of middle-aged shoplifters.

There are two broad categories of explanatory theories accounting for this gender difference. The first relates to innate psychobiological differences; for example, that men are biologically more aggressive. The second relates to a variety of social influences. Whatever the explanation, there

---

Box 2.1 Female offenders

17% of known offenders are women

69% of convicted women (compared with 41% of men) are convicted for theft

Women commit fewer serious and violent crimes than men

Women form less than 4% of the prison population

Cautioning is the main disposal used for female offenders (half of female offenders, a third of males)

Women sentenced for indictable offences are more likely to receive a conditional or absolute discharge (34% female, 15% male) and more likely to be put on probation (19% female, 10% male)

has been a proportionately greater increase in crime in females than in males over the past two decades, especially in young women. Box 2.1 summarises some of the key characteristics of female offenders. The figures relate to 1990 (Home Office 1992).

Classification of crime

A criminal act is a complex episode of behaviour and usually depends on aspects of the offender, the victim and the general circumstances. In the discussion which follows, each category of crime will be considered separately, with particular emphasis on the ways in which a psychiatric disorder in the offender may be relevant. A conventional classification of crime is shown in Box 2.2.

Box 2.2 Classification of crime

Violent offences; from minor assault to homicide
Sexual offences; from indecent assault to rape
Robbery
Burglary
Theft and handling stolen goods
Fraud and forgery
Criminal damage; from minor property damage to arson

Homicide

Homicide is the general term for the killing of one human being by another. Box 2.3 shows how it is subdivided legally.

Murder

Homicide is said to be murder when the offender is of sound mind and discretion (over the age of 10 years), and had malice aforethought (i.e. the intent to cause death or grievous bodily harm). Intent is assumed if the offender was reckless as to the effects of his act, knowing that death or serious harm was a virtual certainty. There is a mandatory sentence for murder, namely life imprisonment; the court has no discretion.

Manslaughter

Homicide is said to be manslaughter when the circumstances, although unlawful, do not meet the full criteria for murder or where there are certain

---

Box 2.3 Legal classification of homicide

Lawful homicide including:
- justifiable killings (e.g. on behalf of the State)
- excusable homicide (e.g. an accident or reasonable mistake)

Unlawful homicide (in common law, "the unlawful killing of any reasonable creature in being and under the Queen's peace, the death following within a year and a day of the deed"). This includes:
- murder
- manslaughter
- killing of infants, which includes child destruction (the killing of a child before birth) and infanticide
- death by dangerous driving

---

mitigating factors. Thus an absence of intent to kill or cause grievous bodily harm would reduce the charge to manslaughter despite unlawful or negligent behaviour. Mitigating factors include:

(1) immediate severe provocation
(2) having an abnormality of mind ('diminished responsibility', Section 2 (1) of the Homicide Act 1957, sometimes referred to as "Section 2 manslaughter")
(3) where the homicide was part of a suicide pact (Section 4 (1) of the Homicide Act 1957).

Killing in self-defence, if accepted by a court, results in acquittal. The court has complete discretion in sentencing a person found guilty of manslaughter. The sentence may vary from absolute discharge to life imprisonment, a psychiatric disposal or a probation order.

Legal criteria for distinguishing murder from other forms of unlawful homicide apply in the Republic of Ireland and in Scotland. The statutory definition of murder in Ireland is broadly similar to that of England, and the crime of manslaughter covers homicides where there may be mitigating circumstances (Doolan, 1991). Diminished responsibility does not exist in Ireland. In Scotland there is no statutory definition of murder, and the Crown has wide discretion to prosecute for either murder or the lesser crime of culpable homicide (Gordon, 1978). Diminished responsibility is one of many factors that might reduce a charge of murder to one of culpable homicide. See Chapter 5 for further discussion of these matters. In Northern Ireland the distinction between murder and manslaughter is similar to that in England and Wales.

General aspects of homicide

Homicide, like most other crimes, is committed predominantly by men. The rate of homicide varies greatly from country to country, and widely between social groups in any one country. The US has one of the highest rates with some 140 homicides per million of population, varying from 12 per million in white middle-class rural communities, to several hundreds per million in deprived black urban communities. In Europe the rates are generally much lower. In England and Wales there has been a slow but steady increase in the homicide rate. There are now about 12 homicides per million of population (683 recorded homicides in 1992, Home Office, 1993). In Scotland (population 5 million) there have been approximately 100 homicides annually in recent years; more than half of them occur in the Strathclyde region. In the Irish Republic there were 42 homicides recorded in 1992, but there are rarely more than ten convictions annually for murder.

In British studies, the victim is known to the offender in approximately three-quarters of homicides; in half of the cases, the victim is related to the offender or is a lover, so that homicide can be said to be predominantly a domestic matter. Each year about 100 men and 25 women are convicted of killing their spouse or lover. About 15% of all victims of homicide are children, the commonest victims being children under one year. Males are generally at more risk than females. The killing of a parent is the rarest of intrafamilial homicide, accounting for less than 5% of all homicides annually. In the UK, matricide appears to be more common than patricide (Green, 1981), although this varies in other countries.

The commonest method of killing is by the use of a sharp instrument (41% in 1992). There is a gender difference for the next most common method; more female victims than male victims are killed by strangulation or asphyxiation. Male victims are more likely to be killed by striking, punching or kicking. The use of a blunt instrument accounts for some 12% of deaths in both sexes, and shooting for 10% overall. Killing by burning, drowning and poisoning make up the remainder.

Anger, jealousy, revenge and threat of separation are among the commonest precipitants and possible motives for unlawful homicide, often complicated by the disinhibiting effects of alcohol or, to a lesser extent, drugs. These factors are common to 'normal' and 'abnormal' homicides (see Box 2.4). Particularly common in the homicide of lovers or spouses is a history of an 'on–off' relationship which becomes provocative for both parties.

Psychiatric aspects of homicide of adults

Homicides may be regarded as 'normal' or 'abnormal' according to the psychiatric state of the offender (see Box 2.4). Psychiatric factors are more

---

Box 2.4 Psychiatric classification of homicides

'Normal' homicides:
- during the course of a crime
- for political reasons
- from "normal" emotions such as anger, jealousy or revenge

'Abnormal' homicides, where the offender has a psychiatric disorder which may include:
- psychosis – functional or organic
- neurosis – including affective disturbance
- personality disorder – including sexual psychopathy
- learning disability

---

often described in female than male homicide. Gibson (1975) found that 68% of female homicides were 'abnormal' (in that the offender was found insane, or convicted of infanticide or manslaughter on the grounds of diminished responsibility) compared with 28% of male homicides. Also, women were responsible for over a third of all the abnormal homicides, but only for 2% of normal homicides (in which the conviction was for murder). Thus men are almost exclusively responsible for 'normal' killing. The presence of a psychiatric disorder is a *clinical* issue, separate from the legal considerations relating to diminished responsibility and insanity (see Chapter 5).

This division is far from perfect; for example, 'normal' revenge may coincide with personality disorder or learning disability. Alcohol or drug intoxication may be present in any category: alternatively, a near delusional state (e.g. of jealousy or erotomania) may be present, alone or in, for example, cases of schizophrenia. The major psychiatric disorders, and the ways they might lead to violence, are described in Chapter 3. In forensic practice, neurotic and personality factors are commonly encountered in homicidal offenders, and some further comment is necessary.

It is often difficult to tease out components of depressive reaction, personality disorder and factors of stress within this group. There is frequently clinical dispute in these cases, as well as the familiar adversarial argument in the courtroom. Women predominate among depressive homicides, and their commonest victim is their child. In depressive states the homicide may be part of a suicide pact with the victim, which the victim resisted. In men the conjunction of depression and homicide tends to occur in an older age group, with their spouse the most likely victim. Depressive reaction is a recognised precipitant of homicides committed by those with unstable personalities in situations of domestic, social or financial stress.

In general, aggressive acts by people with personality disorders may be seen to be either psychologically reactive (and defensive) or wilful and proactive (sadistic). In 'reactive' cases the offence may reflect the temperamental difficulties of the offender, for example, a tendency to a violent response either from a quick temper, or from an over-sensitive nature, or from tension associated with inadequacy and feelings of stress. In those with personality and psychopathic disorder, the affective state (e.g. a depressive 'swing') of the offender may be crucial in the balance between their capacity or failure to cope with rejection or other threat to self-esteem. The link between low self-esteem and sex offending is well known, but has general applicability for violent acts.

Sadistic acts vary in degree, from moderate, to those described by Brittain (1970) as a particular syndrome of the sadistic, and often sexual, murderer. In these rare cases, the man typically appears prim and is often socially isolated, since he has difficulty in all interpersonal relations; he may also have a long-standing interest in weapons, torture and the activities of the Nazi party. He develops sadistic fantasies, for example, of gross mutilation of his victims. He is also particularly likely to act out the fantasies at times when he feels a need to bolster his low self-esteem. A psychodynamic account of extensive experience with sexual murderers is provided by Williams (1964).

Multiple victims

There is evidence for the increasing prevalence of homicides involving multiple victims (see Box 2.5). There is a relative lack of literature, partly because of their rarity and partly because the offenders frequently commit suicide after the killing. However, a typical profile is of a non-psychotic, white male, around 20–30 years of age, of socio-economic group 3–4 , who uses a firearm in a dramatic scenario to express resentment and anger at life's frustrations and his personal difficulties (Levin & Fox, 1985).

Box 2.5 Classification of multiple victim homicide

From one incident:
- atrocities in war
- terrorist activities
- organised crime activities
- "mass murder" (e.g. Jonestown and Waco)
- "spree killing"

Repetitive killings over a period of time:
- professional assassinations
- murders committed by "serial killers"

Both mass murder and serial killing appear to be more common in the US and it is noteworthy that the ratio of approximately 10:1 of black to white perpetrators of single victim homicide in the US is reversed in these multiple victim categories. The perpetrators of serial killings are most commonly white males, aged 20–30 years, tending to be slightly older than most single victim killers. They kill repetitively to satisfy or relieve psychological needs and often present a quiet, conforming appearance. They tend to pick strangers as victims, and subjugation and torture may be an integral part of their acts. Narrative accounts of two extreme cases of homosexual killers are those of Nilsen (Masters, 1985) and Dahmer (Masters, 1993). A comprehensive account based on FBI data is that of Wilson & Seaman (1990).

Some serial killers are psychotically motivated, and in these cases their victims may be prostitutes. The killer may be responding to delusional beliefs. However, these descriptions are based only upon a few infamous serial killers and there are inevitably variations to these caricatures. Women whose behaviours show many of the features of Münchausen by proxy syndrome (see below) may prove to be serial killers. One such case involved the 'consecutive' filicide of at least three and possibly nine children (Egginton, 1989).

Killing of infants and children

The two commonest groups of offenders who kill children are parents or parent substitutes (80% of the total) and sexual offenders. Of children killed under one year old, 60% are killed by their mother. There are two important accounts in the British literature by Scott (1973) and d'Orban (1979).

Infanticide is the killing of a child under the age of 12 months by the mother. The killing of a baby less than one day old is known as neonaticide (Resnick, 1970). The crime of infanticide is dealt with in Chapter 5; the clinical aspects of the behaviour are summarised here. There are two principal 'types' of killing within the infanticide category, each accounting for nearly half of the cases: firstly, a loss of temper associated with a desire to stop intolerable behaviour by the baby – an extension of child battering; and secondly, motives derived from a depressive (possibly puerperal) disorder or a frankly psychotic state, perhaps with delusions of impending catastrophe or of the baby's gross deformity. Other motives in cases where parents are implicated include:

(1) a planned action springing from a desire to get rid of an unwanted child, usually at the time of birth or soon after, and frequently by suffocation after the first cry. In these cases the offender is typically an unmarried mother, under 25 years old, motivated by shame or fear, but who is otherwise law-abiding. She will typically have

successfully hidden the pregnancy from others. These mothers are unlikely to repeat the offence except in the rare case that their offending is part of a general picture of psychopathic behaviour

(2) a desire to punish the spouse (usually the husband) by killing the children – the so-called "Medea complex". This may be a conscious act of punishment, or an unconscious displacement of hostility towards the husband

(3) rarely, the "mercy" killing of a deformed child.

Killing of older infants and children may arise from:

(1) battering, where the motive is a desire to control the infant's exasperating behaviour. Empirically, this "cause" decreases rapidly after the child's fourth year, perhaps as the child can recognise – and is able to escape from – parental tension and wrath

(2) as part of another offence (e.g. loss of control, the death occurring during the course of sexual abuse)

(3) mental illness and the related psychotic beliefs

(4) rarely, sadistic homicide (see below).

Death by dangerous driving

Dangerous driving is responsible for a far greater number of deaths annually than all other categories of interpersonal violence. There were 5217 deaths from this cause in 1990 in England and Wales, including 368 children under 15 years old, according to the Department of Transport (1990), although there is provisional evidence of a small reduction in the overall figure to 4500 in 1991. Approximately 800 cases involved an illegal level of alcohol consumption by either the driver or the victim.

Psychiatric assessments of people charged with dangerous driving are rarely requested; there is little evidence to show an increased incidence of driving offences or accidents among the psychiatrically ill. One explanation is that few psychotic patients are likely to be driving anyway. However, there is good evidence that people suffering from alcoholism and personality disorder, including paranoid thinking, depressive affect, suicidal tendencies and impulsive violence, are much more likely to be involved in accidents (Cremona, 1986). The combination of cannabis and alcohol is demonstrated to have a particularly powerful synergistic effect upon driving ability.

Other assaultive crimes

Offences of assault in descending order of seriousness are shown in Box 2.6. Chance factors, such as the availability of medical care, may determine

---

Box 2.6 Offences of assault

Wounding:
- with intent to cause grievous bodily harm (Section 18, Offences Against the Person Act 1861)
- with no intent to cause grievous bodily harm (Section 20, same Act)

Assault occasioning actual bodily harm (Section 47, same Act)

Common assault

---

whether an assault results in a charge of wounding, attempted murder, or murder.

Child abuse and neglect

The 'battered child syndrome' was first described 30 years ago (Kempe *et al*, 1962). A more neutral term is 'non-accidental injury', which was adopted in 1974 to describe the same facts – that is, of a child who has suffered serious physical assault, generally from parents, foster parents or other carers. Both terms have now been replaced by the broader term 'child abuse and neglect' which encompasses non-accidental injury, child neglect, non-organic failure to thrive, and sexual and emotional abuse. Abuse varies from the most minor of assaults to the most life-endangering. There is overlap at all levels between physical abuse, neglect and sexual abuse (Bentovim, 1977). Box 2.7 shows a classification of physical abuse and neglect.

In all these categories there may appear to be "attachment" of the child to its parents but in cases of abuse this may be anxious, avoidant attachment, possibly desperate, and will arise from necessity rather than from trust. While abuse can occur in any social group and at any socio-economic level, parents or carers who abuse children tend to be young (late teenagers or early 20s) and have generally been found to be living under multiple stresses – for example, impoverished single parents in poor housing who are socially isolated. They commonly come from families in which there has been neglect and abuse over several generations, sometimes associated with psychiatric disturbance, physical disability and illness, and criminality (Rutter & Madge, 1976).

The complex issues of child abuse and neglect necessarily involve many different agencies and professionals. A Department of Health and Social Security document, *Child Abuse – Working Together for the Protection of Children* (1989), presents an admirable overview and comprehensive guidance for such work.

Box 2.7 Classification of child abuse and neglect

Physical abuse:
- severe abuse involving multiple injuries occurring over a sustained period of time
- moderate abuse specifically excluding injury to head or face
- mild abuse typically involving bruises and lacerations

Child neglect:
- severe neglect – characterised by failure of growth as a result of emotional neglect and failure to feed, with emotional misery and hopelessness
- failure to thrive syndrome – associated with a lesser degree of growth retardation and emotional delay (Harris, 1982)
- developmental delay – with social and emotional withdrawal, and impairment of language and communication skills

---

Münchausen syndrome by proxy (MSBP)

This is a relatively uncommon special case of child abuse. It is also referred to as "factitious illness by proxy". The terms refer to the behaviour of a parent or carer, usually the mother, who fabricates symptoms or injures the child, and then presents the child for treatment to a doctor or other medical personnel. There are two components to the aspect of "proxy": the creation of illness in another, and the consequent distress caused by the doctor in the investigation of the puzzling symptoms. The perpetrator will frequently have had nursing experience and the chosen method of causing harm is often by poisoning or suffocation. The name was coined by Meadow (1982, 1989) and is based on its similarities to Münchausen syndrome. Indeed, in approximately a third of cases there is a history of factitious illness behaviour in the mother. As with other aspects of child abuse, identification is dependent upon a judicious level of clinical suspicion. A common characteristic is that the father is emotionally if not physically "absent" and is apparently oblivious to such goings on. The perpetrator, by contrast, often appears to be an exemplary mother who seems to take great concern over the welfare of her children.

Management and treatment present numerous difficulties. There is a grave risk of repetition of the injurious and frequently life-threatening behaviour. It is often difficult to assess with confidence whether all children in the family, and possible future babies, are equally or differentially at risk. There is some evidence for the long-term benefits of individual psychotherapy, in selected cases, but if this is to occur, and the child is to remain in the parent's care, this often requires the availability of a mother and baby unit for a prolonged period. Such a facility is a scarce resource. An excellent overview is provided by Schreier & Libow (1993).

Child abduction

Child abduction, the stealing of a baby or an older child, is a rare offence. The law is contained within the Child Abduction Act 1984. Three main groups have been defined (Box 2.8).

Box 2.8 Child abduction

Abduction by parents – the largest group in custody disputes

Abduction of older children – usually a man with a sexual motive
   (d'Orban & Haydn-Smith, 1985)

Baby stealing – the smallest group, usually carried out by women
   with evidence of psychological disturbance

Child stealing by women

D'Orban (1976) categorised women who steal babies into three groups according to diagnosis and motive. *Comforting offences* were carried out by young women and were motivated by a desire to satisfy their need to look after a young child. They were more likely to take a child they already knew, for example, as baby-sitters, and had a history of their own children being taken into care. There was frequently a background of delinquency and emotional deprivation, and the diagnosis was usually one of personality disorder. Hysterical or immature personality traits were common. *Manipulative offences* were carried out by older women, also with personality disorder but with better social adjustment. The baby was stolen for a particular purpose, for example, to maintain a relationship by claiming the baby was her partner's. Sometimes a baby was stolen to replace one lost by miscarriage, with subsequent fear of desertion. Finally, *impulsive psychotic offences* were carried out during an acute relapse of a psychotic illness, usually schizophrenia, sometimes in response to delusions or as a bizarre and impulsive act. There is a small risk of repetition, particularly in emotionally deprived, hysterical personalities who are preoccupied with their desire to have children.

Non-psychotic women who abduct children are likely to receive a punitive sentence, but those who are suffering from a serious psychiatric disorder are more likely to be admitted to hospital. Most abducted babies are found fairly quickly, and are usually well cared for and unharmed.

Spouse abuse

The term 'spouse abuse' replaces an earlier term 'wife battering', and acknowledges the existence of the complementary syndrome of the 'battered husband'. The term 'battered wife' is used where physical force has been used on the wife by the husband (or cohabitee) in order to oppress and control, involving deliberate repetitive severe assault; the violence may eventually result in death. The incidence is unknown. Estimates vary from 1 in 500 marriages to 1 in 10. The problem of getting a good estimate arises both from the problem of definition (i.e. how much oppression or fighting counts as battering), as well as the intrinsic difficulty of achieving an adequate epidemiological survey. Pizzey (1974) gives a moving account of the range of behaviours subsumed under the term 'battering' from the perspective of a woman's refuge, which she pioneered in this country.

The offending appears to be associated with general factors such as stress, poverty, unemployment and low educational achievement. Equally it is said that it occurs at all levels of society, but that it remains covert in the more well-to-do. The principal characteristics of the abuser are those of possessiveness, sexual jealousy, and a need to dominate and control in emotional, financial and domestic matters. The principal predisposing factor, in general, is a marital relationship in which the battering spouse perceives a threat to his position of primacy. This may happen in a range of different circumstances: for example, the wife, by becoming pregnant, may "threaten" the husband's dependency. Abuse of alcohol by the abuser may be a precipitant, or, less frequently, by the abused. Other precipitants include statements, accusations or behaviour which stimulate the vulnerabilities of the abuser, and there may be an element of conscious or unconscious "victim precipitation" – an issue which is complex in its dynamics. The outcomes vary widely. The wife may tolerate the battering, feeling helpless to act. She may fight back and the violence may escalate, or she may retreat to a refuge. However, up to two-thirds of women return to their abuser within days. Possible alternative outcomes are suicide, or homicide by her husband or of her husband.

Elder abuse

This is defined as violence, neglect or emotional abuse of elderly relatives, often the surviving, widowed, elderly mother. Yin (1985) and Johnson *et al* (1985) provide extended overviews of what not long ago was called "granny bashing". There is an increasing awareness of such abuse, and there may be a real increase in prevalence, related to the growing number of the elderly and changing patterns of social care. Studies in the US have reported prevalence rates of 3% to 5%, mostly of women, and, in many cases, of those over 80 years of age. The offenders are likely to be the son or daughter of the victim. Half the sons have been found to be, themselves, over 60 years of age. The abuser is likely to be under stress from, for example, marital and financial problems, or to abuse alcohol or drugs. He or she proves to be unable to cope with the added stress of looking after the victim – upon whom he or she may still be emotionally or economically dependent. There are likely to be marked unresolved emotional conflicts between the abuser and the abused. A particular contemporary concern in Britain, with the moves towards community care, are recent reports of tyrannical abuse of the elderly, often by unqualified staff, in poorly managed nursing homes (Pitt, 1992).

Sexual offences

A behaviour or a disorder?

Sexual offending is a term which covers a widely heterogeneous group of offending behaviours. Although sex offences comprise less than 1% of offences in the annual criminal statistics (29 500 in 1992), they generate a disproportionate amount of legitimate concern. It is a subject of great human and social consequence because of the increasingly demonstrated effects on victims of the more serious forms of sexual offending. There is gathering evidence that sexual assault may be a contributory factor to a range of psychiatric disorders, including affective disorder, post-traumatic stress disorder, severe personality difficulties, borderline personality disorder and eating disorder, as well as subsequent delinquency. In some cases of sexual offending "the abused becomes the abuser". However, it is not clear to what extent the sexual abuse rather than the whole abusive context contributes to these sequelae.

There are widely divergent views concerning the different component 'causes' of sexual offending. All crimes, and particularly sexual offences, may be seen to depend upon the interaction of features in the offender, the victim and the environment. To quote Chiswick (1983), "the psychiatrist wishing to understand such offences will usually require to free himself of the rigidity of psychiatric nosology . . ." Thus classification by offender psychopathology, by motivation, by type of victim, or by situational factors alone, can at best only provide a partial account of what is invariably a complex act.

"Sexual deviation" is used as a neutral term to describe any sexual behaviour which varies from the statistical norm. *"Paraphilia"* – the descriptive term used in DSM–IV – is subdivided into numerous specific behaviours. *"Perversion"* remains largely the preserve of psychoanalytic workers, but is generally considered to have a judgmental flavour. It implies a theory of meaning underlying the behaviour. There is considerable overlap between sexual offences, paraphilias, sexual deviations and

perversions, but they are not all the same. For example, sadomasochism, fetishism, transvestism, transsexualism, voyeurism and, arguably, homosexuality – all of which may be components of sexual offending – are not, in themselves, offences.

Legal aspects

Sexual offences are classed as offences against the person, and encompass a wide range of legal categories and subcategories. They range from sexual offences against children, including incest and unlawful sexual intercourse, to offences against adults, including rape, indecent assault and homosexual offences. The most common sexual offence, indecent exposure, is not classified as a notifiable offence. A report by the Howard League Working Party (1985) provides an excellent account and overview of sexual offences. Aspects of homosexuality are considered in Chapter 3.

Child sexual abuse

Incidence

Mullen (1990) estimates that 10–15% of female children will have been victims of unequivocal sexual assault, of whom 5–8% will have experienced sexual intercourse, which, under the age of 13 years, is regarded in law as statutory rape. Sexual abuse of male children appears to be a little less prevalent. By contrast, in 1989 there were 5800 cases of child sexual abuse (CSA) on the child protection register, which is very low compared with the prevalence findings of population surveys. It is accepted that sexual abuse of children often does not come to light until years later. The apparently huge increases found in many recent studies probably represent a large component of increased awareness as well as a possible increase

---

Box 2.9 Legal classification of child sexual abuse

Incest
Unlawful sexual intercourse with a girl less than 13 years (it is no
    defence for the girl to consent or for the male to believe her
    to be over 16 years)
Unlawful sexual intercourse with a girl under 16, but over 13 years
Indecency with children (inciting children to perform acts of gross
    indecency upon an adult, or taking, possessing or showing
    indecent photographs or films of a child)
Defilement of girls (e.g. encouraging them into prostitution)
Any other offence (e.g. buggery, indecent assault) where a child
    is the victim

in prevalence. The behaviour is obviously intended to remain secret. The abuser uses tactics to coerce the victim into silence, and population surveys report data based on the long-term memory of the victim. Box 2.9 gives a legal classification of CSA.

Assaults on children occur in a variety of situations ranging from persistent sexual abuse within families to isolated attacks by relatives, people acting *in loco parentis* (e.g. baby-sitters) or strangers. Most, but not all, sexual abuse is perpetrated by men and boys. While it has been traditional to distinguish between extra-familial ('paedophilic') and intra-familial ('incestuous') abuse, one recent study found that half of the incestuous fathers had molested female children outside of the family as well (Abel *et al*, 1988).

Extra-familial sex offending against children

The abusers may be:

(1) adolescent boys, or mentally handicapped males, making clumsy or immature approaches. At least 50% of adult sex offenders are found to have started offending in adolescence. Not infrequently, young adolescents may be victims of abuse themselves, while at the same time they are abusing younger children

(2) males with "primary" or "fixated" paedophilic sexual impulses. These men are not only "conditionally" dangerous (i.e. when an opportunity presents itself), but seek out and create opportunities

(3) people with aggressive personalities, with general psychopathic and possibly fixed sexual psychopathic features, indiscriminately using children as sex objects

(4) susceptible men undermined by stress, mental illness or organic brain disorder, "giving way" to repressed paedophilic impulses normally regarded as alien to them. This group constitutes the so-called "regressed" or "secondary" paedophilic category

(5) stepfathers assaulting their step-children as a reflection of their personality, attitudes, or disturbed family dynamics. In some cases men may have taken on a step-family because of the attractions of the children rather than of those of their partner.

The exclusive paedophile usually remains fixed in his sexual orientation, preferring involvement with either male or female children, and less often with both. As with the aetiological theories of other deviant sexual orientations, there are no universal features which determine a sexual interest in children or young persons. Absent or distant relationships with fathers and over-involvement with mothers are sometimes cited. Sexual abuse in childhood by adults is regularly reported. Some describe how exploratory homosexual or heterosexual behaviour in late childhood or adolescence unaccountably becomes fixed, leaving the paedophile with a lack of comprehension of a sexual interest in an adult of either sex. It is sometimes striking how the persistence of immature sexual behaviour is mirrored in the general immaturity of the individuals, sometimes despite an otherwise stable and successful life. Confirmed paedophiles have little insight into what constitutes a normal adult/child relationship; their lack of acceptance of the deleterious effects of their sexual behaviour on children is very resistant to change, and unless methods of self-control are developed, reoffending is common.

Both intra- and extra-familial abusers typically display distorted perceptions and attitudes (Kennedy & Grubin, 1992). A father or stepfather will report that he only acted out of love for the child; the child loved him above all others; the child acquiesced, encouraged or even demanded increasing sexual contact; the child enjoyed it; he was just educating the child in sexual matters and was doing nothing wrong; the child suffered no physical or psychological damage. These views are maintained even when the facts of the relationship offer no support. Denial or minimisation of abusive behaviour is common. The similarities between paedophiles and sexual abusers have led some authors to the view that sexual abusers in family units are but paedophiles who happen to be able to form adult sexual relationships (Salter, 1988). When they come into contact with a victim of the appropriate age and sex, they adopt a deviant mode of sexual expression. Separated from a family when the abuse is discovered, they may seek out another woman with children to start all over again.

Incest

It is an offence for a man to have sexual intercourse with a female whom he knows to be his daughter, granddaughter, sister (or half-sister) or mother, or for a woman of over 16 years to permit a man she knows to be of such consanguinity to have sexual intercourse with her. Consent is not a defence to the charge. Family relationships which do not involve consanguinity, for example, stepfather/daughter, do not fall within the legal definition in England and Wales. In Scotland, and other jurisdictions, step relationships and in-laws are included within the legal prohibition of incest. The legal definition of incest requires that sexual intercourse (i.e. vaginal penetration) should occur, whereas much intra-familial sexual behaviour falls short of full intercourse.

Father–daughter incest is overwhelmingly the most common, although brother–sister incest is said to be much underreported, and mother–son incest is increasingly recognised. Father–daughter incest usually takes place when the girl is about 10 or 11 years of age or even earlier, with the father initiating sexual "games" apparently stimulated by physical changes in the girl as she approaches puberty. This may proceed to regular sexual intimacies and possibly full intercourse or buggery. The father may switch his sexual attentions to younger daughters as either the victim leaves home or the younger ones become more sexually attractive to him. The behaviour is usually disclosed when the daughter complains – often to the mother – or when there are enquiries about tearfulness, failure at school, or other matters. The mother may be in apparent ignorance of what has been going on; she may even give tacit encouragement or be covertly collusive. Significant marital conflict will frequently be found. Incest may be incorporated into the family patterns with sons imitating their fathers, or even each family member abusing several others irrespective of gender and age.

The father who has an incestuous relationship with his daughter rarely suffers from a psychiatric abnormality, although he frequently shows evidence of personality difficulties and inadequacies. Depressive symptoms will sometimes be found, but these may occur as a consequence of discovery with subsequent police involvement and exclusion from the family home.

Mother–son incest was thought to be extremely rare and only associated with severe mental illness on the part of the mother, but is now thought to be more common than first realised. It is often associated with neurotic states, personality difficulties or occasionally psychosis in the mother.

Consequences of incest. The consequence of father–daughter incest depends upon the personality of the daughter and the quality of the relationship between the father and the daughter. When the daughter has been subjected to repeated abuse by a psychopathic father, the consequences are likely to be much more damaging than where there has been an affectionate bond, however tenuous. Despite numerous attempts to define patterns of behaviour that should alert professionals to the likelihood of child abuse, the presentations are not specific, and few if any clinical states are conclusively diagnostic of abuse (Kolvin & Kaplan, 1988).

Management of child sexual abuse

Typically, disclosure of sexual abuse may first be made outside the family to school authorities, social services, the general practitioner or paediatrician. The first consideration must be the protection of the child from further abuse. The interview procedure for a child suspected of being sexually abused is a delicate matter and has been reviewed by Vizard (1991). For example, there is much dispute about the validity of children's testimony, and specifically of the use of anatomical dolls. All treatment aims to achieve acknowledgement of their acts by the offenders and acceptance of responsibility. Recently developed methods for working with the family, the offender and the victim have been described by a number of authors, including Finkelhor (1986), Bentovim *et al* (1988), Salter (1988) and the Department of Health and Social Security (1989).

In cases of intra-familial abuse, ideally a case conference will be called with the participation of the local social services and the police, as well as other professionals responsible for the child's welfare. A consensus will hopefully emerge concerning immediate protective action, the need for further investigation and a decision regarding the registering of the fact of abuse. It is recommended that a key professional is appointed to coordinate services. Immediate protection, if considered necessary, can be given by the application of a 'place of safety order'. In the longer term, consideration may be given to an interim care order or to wardship proceedings, or placement on the 'At Risk Register'. Decisions will also need to be made about the relative merits of prosecution, and of the involvement of a forensic psychiatrist in the assessment of the abuser. Prosecution will depend upon the seriousness of the offending behaviour, as well as upon judgements regarding the welfare primarily of the child but also of the whole family. These issues are reviewed by Bentovim *et al* (1988) and in a Ciba Foundation publication *Child Sexual Abuse Within the Family* (Porter, 1984). An overview of the treatment issues for the child are contained in a review by Glaser (1991).

Violent sexual assault against adults

The great majority of acts of sexual violence against adults are perpetrated by men against women. However, adult males may be the victims of violent sexual assault by other males (Mezey & King, 1989).

Rape

Rape is defined legally as vaginal intercourse with a woman without her consent and knowing that she did not consent, or being reckless as to whether or not she had consented. The penis only has to penetrate to the slightest degree to constitute rape, and emission is not necessary. Consent is not valid if obtained by fear, fraud, impersonation or by the use of drugs or drink. Husbands in Scotland, England and Wales had been protected from a charge of rape against their wives, but this immunity has recently been removed by a court ruling. The Sexual Offences (Amendment) Act 1976 introduced the present emphasis on lack of consent, replacing the previous focus on the use of force , and of threatening bodily harm. On conviction the maximum sentence is life imprisonment.

Clinical classifications of rapists have generally focused on the nature of the act: whether predominately aggressive, sadistic or sexual. These sub-categories have received some empirical validation (Prentky *et al*, 1988). Rape is predominately an act of violence expressed in sexual terms. It is noteworthy that at the moment of the act many rapists suffer relative impotence and sexual failure, with the majority failing to ejaculate. Few rapes are committed by men suffering from a mental illness. The following classification combines a number of previously described groups (see Bowden, 1978 for an overview).

(1) "Normal" men in abnormal settings. It is asserted that invading soldiers and gangs of youths who commit rape would not do so except under the influence of group pressure, over-arousal and excitement.

(2) Men with a history of violence and egocentric, impulsive, psychopathic behaviour sometimes commit rape at a time of stress or over-arousal, frequently compounded by the intoxicating effects of alcohol and drugs. These offenders show little empathy for their victim. The act is typically not planned. They are likely to have had a life-long inability to relate normally to women, which may reflect severe parenting problems from childhood.

(3) Inadequate men under strain or as a result of threats to status or self-esteem may behave impulsively either with violence or sexual violence, to their later remorse and regret.

(4) Some severely inhibited men become aware of an increasing desire for violent sexual behaviour. They are shy, often phobic, and sexually guilt-ridden. They may begin to act out their desires even though they dislike them. In a small minority there may have been prior acts of exhibitionism.

(5) Men who have developed ego-syntonic, pleasurable fantasies of hurting, mutilating, torturing, raping and killing women. The masturbatory fantasies begin in childhood and reflect a deep-seated hatred of women, and a need to dominate and possess the victim. The fantasies and consequent behaviour are conscious and much dwelt upon. MacCulloch *et al* (1983) have described how fantasies may be "rehearsed" and may progress to sadistic rape or murder.

(6) Children may be raped for similar reasons by men with paedophilic inclinations. Sometimes the rape appears to have been committed opportunistically by psychopathic men in category 2, with no previous history of sexual attraction to children.

(7) Rape may, rarely, be committed as a direct result of a delusional state or hallucinations. More commonly there is a profound character disorder, and drug abuse and alcoholism is common. Some perpetrators show evidence of intense homosexual fears, against which the rape may be seen as a defence, and these may be experienced at a near psychotic intensity. For example, one young man raped after weeks of "argument" in his mind between his homosexual and his heterosexual self.

(8) Some rapes are committed by men with learning disabilities who may be experiencing sexual frustration, and who also have anger and grievance about their general failure to be able to compete and cope with life's challenges.

Most rapists do not score differently to other offenders on personality tests or social skills assessment, nor on intelligence testing. They are mostly indistinguishable from other delinquents and, indeed, the majority will have a history of other (non-sexual) offending. However, penile plethysmography (PPG), which measures changes in penile tumescence, has shown that some rapists are more likely than controls to be sexually aroused by images of rape. There appears to be a very small group of rapists who have high testosterone levels, but most are no different from controls. Thus the two clearest demonstrable characteristics which distinguish some rapists from controls are their sexual arousal by violent sexual acts, and their general criminality and delinquency. Phallometric studies of response to rape imagery may be considered potentially useful in assessment. However, in any given individual, phallometry results need to be interpreted with caution. False negatives may occur, for example, as a result of the wrong imagery being chosen, or by the individual suppressing his responses. Equally, 'positive' PPG results are evidence of arousal to certain stimuli but do not predict future behaviour. Another complicating factor is that rape fantasies and images of the infliction of pain, of spanking and of bondage are not uncommon among the reported fantasies of so-called "normal" men (Crepault & Couture, 1980).

Sexual assault and homicide

Rapists may deliberately kill their victims to silence the victim and avoid detection, or as part of a compulsive sadistic attack, perhaps associated with mutilation of the victim. Rapists who kill show lifelong features of social isolation and a lack of heterosexual relationships (Grubin, 1994). A comprehensive American review, based on an FBI study of 36 convicted, incarcerated sexual murderers, is described by Ressler *et al* (1988). A full account with clinical details of psychodynamic treatment is given by Williams (1964).

Management of sexual offenders

Sex offenders in custody

The more serious sex offenders will receive prison sentences. In England and Wales there are about 3000 men serving prison sentences for sex offences. The Prison Service is finding difficulty in providing suitable accommodation for sex offenders because of the way that other prisoners mete out violent "punishment" to this group of offenders, requiring them to be segregated in protective custody (Rule 43) (see Chapter 9). In statistical terms, adolescents make up a third of the increasing prison population of sexual offenders, who themselves comprise 7% of the total prison population (Home Office, 1990). There is also growing evidence that the great majority of perpetrators of sexual crimes begin their offending behaviour in adolescence, frequently in their early teens or even earlier (Davis & Leitenberg, 1987). Treatment programmes would do well, therefore, to target these age groups before established behaviour and offending patterns set in. There are now established 'treatment packages' in some prisons for sex offenders serving sentences of more than four years. These include attempts to improve social functioning by group and individual psychological approaches, based largely on cognitive–behavioural principles (see Chapter 9).

Psychiatric treatment

The small group of mentally ill sex offenders will require psychiatric treatment of the underlying disorder, in a hospital in the first instance. Where (rarely) the rape has been the direct result of psychotic illness, the patient is more likely to be regarded as safe once the illness is controlled. Those with a learning disability may also benefit from hospital treatment (Day, 1988), although some, especially those in the borderline intelligence group, may find themselves in prison. Relatively small numbers of those who fall into the psychopathic group are usually considered suitable for hospitalisation for both clinical and legal reasons; sexual deviation, in itself, is specifically excluded as grounds for detention under the Mental Health Act 1983. However, about a third of male patients detained in special hospitals have committed a sexually related index offence. Most have a diagnosis of psychopathic disorder. Out-patient NHS treatment for sex offenders has been developed piecemeal by a number of agencies, including regional forensic psychiatry services, often in conjunction with the probation service.

The "success" of treatment depends upon careful selection, which in turn hinges upon comprehensive assessment. Only a minority of offenders are well motivated and these generally have the best prognosis. Treatment should ideally include social skills training, anger management and specific behavioural and cognitive therapies to attempt to modify aggressive behaviour and sexual impulsiveness. There are comprehensive accounts of treatment approaches and the present state of the art by Marshall *et al* (1990), including an account by Pithers (1990) of his influential emphasis on 'relapse prevention' and enhancement of treatment gains, rather than any philosophy of 'cure'. Quinsey (1984) and Hollin & Howells (1991) provide overviews of cognitive–behavioural treatments. A balanced account of clinical work with sex offenders in secure settings is provided by Perkins (1991).

Antilibidinal medication (for example, with cyproterone acetate) may be considered but requires the patient's compliance and consent. Possible side-effects include erectile failure, gynaecomastia, inhibition of spermato-genesis, depression, asthenia, lassitude and weight changes.

Sexual offenders can provoke strong emotional reactions in all of us, but particularly in new and inexperienced staff who will need the sympathetic support of colleagues, preferably with regular supervision. The patient must be able to feel that he can report his aberrant inclinations to the psychiatrist/therapist without the latter "panicking" at the honest sharing of aggressive sexual material.

Prognosis of the violent sexual offender

Soothill *et al* (1976) found that 90% of rapists did not commit a second rape, although 15% were convicted of a further sexual assault and 17% of a violent offence. Re-offending correlated positively with the number of previous offences and inversely with the age of the offender. However, some sexual offenders (for example, offenders against children) are more likely to re-offend. Follow-up needs to be long-term; otherwise, serious underestimation of recidivism is likely to occur. There is some evidence for the reduction of sexual offending while treatment and follow-up supervision and support continues. The achievement of permanent change is more doubtful.

Victims of rape and serious sexual assaults

Victims of rape (male or female) are susceptible to short and long-term traumatic after-effects (Mezey & Taylor, 1988; Mezey & King, 1989). The reactions of victims vary, reflecting not only the nature of the assault or rape but also the psychological characteristics of the victim. Those with a history of psychological, social, sexual or medical problems tend to be less resilient to the effects of such trauma. In general, there is likely to be an immediate period of anxiety with depressive feelings of shock, disbelief, guilt and self-blame, together with memory 'flashbacks' during waking, and re-enactments in nightmares during periods of resolution over weeks or months. However, some 20% will develop chronic anxiety and depressive symptoms, which may occur after a delay of some years. Sexual and interpersonal relationships may become disturbed, with persisting feelings of degradation and rage. The (usually male) spouse of the victim may develop a state of anger and blame with some depressive symptoms.

A better understanding of the predicament and experience of victims will reduce the post-traumatic effects of rape. A calm and sensitive reaction from a trained (usually female) police officer is more effective than an alarmist one. Introduction to a rape crisis centre will provide the opportunity for support and counselling over the immediate acute period, as well as providing contacts for peer support over the longer term. Referral for psychiatric help may be required if the symptoms are severe and persistent.

Buggery

This is defined as anal intercourse with males or females, and anal or vaginal intercourse with animals ('bestiality'). Participants in anal intercourse may be prosecuted unless they are consenting males over the age of 21, and their act is in private. Anal intercourse within a *heterosexual* couple is illegal, at whatever age, including an act between man and wife; the maximum sentence remains life, for both partners, although the law in this area is effectively in abeyance.

Indecent exposure (exhibitionism)

Indecent exposure is an offence; exhibitionism is a paraphilia. In law the offence was originally defined in the Vagrancy Act 1824, whereby "a person who openly, lewdly and obscenely exposes his person with the intent to insult any female should be deemed a rogue and a vagabond". Subsequent amendments and ruling have clarified that it is an offence to expose in public or private places, and "person" in this context means "penis". More generally, it is an offence for a man or woman to expose to anyone (male or female) in a public place.

Incidence

Indecent exposure is said to be a common behaviour but it is classified as a summary offence and therefore does not appear in the criminal statistics. Only a minority of cases are reported, few offenders are detected, and only in some cases does the behaviour lead to prosecution. There were only 1000 convictions for indecent exposure in 1990 in England and Wales (Home Office, 1992). Only 1% are dealt with under the Mental Health Act, and these represent the small group of mentally ill people who are not "true" exhibitionists. Eighty per cent of first offenders are said not to re-offend (Rooth, 1971).

The following characteristics were first described by Lasegue in 1877:

(1) the cases are almost always men, often of previously blameless character
(2) they describe sudden, powerful urges to display their genitals
(3) the urges and behaviour are often repeated and are usually associated with sexual excitement
(4) they expose with little (apparent) attempt to avoid apprehension;
(5) they make no attempt to enter into any kind of relationship with their victim
(6) the exposer finds his own behaviour quite inexplicable.

"True" exhibitionists should be distinguished from those rare cases in which people expose themselves while suffering from severe mental illness (e.g. schizophrenia, mania, organic disorder or learning disability). In some cases, isolated acts of exhibitionism may occur in those under stress or those who are chronically or reactively depressed. Blair & Lanyon (1981) summarise the personality characteristics of exhibitionists as: timidity of character; lack of social skills; difficulty in anger control; poor psychosexual adjustment; and a history of minor criminal offences of a sexual as well as a non-sexual nature. Rooth (1971) described two main groups: the inhibited but apparently normal personality, and those of an overtly aggressive and antisocial type. Bluglass (1980) gave some validity to this typology.

The genital display may be performed from a relatively discreet position – for example, from a car seat at passers-by, such that the victim may be unsure whether the act was intended. The perpetrator may lurk by a tree or a building, and perhaps insist when apprehended that he was merely urinating. It is characteristic of the behaviour that it happens at a distance and that no physical contact takes place; that is, exhibitionism is an "expressive" act, and only very exceptionally is it a prelude to a sexual assault. It is psychologically important to the perpetrator that his anonymity is preserved, although his behaviour puts him at risk of apprehension. However, there is a group of exhibitionists whose behaviour becomes increasingly aggressive, and who proceed to touching ("aggressive toucherism") or sexual assault. One in four exhibitionists seen for psychiatric reports, and followed up for between 8 and 25 years, subsequently had at least one conviction for a contact sexual offence (Sugarman *et al*, 1994). Exhibitionism may be associated with other sexual offences or deviations such as voyeurism, frotteurism and paedophilia, as well as obscene telephone calling (Cordess, 1990). The latter may be regarded as a form of verbal exhibitionism.

Treatment

Theories of aetiology and treatment, as with other sexual offending, range from the biological, through the behavioural and cognitive–behavioural, to the psychodynamic. Useful reviews of the different approaches are provided by Rooth (1980), Gayford (1981) and Snaith (1983). Cognitive–behavioural techniques include social skills training, "teaching" self-control, aversion and "shaming" programmes, and covert sensitisation. Psychodynamic theory may provide insights into the behaviour, but psychoanalytic psychotherapy will be appropriate only for a selected minority (Rosen, 1979). The use of antilibidinal drugs such as cyproterone acetate may be appropriate in those few aggressive exhibitionists whose behaviour is escalating dangerously.

Offences against property

Of all recorded crime, 94% involves offences against property. However, forensic psychiatry is far more engaged in the smaller group of offences against the person. Property offences can be subdivided into acquisitive and destructive offences (Box 2.10).

Box 2.10 Property offences

Acquisitive offences:
- theft and handling stolen goods
- taking and driving away (motor vehicles)
- robbery
- blackmail
- burglary
- fraud and forgery

Destructive offences:
- criminal damage
- arson

Acquisitive offences

Theft (including shoplifting) and handling of stolen goods comprise approximately half, and burglary an additional one fifth, of all recorded offences annually. However, psychiatric illness is only rarely associated with these offences, with the particular exception of shoplifting. The taking and driving away of motor vehicles may be associated with particular personality and developmental difficulties of adolescents, as part of a general pattern of failure at school and general delinquency.

Acquisitive offending and psychiatric disorder

Most stealing is committed by psychiatrically normal people. Some may have psychopathic elements to their personalities and the behaviour will be ego-syntonic, for the purpose of gain. Others may resist but give way to temptation as opportunity presents. A minority will steal for their own psychological reasons and for no identifiable material gain. The prototypic offence of this sort is that of some cases of shoplifting. Only recently has attention become directed towards the prevalence of "white collar" offences and those of big business and of the social establishment. There are a range of such offences that do not form a homogeneous group. They range from fraud by credit cards, fraud of investors and manipulation of financial markets, down to petty theft from places of work. Only rarely will there be cause for the psychiatrist to become involved.

Shoplifting

Bluglass (1990) distinguishes between three groups of shoplifters (Box 2.11). Early studies of shoplifters found a preponderance of women, although more recent studies have shown equal or greater numbers of men. Peak

---

Box 2.11 Classification of shoplifters

Professional shoplifters
Amateur shoplifters
Shoplifting associated with psychiatric disorder

---

ages are in the teenage years and in middle-age (50–60 years) for female offenders. There has been a substantial and steady increase in recorded offences over recent years – as much as 10-fold over a 40-year period.

Psychiatric disorder is a factor in only a small but significant proportion of shoplifters. Gibbens & Prince (1962) estimated that 10–15% of shoplifters were psychiatrically disordered, but later studies have suggested that only about 5% of shoplifters suffer from substantial mental disorder (Gibbens, 1981). Of those who are psychologically disordered, the subgroups shown in Box 2.12 may be identified.

A minority of shoplifters are referred for a psychiatric opinion. On interview, the subject may claim to be unable to remember the actual offence. An attempt should be made to differentiate between conscious denial (lying), genuine confusion or "absent-mindedness", and uncons-

---

Box 2.12 Psychologically disordered shoplifters

Chronically stressed
Chronically depressed
Personality disorder, in association with low mood
Persons suffering with chronic schizophrenia
  • as part of a general deterioration of behaviour, or for survival
  • rarely, in response to voices or delusional beliefs
Persons suffering from chronic physical illness, such as gynae-cological disorders among women, asthma or diabetes
Organic states
  • dementia, depressive pseudodementia or brain damage may cause confusion or disinhibition, leading to "absent-minded" behaviour (also common in normal populations of shoplifters; *British Medical Journal*, 1976)
  • epilepsy – either in the confusional period following an epileptic attack or in association with an abnormal personality
  • the effects of abuse of alcohol or drugs – either to finance the habit, or from impaired concentration due to alcohol, drugs or legitimate medication

cious denial ("psychological amnesia") which may take various clinical forms (e.g. hysterical dissociation). The account of the offence provided by the store detective or shop owner, if available, will give considerable information about the behaviour of the subject at the material time. Where a psychiatric disorder is diagnosed, then a psychiatric recommendation should be made, either for voluntary treatment or as a condition of a probation order. Where there is psychiatric evidence that there was no intent to steal at the time of the act the court may decide not to record an offence. The Crown Prosecutor may (under the Prosecution of Offences Act 1985) choose not to prosecute some offenders, including shoplifters, where it is considered that prosecution will produce adverse effects on the defendant's mental health, and where these outweigh the interests of justice. This more humane approach follows several cases where prosecution for shoplifting has led to the suicide of a vulnerable person.

Treatment may include medication, for example, for a disorder of mood, and counselling and advice, possibly with more intensive psychotherapy in selected cases. There has been an increase in the provision of groups for some shoplifters, using techniques varying from the psychodynamic to self-help. In recidivist cases, simple advice about situational measures may prove helpful; for example, leaving bags outside shops, and only shopping when accompanied by others.

Burglary

Burglary is described as an offence of "ulterior intent", meaning that there has to be an intent over and above that of entering the building (trespassing). The intent may not necessarily be acquisitive, although most such offences are deemed to be so. Burglary made up approximately 24% of all crime recorded by the police in 1992, approximately half of which involved burglary of a dwelling, and half the burglary of other buildings (Home Office, 1993). It is the subject of much personal fear and social concern, which is reflected in the fact that it may attract a sentence of up to 10 years imprisonment. Most of the literature concerning burglary is criminological, and no particular psychiatric condition is known to be associated with this offence. Bennett & Wright (1984) reviewed some of the literature and remarked upon the lack of any clinical perspective. However, burglary seems to be a common feature in drug-dependent offenders seen by psychiatrists.

In the author's experience there is a subgroup of young, adolescent burglars who appear to be drawn to buildings which offer relatively easy access, for no apparent good motive at the time. Once inside, in the words of one young offender, referring to his mixed state of fear and excitement, "anything could happen". This may include nothing, appropriation of goods, ransacking of the interior, or alternatively sexual activity (for example masturbation), urination or defecation, or fire-setting. If the burglar is disturbed, a violent or sexual offence may ensue, which is recorded under the more serious category of crime rather than burglary. There is also a group of "professional" burglars who commit a very large number of individual offences with considerable profits. One of these adolescent individuals gave his occupation, since leaving school, as "house clearance".

Destructive offences

Criminal damage, including acts of vandalism and fire-setting, made up about 16% of all notifiable offences recorded by the police in 1990 (Home Office, 1992). According to the *British Crime Survey* (Home Office Research Study, 1988), only 10% of criminal damage offences are recorded.

There is little psychiatric literature on vandalism. Frequently the behaviour is part of a delinquent pattern involving other antisocial behaviour. Acts of minor vandalism are common among adolescents and are within the norm, unless they become an established pattern of behaviour. Other acts of damage or injury – for example, acts of cruelty to animals – may be ominous signs of likely escalation to more serious offending.

Arson

Arson is clinically better referred to as fire-setting. It is regarded as an act of great seriousness because of its capacity to cause immense damage to life and property. As technical developments improve the prevention and control of accidental fires, there appears to be a general and alarming increase in non-accidental fire-setting (arson) throughout industrialised societies. Only a proportion of arson offences come to prosecution since the circumstances of the act are often obscure and there is ample opportunity for leaving the scene of the crime.

There were 26 500 offences of arson recorded by the police in 1990, with a clear-up rate of only 21% (Home Office, 1992). This figure is just a few thousand less than the total number of sexual offences recorded, and represents about 0.8% of all recorded offences. Official figures certainly underestimate the true rate of actual offending. In the UK, arson appears to be most commonly an offence of males, in a ratio of 9 to 1.

The classification of reasons for arson (shown below) is modified from Lewis & Yarnell (1951), Prins *et al* (1985) and others. The categories are based upon putative motives, some of which are conscious and obvious, and others which are unconscious and need to be more or less inferred. There is necessarily considerable overlap.

(1) Insurance fraud.
(2) Covering the evidence of a crime.
(3) Political motives.

(4) Gang activities for excitement. Arson, as with other offences such as gang rape, may be committed by groups of young people in a state of excitement with no obviously clear motives. It may be led by a disturbed individual, and other members of the group will generally present a low risk of repetition of the offence.

(5) Revenge, self-protection and anger. In this sub-category, which makes up at least half of the total referred for psychiatric assessment, the fire is set for revenge or as a maladaptive expression of anger. This group includes many apparently "normal" people (i.e. of previously good behaviour) in states of great arousal, such as the man who sets fire to the work place from which he has just been dismissed. The few of this group who are psychotic may be responding to psychotic ideas such as a belief that they are being persecuted.

(6) "A cry for help". The fire is set as a way of drawing attention to the plight of the fire-setter. It may be seen in those of inadequate personality or in mentally ill people placed in situations with which they cannot cope.

(7) A desire to feel powerful. The fire-setting is performed to gain a sense of power. The perpetrator sometimes telephones the emergency services, and then may watch the commotion and the arrival of the fire services. He may read about it the next day, and enjoy the feeling of being the cause of such destruction.

(8) A desire to be seen as a hero. The fire is set in order that the fire-setter can appear at the scene and play a "heroic" part. It has been known for firemen to set fires for this purpose.

(9) A fire as a thing of interest. In this group there is a fascination with fire for its own sake, and there may be a history of an excessive interest in fire from the earliest years. However, many children go through a stage of fascination with fire which proves to be only a temporary developmental phase.

(10) Irresistible impulse. These fire-setters are conscious of a repeated urge to set fires but are unable to articulate or understand their motive. They are often isolated, inadequate people. The sub-categories 9 and 10 include those with some of the features of the old category of "pyromania" as described by Esquirol (1885).

(11) Sexual excitement. Surveys of arsonists have found some people who are sexually aroused by fire, but this appears nowadays to be a very small proportion of the total. These offenders are generally regarded as dangerous as long as fantasies of sexual arousal by fire persist, and such fantasies may prove difficult to evaluate.

(12) Depression and tension reducing. The principal motivation for the fire-setter is the relief of despondency and tension by the act of setting a fire. The group has features of the irresistible impulse group and the "cry for help" group.

(13) Psychotic illness. In a small minority of cases the offender may suffer from a psychotic illness. The act of fire-setting may be the direct result of delusions or hallucinations, but is more frequently an indirect effect of chronic illness, with attendant general deterioration of personality and judgement.

Psychiatry has a long history of involvement in the assessment of fire-setting and fire-setters, and this continues to be the case since the majority of apprehended arsonists are referred for a psychiatric assessment. Historically there has been an assumed association between sexuality and fire-setting. The basis of this belief is drawn largely from the psychoanalytic literature and has not received empirical validation. No particular psychiatric diagnosis is associated with fire-setting, although acute and chronic alcohol abuse is frequently implicated. Full assessment, as with other serious offenders, includes a history from the offender, assessment of mental state at interview and at the material time, a study of witness accounts (if any), and all previous medical and social records. The assessor will attempt to assess dangerousness, based on a number of factors including the history of previous destructive behaviour – of fire-setting and other offending – and the presence or absence of clear precipitants. It will inevitably involve a degree of intuition, since we are relatively ignorant about the specific factors and variables which might enable us to predict future fire-setting.

There is little evidence for the place of specific interventions in the management of most fire-setters, although some aversive and other behavioural techniques have been described. Most arsonists are managed within the penal system. Treatment and management, where appropriate, is largely a question of providing firm boundaries and consistency either in residential educational settings for juveniles, or in in-patient settings for adults. Treatment programmmes in assertion and social skills training are also sometimes used (Harris & Rice, 1984; Jackson *et al,* 1987). Where mental illness plays a predominant part in the fire-setting of adults, there can be optimism with regard to prognosis as long as the illness can be successfully treated and managed.

Dangerousness of fire-setters. Lewis & Yarnell (1951) found that 30% of arsonists re-offended, a rate similar to that found more recently by O'Sullivan & Kelleher (1987). However, many will commit other types of offences (Soothill & Pope, 1973). Sapford *et al* (1978) found that, of imprisoned arsonists serving short sentences (less than five years), only 2% committed further arson, compared with 20% of arsonists serving longer terms. Both groups were found to be likely to commit other destructive offences in the follow-up period (e.g. property damage, sexual offences and crimes of violence), which is evidence of an overlap between different destructive behaviours.

Prediction of future dangerousness is notoriously difficult, particularly with juvenile fire-setters. The clinician must be guided by the general principles set out by Scott (1977), including details of the offence, past behaviour and personal history, and the present and future likely protective factors. Adult fire-setters appear to constitute a far more heterogeneous group than juveniles in terms of motives, dynamics and psychopathological characteristics. Studies have tended to be of highly selected samples which have generated different versions of the "typical" arsonist. These range from a "hobo" type, with a drinking problem, no occupation and a wandering way of life, to those individuals who are sufficiently engaged in relationships, work, or society to have a target for their frequently vengeful fire-setting.

Victimology

The central significance of trauma and of victimisation in forensic psychiatry is forcefully stated by Gunn & Taylor (1993), who offer a definition of forensic psychiatry as "the prevention, amelioration and treatment of victimisation which is associated with mental disease". Such victims fall into two main categories:

(1) The victim of, for example, violent offences or rape – either after one episode of victimisation or after serial victimisation. A specific rape trauma syndrome, for example, has been described.
(2) Mentally disordered offender patients who may be victims:
    (a) of childhood physical, sexual or emotional abuse
    (b) (by definition) of mental ill-health and the disruption to their personal and family lives which this may entail
    (c) as a consequence of (a) and (b), secondary victimisation may also include further abuse and harsh treatment, as well as poverty and social marginalisation (e.g. excessively punitive societal responses)
    (d) of their own offending behaviour (most obviously in the cases of those who kill their children or their spouse).

Some victims, for example, the survivors of childhood abuse or neglect, may suffer a range of psychological sequelae, or become offenders in later life. Others may develop the symptoms of post-traumatic stress disorder (PTSD).

The familiar clinical phenomenon of the abused becoming the abuser (termed "identification with the agressor" in the psychodynamic literature) has been demonstrated in numerous recent empirical studies. Also, research has shown an increased incidence of violence among victims of PTSD. For example, in a study of over 1000 male offenders, those suffering from PTSD were found to be five times more likely to commit acts of serious violence (Collins & Bailey, 1990).

Thus the whole field of forensic psychiatry is essentially concerned with victims and survivors as well as offenders. More specifically, the principles of the treatment of traumatic stress with an emphasis upon both psychological and physiological aspects of PTSD are described by Ochberg (1988). He argues that the experiences of the victims of interpersonal violence are qualitatively different from those of other victims (e.g. of natural disasters) in that they frequently suffer from greater degrees of shame, self-blame, morbid hatred and a sense of grievance: other consequences include feelings of defilement and sexual inhibition. The subject is vast and fast-growing, and the reader is directed to specialised texts for a fuller account.

References

Abel, G., Becker, J., Cunningham-Rathner, J., *et al* (1988) Multiple paraphilic diagnoses among sex offenders. *Bulletin of the American Academy of Psychiatry and the Law*, **16**, 153–158.

Bennett, T. & Wright, R. (1984) *Burglars on Burglary*. Gower.

Bentovim, A. (1977) *First Steps Towards a Systems Analysis of Severe Physical Abuse to Children in the Family*. First report from Select Committee on Violence in the Family, **3**, 659–669.

——, Elton, A., Hildebrand, J., *et al* (1988) *Sexual Abuse in the Family*. Bristol: Wright.

Blair, C. D. & Lanyon, R. I. (1981) Exhibitionism: aetiology and treatment. *Psychology Bulletin*, **89**, 439–463.

Bluglass, R. (1980) Indecent exposure in the West Midlands. In *Sex Offenders in the Criminal Justice System* (ed. D. J. West), pp. 171–180, Cropwood Conference Series no. 12, Cambridge.

—— (1990) Shoplifting. In *Principles and Practice of Forensic Psychiatry* (eds R. Bluglass & P. Bowden), pp. 787–795. Edinburgh: Churchill Livingstone.

Bowden, P. (1978) Rape. *British Journal of Hospital Medicine*, 286–290.

British Medical Journal (1976) The absent minded shoplifter. **1**, 675–676.

Brittain, R. P. (1970) The sadistic murderer. *Medicine, Science and the Law*, **10**, 198–207.

Browne, F. (1992) Unquiet days in Belfast. *Journal of Forensic Psychiatry*, **3**, 207–209.

Chiswick, D. (1983) Sex crimes. *British Journal of Psychiatry*, **143**, 236–242.

Collins, J. & Bailey, S. (1990) Traumatic stress disorder and violent behaviour. *Journal of Traumatic Stress*, **3**.

Commissioner Garda Siochana (1993) *Report on Crime 1992*. Dublin: Stationery Office.

Cordess, C. (1990) Nuisance and obscene telephone calls. In *Principles and Practice of Forensic Psychiatry* (eds R. Bluglass & P. Bowden), pp. 677–682. Edinburgh: Churchill Livingstone.

Cremona, A. (1986) Mad drivers: psychiatric illness and driving performance. *British Journal of Hospital Medicine*, **35**, 193–195.

Crepault, C. & Couture, M. (1980) Men's erotic fantasies. *Archives of Sexual Behaviour*, **9**, 565–581.

Davis, G. E. & Leitenberg, H. (1987) Adolescent sex offenders. *Psychological Bulletin*, **101**, 417–427.

Day, K. (1988) A hospital-based treatment programme for male mentally handicapped offenders. *British Journal of Psychiatry*, **153**, 635–644.

Department of Transport (1990) *Road Accidents Great Britain 1990: The Casualty Report*. London: HMSO.

Department of Health and Social Security (1989) *Child Abuse – Working Together for the Protection of Children*. London: HMSO.

Doolan, B. (1991) *Principles of Irish Law* (3rd edn). Dublin: Gill & Macmillan.

D'Orban, P. T. (1976) Child stealing: a typology of female offenders. *British Journal of Criminology*, **16**, 275–281.

—— (1979) Women who kill their children. *British Journal of Psychiatry*, **134**, 560–571.

—— & Haydn-Smith, P. (1985) Men who steal children. *British Medical Journal*, **90**, 1784.

Egginton, J. (1989) *From Cradle to Grave*. London: W. H. Allen.

Esquirol, J. E. D. (1885) *Mental Maladies, Treatise on Insanity*. London: Hafner.

Finkelhor, D. (1986) *A Sourcebook on Child Sexual Abuse*. London: Sage.

Gayford, J. J. (1981) Indecent exposure: a review of the literature. *Medicine, Science and the Law*, **21**, 233–242.

Gibbens, T. C. N. (1981) Shoplifting. *British Journal of Psychiatry*, **138**, 346–347.

—— & Prince, J. (1962) *Shoplifting*. London: Institute for the Study and Treatment of Delinquency.

Gibson, E. (1975) *Homicide in England and Wales 1967–1971*. Home Office Research Study No. 31. London: HMSO.

Glaser, D. (1991) Treatment issues in child sexual abuse. *British Journal of Psychiatry*, **159**, 769–782.

Gordon, G. H. (1978) *The Criminal Law of Scotland*. Edinburgh: Green.

Green, C. M. (1981) Matricide by sons. *Medicine, Science and the Law*, **21**, 207–214.

Grubin, D. (1994) Sexual murder. *British Journal of Psychiatry*, **165**, 624–629.

Gunn, J. & Taylor, P. (1993) *Forensic Psychiatry: Clinical, Legal and Ethical Issues*. London: Butterworth Heinemann.

Harris, G. T. & Rice, M. E. (1984) Mentally disordered fire setters: Psychodynamic versus empirical approaches. *International Journal of Law and Psychiatry*, **7**, 19–34.

Harris, J. C. (1982) Non-organic failure to thrive syndomes. In *Failure to Thrive in Infancy and Early Childhood* (ed. P. J. Accado), pp. 150–159. Baltimore: University Park Press.

Hollin, C. & Howells, R. (1991) *Clinical Approaches to Sex Offenders and Their Victims*. Chichester: John Wiley.

Home Office (1990) *Criminal Statistics, England and Wales*. London: HMSO.

—— (1992) *Gender and the Criminal Justice System*. London: HMSO.

—— (1993) *Criminal Statistics, England and Wales*. London: HMSO.

Home Office Research Study (1988) *British Crime Survey*. London: HMSO.

—— (1992) *British Crime Survey*. London: HMSO.

Howard League Working Party (1985) *Unlawful Sex*. London: Waterlow.

Jackson, H. F., Glass, C. & Hope, S. (1987) A functional analysis of recidivist arson. *British Journal of Clinical Psychology*, **26**, 175–185.

Johnson, T. F., O'Brien, J. G. & Hudson, M. F. (1985) *Elder abuse: an Annotated Bibliography*. Westpoint, CT: Greenwood Press.

Kempe, C. H., Silver, F. N., Steele, B. F., *et al* (1962) The battered child syndrome. *Journal of the American Medical Association*.

Kennedy, H. & Grubin, D. (1992) Patterns of denial in sex offenders. *Psychological Medicine*, **22**, 191–196.

Kolvin, I. & Kaplan, C. A. (1988) Sex abuse in childhood. In *Recent Advances in Clinical Psychiatry* (ed. K. Granville-Grossman), pp. 227–243. Edinburgh: Churchill Livingstone.

Koss, M. P., Gidycz, C. A. & Wisniewski, N. (1988) The scope of rape: incidence and prevalence of sexual aggression and victimisation in a national sample of higher education students. *Journal of Consulting and Clinical Psychology*, **55**, 162–170.

Levin, J. & Fox, J. A. (1985) *Mass Murder*. New York: Plenum.

Lewis, N. D. C. & Yarnell, H. (1951) *Pathological Firesetting (Pyromania)*. Nervous and Mental Disease Monograph 82. New York: Coolidge Foundation.

MacCulloch, M. J., Snowden, P. R., Wood, P. J. W., *et al* (1983) Sadistic fantasy, sadistic behaviour and offending. *British Journal of Psychiatry*, **143**, 20–29.

Marshall, W. L., Laws, D. R. & Barbaree, H. E. (1990) *Handbook of Sexual Assault*. London: Plenum.

Masters, B. (1985) *Killing for Company*. Jonathan Cape.

—— (1993) *The Shrine of Jeffrey Dahmer*. London: Hodder & Stoughton.

Meadow, R. (1982) Münchausen syndrome by proxy. *Archives of Disease in Childhood*, **57**, 92–98.

—— (1989) Münchausen syndrome by proxy. *British Medical Journal*, **299**, 248–250.

Mezey, G. & Taylor, P. (1988) Psychological reaction of women who have been raped. *British Journal of Psychiatry*, **152**, 330–339.

—— & King, M. (1989) The effects of sexual assault on men: a survey of 22 victims. *Psychological Medicine*, **19**, 205–209.

Mullen, P. E. (1990) The long term influence of sexual assault on the mental health of victims. *Journal of Forensic Psychiatry*, 1, 13–31.

Northern Ireland Office (1993) *A Commentary on Northern Ireland Crime Statistics 1992*. Belfast: HMSO.

Ochberg, F. M. (1988) *Post Traumatic Therapy and Victims of Violence*. New York: Brunner/Mazel.

O'Sullivan, G. H. & Kelleher, M. J. (1987) A study of fire setters in the south west of Ireland. *British Journal of Psychiatry*, **151**, 818–823.

Perkins, D. (1991) Clinical work with sex offenders in secure settings. In *Clinical Approaches to Sex Offenders and Their Victims* (eds C. Hollin & K. Howells). Chichester: John Wiley.

Pithers, W. D. (1990) Relapse prevention with sexual aggressors: A method of maintaining thereapeutic gain and enhancing external supervision. In *Handbook of Sexual Assaults* (eds W. L. Marshall, D. R. Laws & H. E. Barbace). London: Plenum.

Pitt, B. (1992) Abusing old people. *British Medical Journal*, **305**, 968–969.

Pizzey, E. (1974) *Scream Quietly or the Neighbours will Hear*. Harmondsworth: Penguin.

Porter, R. (ed.)(1984) *Child Sexual Abuse within the Family*. London: CIBA Foundation/Tavistock.

Prentky, R. A., Knight, R. A. & Rosenburg, R. (1988) Validation analyses on a taxonomic system for rapists: disconfirmation and reconceptualisation. In *Human*

Sexual Aggression: Current Perspectives (eds R. A. Prentky & V. L. Quinsey), Annals of the New York Academy of Sciences, vol. 528.

Prins, H., Tennant, G. & Trick, K. (1985) Motives for arson (fireraising). *Medicine, Science and the Law*, **25**, 275–278.

Quinsey, V. L. (1984) Sexual aggression: studies of offenders against women. In *Law and Mental Health, International Perspectives I* (ed. D. Weisstub), pp. 84–121. New York: Pergamon.

Resnick, P. J. (1970) Murder of the newborn: a psychiatric review of neonaticide. *American Journal of Psychiatry*, **140**, 36–40.

Ressler, R., Burgess, M. & Douglas, J. (1988) *Sexual Homicide: Patterns and Motives*. Lexington: Lexington Books.

Rooth, F. G. (1971) Indecent exposure and exhibitionism. *British Journal of Hospital Medicine*, 521–533.

—— (1980) Exhibitionism: an eclectic approach to management. *British Journal of Hospital Medicine*, 366–370.

Rosen, I. (1979) Exhibitionism, scopophilia and voyeurism. In *Sexual Deviation* (ed. I. Rosen), pp. 139–194. Oxford: Oxford University Press.

Rutter, M. & Madge, N. (1976) *Cycles of Disadvantage: a Review of Research*. London: Heinemann.

Salter, A. C. (1988) *Treating Child Sex Offenders and Victims: a Practical Guide*. London: Sage.

Sapford, R. J., Banks, C. & Smith, D. D. (1978) Arsonists in prison. *Medicine, Science and the Law*, **18**, 247–254.

Schreier, H. & Libow, J. (1993) *Hurting for Love – Münchausen Syndrome by Proxy*. New York: Guilford.

Scott, P. (1973) Parents who kill their children. *Medicine, Science and the Law*, **13**, 120–126.

—— (1977) Assessing dangerousness in criminals. *British Journal of Psychiatry*, **131**, 127–142.

Scottish Office (1994) *Statistical Bulletin: Recorded Crime in Scotland 1993*. Edinburgh: Scottish Office Statistical Service.

Snaith, P. (1983) Exhibitionism: A clinical conundrum. *British Journal of Psychiatry*, **143**, 231–235.

Soothill, K. L. & Pope, P. J. (1973) Arson. A twenty year cohort study. *Medicine, Science and the Law*, **13**, 127–138.

——, Jack, A. & Gibbens, T. C. N. (1976) Rape: a 22-year cohort study. *Medicine, Science and the Law*, **16**, 62–69.

Sugarman, P. Dumughn, C., Saad, K., *et al* (1994) Dangerousness in exhibitionists. *Journal of Forensic Psychiatry*, **5**, 287–296.

Vizard, E. (1991) Interviewing children suspected of being sexually abused: a review of theory and practice. In *Clinical Approaches to Sex Offenders and Their Victims* (ed. C. Hollin & K. Howells). Chichester: John Wiley.

West, D. J. & Farrington, D. P. (1977) *The Delinquent Way of Life*. London: Heinemann.

Williams, A. H. (1964) The psychopathology and treatment of sexual murders. In *The Pathology and Treatment of Sexual Deviation: a Methodological Approach* (ed. I. Rose), pp. 351-377. Oxford: Oxford University Press.

Wilson, C. & Seaman, D. (1990) *The Serial Killers: A Study in the Psychology of Violence*. London: Allen & Unwin.

Yin, P. (1985) *Victimisation of the Aged*. Springfield, Illinois: Thomas.

3 Crime and mental disorder
II. Forensic aspects of psychiatric disorder
James Higgins

Schizophrenia • Affective disorder • Antisocial personality disorder •
Neurotic disorders • Learning disability • Organic states • Substance
misuse • Special syndromes • Minority groups

The relationship between psychiatric disorder and criminal behaviour is far from straightforward. Few psychiatric patients are offenders, and few offenders have a psychiatric disorder (Gunn, 1977a). The relationship may be examined in two ways. Firstly, we can look at offences and offenders, and ask what psychiatric pathology can be observed in association with particular types of offences and with particular offender groups. Secondly, we can ask what features of an individual suffering from a psychiatric disorder might bring that individual into contact with the criminal justice system, and how likely this is to occur. The first question has been discussed in Chapter 2, where the limitations of the approach have rightly been emphasised.

The second perspective is the subject of this chapter. The issues are complex. What do we mean by "an individual with a psychiatric disorder"? Is it a person who considers he has a psychiatric problem and desires or insists upon treatment, or a person treated by a general practitioner for minor psychological symptoms, or someone treated by a psychiatrist as an out-patient or in-patient? When do below-average intellectual abilities, minor adverse personality characteristics, minor neurotic conflicts, or harmful drinking or drug-taking patterns reach the level of a psychiatric disorder? In a psychiatric clinic out-patient sample, Guze *et al* (1974) found that only 4% of attenders had a record of a relatively serious offence, and that personality disorder and alcoholism were by far the most common diagnostic categories. Serious functional psychoses were completely absent. Perhaps this is explained by early diversion from the criminal justice system of offenders who are seriously mentally ill. Such individuals are not recorded in criminal statistics, and a significant relationship may thereby be concealed.

The purpose of stressing the difficulties in examining the relationship between mental abnormality and offending is to emphasise the complexity of the issues. It is important to avoid superficial and over-simplistic premises: for example, that all offenders must have psychological problems or even a psychiatric disorder; that people who commit rare, serious or bizarre offences must be psychiatrically disordered; that those with psychiatric disorder are prone to committing offences; or that those with particular psychiatric syndromes are likely to act in a particular antisocial way. It is preferable to see each mentally disordered offender as a rare individual from a unique social and cultural network, with particular advantages or disadvantages, who has acted in a particular way against people or property, at a particular time, in particular circumstances. He has been detected by the police, subsequently charged, and referred for a psychiatric assessment during which it has been discovered that there is sufficient psychopathology to constitute a diagnostic entity. The examining psychiatrist might then be able to attempt an explanation of what has taken place. But the 'softer' and the more minor the form of psychiatric disorder, the less likely is the emphasis to be on psychopathology than on social and psychological factors which contribute to the generality of offending. Even severe psychopathology, for which treatment in hospital may be advised, will rarely provide a complete explanation for the offending behaviour.

With these cautionary observations the reader should consider the following account of offending behaviour in different psychiatric disorders. Whether or not the psychiatric disorder leads the police or court to deal with the offender in a special way is an entirely separate issue which is discussed in Chapters 4 and 5.

Schizophrenia

Research provides limited answers to some important questions. Does having schizophrenia lead to a greater risk of offending? What sort of offending might this be, and at what stage of the illness might it occur? What clinical features are important, and what steps can be taken to prevent, or at least diminish, the risk of similar behaviour in the future?

Most research studies deal principally with cohorts of people with schizophrenia selected in specific ways. They often omit details which enable comparisons to be made over time and in different countries. They concentrate on the most serious offences and the most easily studied populations, namely those on remand or serving a sentence in prison, or those detained in a secure psychiatric hospital. The relationship found between schizophrenia and offending depends on the nature of the sample under study.

Relationship to offending behaviour

People with schizophrenia show a similar rate of offending in general as the rest of the population (Lindqvist & Allebeck, 1990). Although they are more likely to commit a crime of violence, this will usually be minor in degree. They are more likely than other offenders to be detected and arrested (Robertson, 1988). When samples of discharged patients with schizophrenia are examined, we find rates of violent offending that are significantly higher than in the general population (e.g. Zitrin *et al*, 1976). This may be because more people with schizophrenia are in the community, and therefore "available" for offending, than previously. For first admissions with schizophrenia, violence preceding admission is common (Humphreys *et al*, 1992). Similarly, among psychiatric in-patients, the highest frequency of violent incidents is found in those patients with schizophrenia (Noble & Rodger, 1989).

In prison remand populations, a person with schizophrenia is six times more likely than other prisoners to be facing a charge for violence (Taylor & Gunn, 1984). Among convicted prisoners serving sentences, Gunn *et al* (1991) reported that 1.5% suffered from schizophrenia.

The risk of violence by people with schizophrenia must be acknowledged, but put into proper perspective. Schizophrenia (27 cases) was the largest single category of psychiatric disorder in 100 homicides by mentally disordered people identified in a recent report (Confidential Inquiry into Homicides & Suicides by Mentally Ill People, 1994), compared with a total of approximately 1000 homicides in England and Wales during the same period. In a community survey in the US, Swanson *et al* (1990) found that any psychiatric diagnosis was associated with assaultive behaviour, but that rates were higher in those with alcohol and drug problems than in those with schizophrenia.

Patterns of clinical presentations

Patients with schizophrenia who offend fall into two broad categories, with some overlap. The first category consists of acutely ill patients with positive symptoms who act in response to delusional ideas, to redress a perceived wrong or to deal with a perceived threat. The link between the abnormal mental experiences and the offence is usually quite obvious. Patients with paranoid schizophrenia, in particular, may commit occasional but often well planned and serious violence.

In the second category of patients, some positive features of the illness are present but they tend to be less prominent. The significant features in this group are negative symptoms – the ravages of a more chronic and disabling illness. The offence is committed inadvertently or neglectfully, when confronted or thwarted, when no other alternative seems available, or even quite deliberately to achieve ends such as survival in the community, admission to hospital or prison, or prevention of discharge from hospital. In contrast, and much less frequently, a chronically ill patient may show a sudden and unexpected eruption of violence due to reactivation of an old delusional idea, the sudden emergence of a new highly arousing one, or some other new mental phenomenon.

Clinical features of forensic importance

Although there have been attempts to identify what specific features of schizophrenia might motivate offending behaviour, it is not possible to make any definitive statements. Certain constellations of symptoms are more worrying than others, but no particular abnormal mental experience is of special value in predicting future offending behaviour. Indeed, it is remarkable how rarely patients act aggressively in the face of beliefs and experiences which give concern to others. Equally, any delusional idea, hallucinatory experience or other abnormal mental phenomenon may provide the focus for behaviour which could result in an offence. Each patient must be assessed individually. The assessment is not just of mental state, but also the availability and features of a specific victim, and whether there are social and environmental factors which might increase or reduce the risk. These are now considered in turn.

The illness

(1) *Level of arousal or distress.* Abnormal mental experiences affect patients in different ways. A patient who is manifestly distressed by them, who is anxious, uncertain, perplexed, threatened or frightened, is more likely to act in an unpredictable way, either spontaneously or when confronted. Conversely, an emotionally blunted individual with deterioration of personality may be able to cope, with apparent equanimity, with ideas and experiences which would seem to warrant offensive or defensive action. There has been interest in determining at what stage of a schizophrenic illness violent behaviour occurs. Early in the illness, when starting to experience uncertainties about himself and others around him, about his place and purpose in the world, and while still retaining a relatively undamaged capacity for normal affective responses, he may become irritable and uncertain and act aggressively towards others. Usually the persistence of normal aspects of personality acts as a brake on aggressive behaviour, especially in those not habitually prone to using violence to resolve interpersonal difficulties.

Progression of the illness, with elaboration and crystallisation of abnormal ideas, together with increasing damage to other aspects of the personality, might provide more fertile ground for acting on delusional ideas (Taylor, 1985). As the illness develops further, encapsulation and emotional blunting supervene and may again reduce the risk. Hafner & Boker (1982) provided some support for such a progression. In their sample of schizophrenic homicides in West Germany between 1953 and 1964, only 3% of offenders killed within one month of the start of their illness, 84% had been ill for more than one year, and 55% for over five years. The patients were usually well known to the psychiatric services.

As a general principle it is prudent to pay particular attention to the patient's degree of arousal, to estimate how close he seems to be to loss of control, and how close he thinks he is to loss of control. It is essential to consult those who know him well for any new attitudes or behaviours which might indicate impending loss of control.

(2) *Delusional ideas.* Delusional ideas often motivate an act. Half of the cohort reported by Wessely *et al* (1993) had acted on their delusions, although violent acts were uncommon. Hafner & Boker (1982) found that delusions were present in 89% of their sample of violent schizophrenic offenders, compared with 76% of the schizophrenic controls; delusions of infidelity and infatuation were particularly common. Delusions of being directly threatened are obviously important, particularly when the threat is specifically ascribed to an individual. Delusions of poisoning have also been described in relation to violence (Mawson, 1985). In a study of first schizophrenic episodes (Humphreys *et al*, 1992), half of the cohort acted violently in response to delusions (usually of poisoning) or hallucinations.

Violence seems particularly likely when the patient's response to these delusions (often bizarre) is ignored by the recipient. Delusional ideas with marked religious components, or those concerned with the occult or with an omnipotent or cataclysmic quality, have an ominous ring. Strong emotional investment in such ideas, often after a period of considerable deliberation, sometimes permits the overriding of taboos against violence towards close relatives or neighbours. The violence may be carried out in the victim's supposed best interest, or in the expectation that it will produce no real harm and might resolve issues of cosmic significance.

The particular risk of violence from jealous men, in this context those with delusions of jealousy in the setting of a schizophrenic illness, have been described by Mowat (1966). Other delusional ideas arising in schizophrenia, de Clerambault's syndrome (erotomania, see later), and Capgras' syndrome (delusion of doubles) are occasionally reported as resulting in violent behaviour.

(3) *Other phenomena.* Command hallucinations or other overwhelming hallucinatory or passivity experiences are worrying developments. Patients reporting these, especially if concerned about their ability to resist them, must be treated very seriously. Sadly, such phenomena are likely to be revealed only after the event and may even be denied beforehand. Their existence may be suspected by sudden changes in attitude and behaviour associated with obvious autonomic features of arousal. Self-destruction may be seen by the patient as the only solution; attempted suicide by fire resulting in a charge of arson.

Features of the victim

There has already been reference to the importance of a readily available victim. Assaultive crimes by people with schizophrenia are similar to most assaults. For the most part these assaults are against victims they already know: wives, children, relatives, friends or neighbours. Perhaps in the killing of parents they may be exceptional (Gillies, 1976). The assault of strangers by people with schizophrenia is, in fact, a rare event. The most commonly assaulted stranger is the arresting police officer after a public order offence.

In assessing the likely risk to a victim, it is essential to explore the delusional ideas very carefully (an assessment analogous to that of risk of suicide). The better a specific victim can be identified, the more specific the threats that have been made, and the clearer that future action has been contemplated or planned, then the more serious the risk to the victim. The real or perceived response of the victim to early approaches is also important. The response may be considered by the patient to be provocative, either because it is aggressive in self-defence or through fear, or because it was evasive and ambivalent.

Situational factors

The concept of high expressed emotion explains the effects that certain attitudes and behaviours of relatives can have on the patient's mental state. Increasing tension, anger and frustration may result in emotional outbursts and violence. In hospital or other residential settings, institutional factors are equally important (Powell *et al*, 1994). An overcrowded, over-restrictive ward, impoverished in occupational and recreational resources, may prove too unsettling and stimulating for an actively psychotic patient. Certain times of day and certain ward activities are well recognised as the most unsettling; getting up, washing, meals and medication times are the most widely reported occasions when aggressive behaviours occur. Those looking after highly aroused and acutely ill patients should be aware of these features, and not see intensive social interactions as a necessary goal in the early stages of treatment. It is unfortunate that disturbed behaviour is so readily ascribed to features in a patient, rather than the quite unsuitable setting in which he may be treated.

Substance misuse is a recognised feature of much offending behaviour, and many mentally ill people are intoxicated when they commit offences. The interaction between substance misuse and schizophrenia is complex and the magnitude of the problem underestimated (Smith & Hucker, 1994). Alcohol or drug misuse may be a precipitating factor, related to the onset or relapse of the illness. In a sample of acutely psychotic patients admitted to hospital, more florid symptoms were found in those with cannabis-positive urine analyses than in others (Mathers & Ghodse, 1992). Substances may have been taken in increasing quantity as the most readily available and effective tranquilliser for disturbing abnormal mental experiences. They may be used to give "Dutch courage" to act upon delusional ideas. A careful assessment is required to evaluate the part played by alcohol or drugs for diagnostic, management and predictive purposes.

Box 3.1 Schizophrenia and offending

Minor offences are more common than serious offences
People with schizophrenia are overrepresented among violent
  offenders and violent in-patients
Violence may occur in acute or chronic phases of illness
Acting on delusions is common in schizophrenia
Individual phenomenology, situational factors and features of the
  victim may all contribute to violence
Substance misuse is commonly a contributory factor

It is essential to review the availability or possession of lethal weapons
by the patient and to consider why a particular weapon was chosen; this
may have been on impulse or as a considered decision. Sometimes the
patient may have carried the weapon as a result of his illness or as a
feature of his cultural or subcultural mores.

Personality and treatment considerations

Consideration of personality features is important in understanding the
interplay of factors producing offending behaviour. This is necessary in
planning effective treatment and aftercare. The interplay of personality
features and schizophrenia is complex, and the following issues are
relevant.

Premorbid delinquency

An individual who subsequently develops schizophrenia may have the
premorbid characteristics and social and cultural background of a 'normal'
delinquent. When the illness supervenes, there is usually a change in the
observable behaviour and this may result in a different type of offending.
Treatment of the schizophrenia, and restitution of as near normal functioning as possible, is unlikely to affect the pre-existing pattern of offending,
especially if this is ingrained and receives cultural reinforcement. Care is
therefore required in assessing the effects of the illness, what treatment is
required, and where this should take place. In general, a schizophrenic
offender's need for assessment and treatment in hospital should be
determined solely by his mental state at the time of the examination.
Occasionally, continuing treatment of a well-stabilised, optimally-treated
and compliant schizophrenic offender is practicable in prison. Psychiatric
treatment, however, is much more than the use of medication. Prison is
a stressful environment for a psychologically robust individual, let alone
one who is mentally ill. Regimens in prisons do not tolerate behavioural

quirks and usually the only measure is one of containment. The organisation of prisons can lead to a mentally ill prisoner becoming 'lost' to care.

On the other hand, suffering from schizophrenia which is well under control should not provide an automatic escape from the results of wilful and deliberate offending in a patient who shows good social adjustment. To summarise, any person with schizophrenia in custody should be transferred to hospital for assessment and treatment, unless there is a cogent case for a contrary approach.

Premorbid schizoid features

In some youths or young adults, offending may be unexpected in the light of the person's social and subcultural background. It may appear to arise from a gradual development of schizoid personality characteristics, usually starting in early adolescence, with the suggestion of underlying psychosis. A careful assessment of such individuals is necessary, preferably in hospital, and probably involving a trial of treatment with neuroleptic medication. This is easier to implement if the individual is willing to accept such a course. If the offence is minor there may be difficulty in justifying compulsory detention and treatment in hospital. It is, however, very important to make the best assessment and to institute treatment quickly to prevent further deterioration. When such diagnostic difficulties persist in more serious offenders, and admission to hospital is not considered appropriate, the sentence of the court is often a disproportionately lengthy period of imprisonment, if only because of the psychiatric uncertainty and possible risk. Such individuals often emerge later in prison with a florid psychotic illness. The subsequent management of such potentially dangerous and damaged individuals, in prison, in hospital and in the community, requires much careful planning.

Schizophrenia and personality deterioration

Undue emphasis is sometimes given to adverse personality characteristics, when all the evidence indicates that these have arisen solely as a result of a chronic schizophrenic illness. Deleterious effects on personality are well recognised features of schizophrenia and it seems unnecessary to apply an additional diagnosis of personality disorder. Perhaps the reason for this preoccupation with features of personality lies in frustration at the inability to manage, with the facilities available, that group of petty recidivist, chronically psychotic, socially disadvantaged and friendless individuals, almost invariably of no fixed abode, who have been succinctly described by Rollin (1969) as "incorrigible in penal terms and untreatable in medical terms". Changes in the philosophy of psychiatric care have led to the closure of facilities which can provide long-term care for such individuals. Unfortunately, the necessary alternative community facilities are rare, or patients decline to use them. Surely it cannot be intended that prisons should once again become the principal providers of care for people with chronic schizophrenia, arrested by the police because of their manifestly dilapidated and deteriorating state, or because of minor offences committed to survive in the community.

Schizophrenia in sentenced prisoners

Finally, imprisonment does not predispose or protect an individual from developing a first episode of schizophrenia. The majority of such illnesses are unremarkable in nature. Substance misuse is, however, now endemic in prisons, and psychosis may be attributed to drug-taking. Sometimes the drug-taking history is unconvincing, or it follows the onset of psychosis, or the psychosis persists after a drug-free period, or reappears when there has been no further drug misuse. The management of such a sentenced prisoner with an acute psychosis should be a relatively straightforward matter. He should be transferred under Section 47 of the Mental Health Act 1983 to a hospital offering the degree of security required by his mental state and behaviour and by the perceived risk to the community (see Chapter 7). If the sentence is a long one, imposed for a serious offence, a secure unit is appropriate, but when the sentence is short and the offence petty, there is often an unfortunate reluctance by local psychiatric hospitals to agree to a transfer.

The management of prisoners with schizophrenia who are serving long sentences, particularly life imprisonment, poses particular difficulties. Ideally such a prisoner should be transferred to hospital for treatment of his mental illness. If treatment is successful, he must be remitted to prison; indeed, the patient may bitterly object to continued detention in a psychiatric hospital and may act out accordingly. If the prisoner then stops taking medication on return to prison, the cycle of transfer to hospital will be repeated. For some mentally ill life-sentenced prisoners, release is often much delayed, not because of risk to the public, or for reasons of retribution and deterrence, but because of the emergence of a psychiatric disorder which did not exist at the time of the index offence. Such prisoners are subjected to a form of double jeopardy, and it requires flexibility by the Home Office and psychiatric hospitals to circumvent it.

Affective disorder

The clinical features of the two main syndromes of affective disorder, depression and hypomania, determine what types of offending behaviour may be likely. However, research in this area is limited and its interpretation is bedevilled by uncertainties in the criteria used to classify depression over time and in different countries, and because the samples of hypomanic patients who have committed antisocial acts are very small.

Depression

Assessment of the nature, severity and relevance of depressive symptoms in forensic settings presents particular difficulties. Depression after arrest might incorrectly be seen as reactive to circumstances. A criminal act and its aftermath may have a cathartic effect or be seen by the perpetrator as justified punishment, both resulting in deceptive presentations of calmness and detachment. Increased alcohol consumption is occasionally a major feature of a depressive disorder, and this may be seen as a prominent component in the explanation of the offender's behaviour. A careful history is therefore required, not only to detect depression but to delineate its exact nature, to ensure that the most appropriate treatment approach is taken, and that the anticipated outcome is realistic. Overreliance on the effects of antidepressant medication without proper regard for personality features and the effects of social circumstances can result in therapeutic over-optimism, only to be followed by frustration and disappointment.

Relationship to offending behaviour

(1) *Violence.* One in six people with manic–depressive disorder kill themselves. Violence to others is much rarer; only six in 100 000 people with the disorder were seriously violent to others (Hafner & Boker, 1982). However, there has been very little published research on the subject of violence and mania. Violence by people with depressive disorders is usually directed towards close family members: husbands towards wives and children; mothers towards children. The classical picture is that of psychotic depression with delusional ideas of unworthiness, self-criticism, failure, poverty and physical illness. The resultant suicidal ideation is then extended to include the killing of close family members in an extended suicide, the patient believing that if the family members were dead they would not have to endure the additional distress, humiliation and stigma of a suicide in the family. Only a proportion of such depressive killers come to court because many succeed in committing suicide (West, 1965).

Some authors have questioned this simple picture of altruistic suicide, emphasising the frequency of insoluble conflicts in a chronically unhappy relationship, particularly with men who kill their partners. These may result in mounting tension, anger, frustration and even jealousy, which then explodes into lethal violence, often precipitated by a final but unremarkable event (Parker, 1979). In such cases, although depression is a prominent feature and may even be severe, the clinical picture is of a non-psychotic depressive episode in a personality with features vulnerable to, and perhaps contributing to, chronic marital disharmony.

Predicting which depressed women will kill their children, and husbands their wives, cannot be based on any particular feature of mental state but is analogous to the assessment of a potentially suicidal patient. Every seriously depressed individual, psychotic or otherwise, should be asked about homicidal intent, particularly if there are vulnerable potential victims. Sadly, many cases will present with the killing and subsequent failed suicide, but it has been observed that the most likely time for such an outburst of violence, in depressed patients already known to psychiatric services, is some months after discharge from hospital, when drive has returned but the illness remains incompletely resolved (Hafner & Boker, 1982).

(2) *Shoplifting*. Shoplifting has been regularly reported in association with depression. Gibbens *et al* (1971), for a large sample of female shoplifters assessed on bail, described 5% who required psychiatric treatment, 24% suffering from depressive disorder and 2% with a manic–depressive illness. In another sample of women remanded in custody, 4% were subsequently admitted to hospital, a third of those with a manic–depressive illness. These proportions are very small, and while the diagnostic status of the manic–depressive cases is clear, Gibbens *et al* (1971) is less specific about the nature of the depressive disorders. A presentation with mixed clinical features is commonly found in the psychologically disturbed female shoplifter (Gudjonsson, 1990). Typically she harbours suppressed and unexpressed emotions about the changes in her life in her middle age, frustration at her lack of opportunity, and the unrewarding nature of changing family relationships. She may have experienced a series of disturbing life events, or physical illness. Hostility and anger are often as prominent as depression, and biological features may not always be present. Simple treatment with antidepressants is thus rarely successful. A full account of other aspects of shoplifting is discussed in Chapter 2.

(3) *Other forensic presentations*. Depression may result in attempted suicide by fire, and a charge of arson may follow. A minor sexual offence by a depressed man may be best understood as the result of sexual regression, but occasionally it is difficult to avoid the view that it has a symbolic self-destructive quality (see Chapter 2).

Hypomania and mania

Hypomania presents in forensic practice more frequently than depression. Elated, overactive, grandiose, irritable, paranoid and sexually disinhibited individuals, perhaps misusing alcohol, act in ways which are embarrassing, disruptive, intolerable or threatening. If the behaviour is not seen as an obvious manifestation of mental illness, it may result in criminal prosecution.

Some hypomanic patients, especially those with a low-grade grumbling illness associated with chronic alcohol misuse, present particular problems in diagnosis. The affective illness is sometimes missed on remand, mistaken emphasis being given to the drinking problem. The illness may also pass unreported during a short period of imprisonment, provided the level of importunate behaviour is not sufficiently irritating to raise the suspicion of anything other than the 'personality disorder' which the individual is thought to possess. The best way of avoiding such errors is not so much a careful mental state examination, which may be inconclusive, but a careful review of previous medical records that usually exist in abundance. Clear-cut episodes of affective illness may then be seen (depressive as well as hypomanic). The correct diagnosis, however, often does not make management any easier. It is difficult to break the cycle of brief and unrewarding hospital admissions followed by default from aftercare, and a return to alcohol misuse and subsequent offending.

Relationship to offending behaviour

(1) *Petty offending.* Traditionally the pattern of offending in hypomania has been described as quite minor: drunkenness, minor violence and threats of violence, deception and misrepresentation, inappropriate and importunate sexual behaviour. Many manic patients, although acting in ways which could attract a charge, are so obviously behaving out of character and are so obviously mentally ill that they are diverted from the criminal justice system and taken directly to hospital. On the other hand, those who are more chronically disabled by the illness, often with a history of petty recidivism and alcoholism, and who have not responded to or cooperated with psychiatric treatment in the past, tend to appear before courts because there does not seem any better way of dealing with their persistently disruptive behaviour. Hospitals are reluctant to admit them because of the difficulty of containment and compliance experienced in the past. The lengthy remand period in prison, perhaps amounting to the length of sentence which can be imposed, is often taken up with negotiations over finding a place in hospital.

(2) *Serious offending.* The work of Wulach (1983) provides a contrast. He described 100 manic offenders in custody, 13% of whom had committed serious offences, death by dangerous driving, arson and rape. This sample is clearly a much more selected one, but it serves to indicate that manic people do commit more serious offences, as experience of working in a regional secure unit will readily confirm.

(3) *Female offenders.* Women with bipolar illnesses consisting of short and rapid cycling episodes pose particular difficulties. Within a brief period they can present to psychiatrists with depression and self-injury, resulting in a short and unsatisfactory admission to hospital, or they present to the police as irritable public nuisances, often intoxicated. Their volatility of mood is frequently ascribed to an hysterical personality disorder, with or without substance misuse; each episode is seen as a response to the social

---

Box 3.2 Affective disorders and offending

Offending is less common than in other functional psychoses

Violent offending in depressive disorder is rare but may be serious

In severe depression, enquiry should be made about homicidal ideation

A family member is the usual victim in altruistic homicides

Shoplifting, particularly in middle-aged offenders, may be associated with depressive disorder

Offending is more common in mania and hypomania than in depression, and may be serious

Rapid-cycling bipolar disorder may be missed in offender patients

---

or interpersonal problems with which they are often burdened. Again, a longitudinal perspective is often valuable. Periods of unexpected stability may be seen on mental state examination, together with features hinting at a primary affective disorder. Treatment is often rewarding if the illness is not too chronic or if adverse behavioural patterns are not too entrenched.

Schizoaffective illness

Reference to this diagnosis rarely appears in the forensic literature. D'Orban (1979), in his study of women who killed their children, does mention a few patients with such an illness, presumably schizodepressive in type. Occasionally a typical manic illness supervenes in an individual with a chronic paranoid illness or a markedly paranoid personality, the new affective features producing an additional dimension to previous aggressive behaviour. The affective symptoms are likely to respond readily to treatment, but with little benefit to the underlying paranoid personality.

Treatment considerations

The treatment of forensic patients with affective disorders differs little from that in general psychiatric practice. However, two specifically forensic points are worthy of discussion. Firstly, no matter how typical the illness and the speed of its response to physical treatment, a depressed patient who has committed a seriously violent act or a homicide will require much psychotherapeutic assistance. This is needed to allow the patient to come to terms with what is often a personal and family tragedy, particularly as there is retention of an intact personality structure. Secondly, as has been described, the depressive illnesses are often not typical, with personality features playing a prominent part. Both considerations make the appropriate placement of a depressed serious offender a difficult problem. Rapid response to treatment, which in a non-offending patient would indicate a prompt discharge from hospital, might not meet the needs of the patient and the family or the expectations of the public. A surprising proportion of offenders found to be of diminished responsibility, said to be due to depression, are sent to prison rather than to hospital (Dell & Smith, 1983).

Treatment of recurrent or chronic hypomania in an unstable individual is difficult, whether the instability is independent or a result of the illness. Lithium is often unsuitable as a prophylactic because of anticipated poor compliance. A depot neuroleptic might be preferable and is occasionally effective, but the characteristic long-term side-effects may be more prominent in hypomania than in schizophrenia.

Antisocial personality disorder

People with abnormalities and disorders of personality form a large proportion of patients seen in forensic psychiatry. This section is concerned with the relationship between personality disorder and offending behaviour, with particular emphasis on antisocial personality disorder. Conceptual understanding of personality and its disorders is unresolved and controversial. It is not possible to discuss here those conceptual problems; there have been recent reviews by Freeman (1993) and Tyrer & Stein (1993) to which the reader is referred. There are two particular pitfalls in forensic psychiatry in respect of personality disorder. First is the missing or making of such a diagnosis in the absence of a properly obtained history and appraisal of other information. Second is the tendency to be misled by stereotypes or caricatures, so that a diagnosis of personality disorder is made on the basis of little more than one criminal act simply because the latter is particularly grave or horrific.

Clinical and legal concepts

Before discussing the relationship between personality disorder and offending, it is important to try to make sense of a confusing terminology. 'Psychopathic disorder' is a term that has come to be used in at least two quite separate ways. As a clinical term it is the rather outdated equivalent for what we would today call 'antisocial personality disorder'. However, the term has also acquired a pejorative connotation, particularly when a patient is identified as "a psychopath" or as "psychopathic". The implications are that the patient is untreatable, has no proper place in a hospital and is disliked by clinical staff. It is often employed in order to reject patients for treatment and for this purpose may be deliberately applied to patients with other psychiatric disorders such as schizophrenia or hypomania (Coid, 1988). For all these reasons it is best to avoid 'psychopathic disorder' as a clinical term.

The term will not, however, disappear, because it is part of English law. Psychopathic disorder is one of the four categories of mental disorder in the Mental Health Act 1983 for which compulsory admission may be appropriate (see Chapter 10). Forensic psychiatrists are divided in their views as to whether or not psychopathic disorder should remain in mental health legislation (Cope, 1993). In Scotland, although the words 'psycho-pathic disorder' do not appear in its legislation, a phrase almost identical to the English definition does. Legally, psychopathic disorder is:

> "a persistent disorder or disability of mind (whether or not including significant impairment of intelligence) which results in abnormally aggressive or seriously irresponsible conduct on the part of the person concerned." (Section 1(2), Mental Health Act 1983)

The Butler report (Home Office & Department of Health and Social Security, 1975) provides a useful historical account of the concept of 'psychopathic disorder'. The 'psychopath' and his ancestor in legislation, the 'moral imbecile', represent one aspect of the way the law has tried to exercise control over unacceptable behaviour. In its legal use the term has no specific clinical meaning. It does not mean a unitary condition, but is a generic term which might apply to any disorder (provided it is persistent) which results in antisocial conduct. When using the legal term 'psycho-pathic disorder', the psychiatrist should specify the nature of the clinical disorder present.

In practice, it is preferable to avoid using the term except in its legal context. However, even that dictum would not end the confusion because of the equally inadequate diagnostic basis of the alternative, 'antisocial

---

Box 3.3 Antisocial personality disorder and offending

The term 'psychopathic disorder' should only be used as a legal category

Personality disorders in forensic psychiatry are usually mixed in type

Diagnosis should be based upon longitudinal assessment and information from other sources

A wide range of abnormal personality traits contribute to offending behaviour

Substance misuse is a commonly associated finding

There is an increased likelihood of other psychiatric symptoms and disorders

Features of borderline personality disorder are common in female offenders in secure settings

personality disorder'. Dolan & Coid (1993) have reviewed the varied diagnostic approaches to antisocial personality disorder and their particular shortcomings in forensic practice. Offenders with personality disorders rarely seem to fit neatly into a single type of personality disorder, be it antisocial, schizoid, paranoid or any other. Coid (1992) found a mean of over three categories of personality disorder per patient in a sample of special hospital patients detained in the legal category 'psychopathic disorder'. Rather than stretching an ill-fitting category of personality disorder, it is preferable to describe the particular manifestations of disordered personality seen in the patient.

Personality disorder and offending

In the account that follows we will review the most prominent and broadest constellations of abnormal personality traits, and consider the types of offending behaviour that commonly follow. These are identified for descriptive purposes as "immaturity", "inadequacy", "hostility and aggression" and "abnormal sexuality". These are not used as scientific terms, but simply to describe the behavioural traits most commonly encountered.

Immaturity

By the term 'immature' we refer to the persistence of attitudes and behaviour associated with younger age, particularly egocentricity, emotional lability, lack of foresight, impulsivity and the need for instant reward or gratification; all are features more characteristic of a child than an adult. Such characteristics can bring individuals into conflict with various social agencies because of their self-serving, predatory or exploitative consequences. Resulting offences are usually minor but may be more serious: robbery; rape without particular sexual or aggressive psychopathology; arson for revenge or to disguise offending; and violence as an impulsive or ill-considered solution to conflict. Alcohol is often a disinhibiting factor. Adolescent or young adult males frequently show excitement-seeking and self-interested behaviour, but with age it usually declines. However, it may be found to persist, often well into middle-age, in those who follow a habitually criminal lifestyle. A common sequence is for overt offending to cease in the early 20s, the consequences of immature traits then transferring from the macrosocial sphere of the community to the microsocial sphere of the family, with all the long-term consequences for partners and children.

Inadequacy

Some petty recidivist men and women show a striking inability to organise their lives in an effective way. Their relationships are shallow and evanescent, exploitative or exploited. Their offending, mostly petty property offences, repeatedly takes place in an attempt to survive, or at least this is the explanation usually proffered. Non-payment of fines or non-compliance with probation eventually results in imprisonment.

Chronic substance misuse is common, principally alcohol and minor tranquillisers, the latter often prescribed for persistent feelings of depression and anxiety. Sexual and physical abuse of children may be found in the disorganised and disjointed family units such individuals form. In such vulnerable women, prostitution is another way of coping.

Hostility and aggression

Well integrated personalities. Some individuals with otherwise relatively well integrated personalities may use aggression as a tool, the extent of any violence dispensed being carefully titrated to achieve desired ends. Professional criminals or "single issue fanatics", such as terrorists or other ideologically motivated individuals, may demonstrate a wealth of evidence of adequate functioning in almost all other aspects of their lives. Their inability to empathise with the targeted individual or innocent stranger is a striking flaw in an otherwise unremarkable personality.

Habitually violent offenders. Habitually violent offenders are quite different, often with sensitive, paranoid and rather primitive personalities. They are anxious, ill-at-ease and quick to perceive a slight; they feel themselves constantly under threat, often to the extent of carrying a weapon for "self defence". Their violence is inappropriate, disproportionate and ineffective in achieving their aims, regularly generating the sequence of responses from others which they claim to have been present in the first instance.

Paranoid personalities. The severity and persistence of paranoid ideation in some individuals can lead to the suspicion that there is a psychotic element but, in the absence of other features of psychosis, the paranoid ideas are better described as overvalued. The usual basis for this over-sensitivity lies in low self-esteem, often despite marked protestations to the contrary. Low self-esteem is often understandable in the context of their damaging childhood and early adolescent experiences. Such individuals are habitually highly aroused, often misusing what tranquillisers are readily available, particularly alcohol. Their mood is very dependent on their perception of their immediate social circumstances, which they attempt to control by dominating those around them. In such a constellation of characteristics, possessive jealousy in their relationships is not unexpected. Regular violence towards partners is common and occasionally fatal; mounting suspicion, coupled with the disinhibiting effects of large amounts of alcohol or drugs, provides a lethal combination.

Over-controlled personalities. For some violent offenders, it is said after the serious assault or homicide that it was totally out of character, because they are the meekest and most non-violent of men. On investigation the history is of an inability to handle assertiveness and aggression in an effective way. In a close or over-involved relationship that they cannot give up for fear of further loss of self-esteem, they seek to accommodate their partner at every turn, repressing the feelings of anger at perceived slights, rejections, and manipulations. These over-controlled personalities struggle to contain hostile feelings, revealing them only obliquely as depression, anxiety or hypochondriacal preoccupations. One incident then breaches the dam. It may be very minor, no different from many that have gone before. Alcohol, drug misuse, tiredness, physical illness or an unexpected life event outside the relationship may serve to act as the precipitant. The violence is often extreme, the memory of inflicting it often hazy or non-existent. The aftermath is profound remorse, bland post-cathartic serenity, or even denial of complicity. The problem having been resolved, the pre-existing style of personality functioning is likely to reassert itself, and therapy is thereby rendered difficult. A further outburst of such violence is unlikely, unless a similar relationship is formed.

Abnormal sexuality

This topic is considered in more detail in Chapter 2. Some general points are given here. It is incorrect to assume that all sexual offences are primarily the result of sexual psychopathology. Aggression and desires to shock, frighten, exploit, degrade, hurt and even kill are often intimately involved with sexual feelings. Aggression may play the major part in offences which superficially appear to be sexual. For example, some male exhibitionists manifest a pattern of frustration, disappointment and compulsion, exposing only at times of stress and often with covert or overt aggressive intent.

Many instances of the most serious sexual offences (i.e. rape and rape/homicide) are principally offences of violence. The motivation, consciously or subconsciously, is often despoilation, revenge, destruction, or release of tension rather than sexual gratification. The psychopathology is usually that of unresolved aggressive feelings about significant female figures, often the mother, for whom the victim becomes a surrogate, or even a representation of all women. There is often a history of factors such as a cold and affectionless upbringing by unloving parents, a violent father and an over-involved mother, institutional rearing, sexual abuse, persistent uncertainties about sexual orientation, all in a setting of marked psychological disturbance and low self-esteem.

Homosexuality

Only a small subgroup of homosexual men, like a similar subgroup of heterosexual men, have such difficulties in their relationships or in control of their sexual behaviour that they act in an antisocial way. It is thus not homosexual activity which is illegal, but how, where and with whom it is performed. Accordingly, as with heterosexual offences, it is sexual behaviour which is coercive, public, or with minors which is illegal; the psychopathology associated with those features is important.

Treatment considerations

The above description demonstrates the difficulties in classifying personality disorder into subtypes and in separating personality disorder from neurosis. Such nosological endeavours have their place but, when dealing with offenders who present with neurotic difficulties and show evidence of personality abnormality, it is unusual for a distinct subtype of personality disorder to be identified. It is more common to find a series of characteristics or behaviours of varying severity which demonstrate the individuality of the offender rather than a manifestation of a particular type of personality. These individual characteristics and their origins and development have to be assessed when considering treatment and prognosis. A diagnosis of personality disorder does not grant immunity from developing other psychiatric illnesses; just the reverse seems to apply (Vize & Tyrer, 1994). Affective, paranoid, neurotic and somatic symptoms are common in this group and may be severe enough to warrant a separate diagnosis.

A simple diagnostic category, particularly psychopathic or antisocial personality disorder, says little about the individual, and leads to therapeutic nihilism. This is not to minimise the diagnostic difficulties, nor to overstate the effectiveness of treatment for those with marked personality difficulties. However, unless the presenting problems are analysed carefully, no treatment strategy can be formulated. Such a strategy may be as simple as bailing the patient out at times of stress and distress, dispensing medication for a short period, or offering a brief admission to hospital. Long-term psychotherapeutic support may be indicated and welcomed by a capable individual. More specific deficits may be tackled by various models of group or individual psychotherapy in settings determined by the degree of structure and security required, the motivation of the patient and his capacities. Expectations of outcome need to be realistic and, usually, modest; an approach based on limited expectations of success, as with other chronic psychiatric illnesses, is more appropriate.

Borderline personality disorder

This term, with its shared origin in psychoanalysis and hospital psychiatry, has proved useful in describing a group of individuals with marked impairment of sense of self-worth and role who form damaged and volatile relationships with others. Jackson & Tarnopolsky (1990) provide an excellent review. People with borderline personality disorder are impulsive, destructive and self-destructive, experience bouts of despair, anomy, neurotic decompensation and even brief psychotic episodes characterised by partial loss of contact with reality, concreteness of thinking and paranoid ideation. The forensic importance of such people is in their capacity for bizarre and violent acting-out under stress, resulting in serious offences including sexual offences and arson. When such people are in hospital or prison, acts of serious self-harm and arson are common.

Early damage to personality development, perhaps associated with sexual abuse, are common aetiological findings. Treatment is notoriously unrewarding; many such patients are repeatedly imprisoned but a proportion, particularly women, may spend lengthy periods in secure hospitals. In a study of self-mutilating women in Holloway remand prison, Wilkins & Coid (1991) found high rates of diagnoses of personality disorders, particularly of a borderline type. Neuroleptic medication (or sometimes lithium) may induce a period of stability, but sometimes long-term containment may be the only realistic treatment option. Treatment approaches have been comprehensively reviewed by Tantam & Whittaker (1992).

Neurotic disorders

It is not common to find offending behaviour in association with a condition that fully satisfies the diagnostic criteria in ICD–10 for neurotic, stress-related and somatoform disorders. That is not to say that neurotic symptoms are not common in offenders; they are, but causal connection with an offence is more likely to be found in an alternative psychiatric diagnosis (e.g. personality disorder, affective disorder or substance misuse). There is, of course, a close link between personality disorder and neurotic symptoms. The preferred diagnosis may depend on whether a longitudinal (in the former) or transverse approach (in the latter) is adopted. Equally it may appear to depend on whether treatment is, or is not, recommended.

Neurotic conflicts (as distinct from disorders) may play a speculative part in just about every type of offence – as they may in any example of abnormal behaviour. Such conflicts have been implicated in shoplifting, fire-raising and sex offending, all of which are further discussed in Chapter 2. West (1988) provides a perceptive review of individual psychopathology and its relationship to crime. The factors that determine whether an offender with neurotic conflicts will receive treatment are complex and often depend on non-clinical issues. For the psychiatrist, decisions about treatment should, as ever, be made on clinical grounds according to the nature of the disorder and whether, even in the absence of an offence, it reasonably warrants treatment.

Learning disability

The range of learning disabilities is wide, and is conventionally divided into four groups: profound, severe, moderate and mild. The first three almost invariably have organic pathology or genetic abnormality, and are evenly distributed throughout the population. On the other hand, mild learning disability, with IQ ranging from 50–70, is unequally distributed and usually lacks gross organic pathology, although there may be features of more subtle and limited brain damage. Mild learning disability predominates in the poorer socio-economic groups and is accompanied by all attendant disadvantages: substandard housing, poor child-rearing practices and health care, and educational under-achievement.

People with learning disabilities show a wide range of social skills and competence, their abilities very much dependent upon their background. Offending by those with severe disabilities is very rare. In contrast, offending by the mildly learning disabled merges imperceptibly with that by those of normal intellectual ability and shares most of its features. While mild learning disability obviously confers particular disadvantages, it is frequently difficult to separate features specific to limited intellectual ability from those which are the consequence of adverse social conditions.

Learning disability and offending behaviour

It must be emphasised that the majority of people with a mild learning disability lead unremarkable lives, either independently or with the support of a caring family or relatives. However, when such protective social factors are absent, or when they are withdrawn, or when some unexpected adverse life event supervenes, the individual may decompensate.

Commonly occurring psychological features associated with learning disability indicate why an individual might be vulnerable and how he or she might offend. Inadequate or faulty socialisation, impaired self-control or capacity to resist temptation, naïvety and gullibility, and lack of comprehension of social norms or of how others might view behaviour are all common features. These may be aggravated by a limited ability to verbalise affection, dissent, anger or frustration. Other impairments such as immature or disinhibited sexuality, poor capacity to manage financial affairs, low self-esteem and poor self-image may cumulatively contribute to offending behaviour.

The significance of organic features is difficult to assess. Gross generalised brain damage, with consequent effects on intellectual performance, emotional stability and judgement, is more likely to be associated with severe learning disability. More subtle organicity, minimal brain damage or attention deficit disorder are presumably due to intrauterine effects, prematurity or other perinatal insults and may be associated with soft neurological signs, intellectual impairment, childhood hyperactivity and behaviour disorder, and later with aggression. Physical abnormalities such as unusual appearance or deficits of hearing and speech can lead to ridicule, further reducing self-esteem and exacerbating other disadvantages. Epilepsy may be found in all degrees of learning disability, but its significance will be considered separately later.

Box 3.4 Learning disability and offending

Offending is more likely in mild and moderate than in severe learning disability

Offending is more likely in association with family, social and environmental disadvantage

Offences are broadly similar to those of offenders without learning disability

Some evidence exists for increased rates of sex offending and fire-raising in the learning disabled

Learning disability together with antisocial personality features carries a high risk for offending

There has been a recent fall in the use of compulsory admission for people with a learning disability

---

Offences

The general similarities in offending patterns of the mildly learning disabled and those of normal ability must be stressed; property offences constitute the vast majority. There are, however, some differences. Offenders with a learning disability are more likely to commit a wider range of offences than those of normal abilities and there is some evidence that they have higher rates of recidivism (Robertson, 1981). Serious violence is less common, but arson and sexual offences were both overrepresented in hospital-based cohorts (Walker & McCabe, 1973; Day, 1988).

Property offences are often committed with a lack of forethought and are opportunistic. Offenders with learning disability who steal often do so in the company of others of normal intelligence. They are frequently used as look-outs or are given a role which carries the greatest risk of being caught. If he is associating with those chronologically, but not intellectually or emotionally, younger than himself, the older offender with a learning disability will frequently be regarded as the ringleader, particularly when he may be the only member of the group old enough to be charged with an offence. Offending may be associated with periods of stress, petty theft or damage to property being a displacement activity or a symbolic act signifying an inability to communicate feelings to those with whom he is living or is emotionally involved.

Sexual offending

Both male and female learning disabled commit a disproportionate number of sex offences (Day, 1990). In women the offence is usually that of prostitution in the setting of social deprivation and personal disorganisation, where it may perhaps be the only available source of funds. Such women are also exploited in casual sexual relationships, sometimes within their family unit. The overrepresentation of sex offending in men with a learning disability is real and not simply a reflection of differential rates of arrest and conviction (Day, 1994). The learning disabled male suffers a number of disadvantages in his relationships with females. He may not understand his own sexuality or comprehend the rules of sexual conduct. He is unlikely to attract a mature adult sexual partner and will tend to associate with females of his emotional, rather than chronological, age.

Fortunately, most unwanted approaches will simply be seen as clumsy exploratory behaviour. If not threatening or repeated, they will result in a rebuff by the victim, a warning by parents or a caution by the police. More serious offending is seen in the seriously personality disordered person with a learning disability. Impulsivity, poor self-control and an inability to appreciate fully the gravity of what has been done contribute to a poor prognosis. For minor offenders, sex education and counselling is indicated. For repeated activity of a moderately serious degree, these approaches together with antilibidinal chemotherapy may be successful. For the rare, very serious case, protracted detention in hospital is often required for the protection of women or of young children of either sex.

Fire-raising

Fire-raising by those with learning disability is predominantly the activity of the late adolescent or young adult male. Such acts by the learning disabled, as by others, often appear to be motiveless (Lewis & Yarnell, 1951), although it may be a means of communicating distress, anger or revenge (Jackson *et al*, 1987) (see Chapter 2). Making false fire calls, loitering around fire stations and ambitions to become a fireman may be associated with a pathological interest in fires.

Fire-setting by women is generally less common. Tennent *et al* (1971) showed that fires tend to be set by severely disturbed young women with an intellectual level at the borderline of disability and the lower range of normal ability. They have a long history of emotional difficulties at home, running away, self-mutilation, criminal damage and promiscuity. Sexual abuse at home is sometimes described or suspected.

Psychiatric treatment poses particular difficulties. A first fire which is small and non-threatening, and in which action can be taken to remedy the precipitants, may not require the patient to be admitted to a hospital. Repeated episodes by a learning disabled person, and for which no motive is offered, usually require detention in a secure setting. Whether this is a prison or a special hospital will depend on the degree of disability and optimism about response to treatment; criteria for detention on the grounds of mental impairment must be satisfied (see Chapter 10). Improvement of general social and personal performance and a lack of interest in fire-setting in a structured environment, however, rarely gives convincing indication of the likelihood or otherwise of further fire-raising on release; indeed, the stress of a move after a long period of secure in-patient care may be sufficient to provoke another fire-raising attempt.

Recidivism and treatment

Walker & McCabe (1973) found that, of almost 1200 patients detained under a hospital order, only 4.5% of the learning disabled were convicted of serious violence, compared with 20% of the mentally ill. However, on subsequent follow-up only 4% of the mentally ill had been severely violent again, compared with 9% of those with a learning disability. The mildly learning disabled who commit serious offences often have the constellation of adverse personality and social characteristics associated with serious offending in those of normal ability (Lund, 1990). The Mental Health Act 1983 reflects this, and there is a marked similarity in the criteria for detention under psychopathic disorder and mental impairment (see Chapter 10). Compulsory admission rates for people with a learning disability have declined drastically over the last two decades (Lund, 1990; Langton *et al*, 1993). When assessing a personality disordered offender of significantly limited intelligence, it may be quite arbitrary under which legal category (psychopathic disorder or mental impairment) admission to hospital takes place. But as has been suggested above, in serious offenders who have antisocial characteristics, the presence of learning disability worsens the prognosis and increases the subsequent risk. Hospital-based units for offenders with a learning disability have been described by Day (1988), Smith (1988) and Mayor *et al* (1990).

Organic states

Three issues are worthy of brief discussion: criminal behaviour resulting from personality changes in a dementing illness or other forms of brain damage; the relationship between epilepsy and crime; and the significance of electroencephalographic abnormalities in delinquent behaviour.

Personality change

Personality change is a frequent early feature of dementia, and where there are no obvious neurological features the underlying condition may remain undiagnosed for a considerable time. Offending by people with this condition is rare. Sex offences against children are traditionally cited, but the vast majority of the elderly who come before the courts are graduate offenders committing the commonest type of offence, namely theft. Non-progressive damage as a result of head injury or other cerebral insult may result in personality changes with disinhibition and consequent offending.

Although very much less common than dementia of Alzheimer's type, the personality changes in Huntington's chorea have generated much forensic interest. Antisocial behaviour often appears before any sign of neurological or psychiatric disturbance in Huntington's chorea. Oliver (1970), in a series of 100 cases of Huntington's chorea, found 38 patients who had exhibited antisocial behaviour, violence, inappropriate sexual behaviour, cruel and callous behaviour, often against the background of membership of a chronically disorganised and disturbed family. It is therefore not surprising that antisocial behaviour is also seen in non-affected relatives.

Epilepsy and criminal behaviour

Much has been written about the relationship between epilepsy and crime. Gunn (1977b) found the prevalence of epilepsy among prisoners to be twice that of the general population, but not greatly different from the rate found in the most disadvantaged socio-economic groups. Contrary to popular misconceptions, there was no excess of violent crimes in epileptic prisoners. The rate and type of offending in epileptics is similar to those of offenders in general. Therefore, the most likely explanation for the raised prevalence of epilepsy in prisoners is that epilepsy and offending are not causally related but that they share the same social and biological disadvantages which predispose to imprisonment (Whitman et al, 1984). Violence resulting directly from epileptic activity is rare (Hindler, 1989). It is usually confused, non-goal directed activity in the post-ictal phase when the subject is being restrained. Ictal violence is even less common, although studies in clinical settings may underestimate its frequency. Offending as a result of epileptic automatism is also rare but is of medico-legal interest, for under current legislation such automatism amounts to insanity (see Chapter 5). The clinical and medico-legal aspects of all forms of automatism have been extensively reviewed by Fenwick (1990).

Electroencephalographic abnormalities and crime

Correlations of abnormalities of the electroencephalogram (EEG) with personality disorder and associated delinquency and violence have been described for many years. Persistence of an excess of slow wave activity is seen as a maturational defect mirroring delayed psychological matur-ation. However, such EEG findings are also widely distributed in the normal population and no reliance can be placed on them as an isolated feature.

Substance misuse

There are complex relationships between substance abuse and criminality. These relationships, although marked, are not directly causal, since premorbid personality characteristics, social and family background, provocative situational factors and even individual susceptibilities all play a part. Alcohol and drugs produce toxic effects and dependence syndromes, both of which make offending behaviour more likely to take place and to be detected. However, features of maladjustment and delinquency and offences of a non-drug and non-alcohol related nature regularly precede drug and alcohol-related offences. Moreover, abstinence does not abolish offending, although it may reduce its frequency and alter its nature. A substantial proportion of substance-misusing offenders are not using alcohol or drugs at the time of committing their offences.

Alcohol

Alcohol misuse plays a significant part in various types of offences: in both perpetrators (55%) and victims (53%) of violence; in rapists (34–72%); in sexual offences against children (49%); and in all types of intrafamilial abuse and neglect (Wolfgang & Strohm, 1956; Rada, 1976; Coid, 1986). A substantial proportion of property offences are committed to generate funds for an expensive alcohol habit, but as heavy drinking is common in young men, the group which commits the most offences, the exact significance of this feature is uncertain.

Care must be taken in drawing conclusions about causation from studies of selected samples of offenders. This applies particularly to prison populations of either serious offenders or repeated petty offenders. Both these groups will inevitably be found to have high rates of alcohol use, perhaps because it might have been stressed at trial as an explanation or a mitigating factor for violence, or because the serious social effects of dependence are those which can lead to imprisonment. Persilia *et al* (1978) have shown that 70% of habitual criminals in the community misuse alcohol.

What can be said about any specific relationship between alcohol and any particular type of offence? Two special groups require mention: habitual drunken offenders, and those suspected of having a pathological susceptibility to alcohol, even in small amounts. There are repeated drunken offenders, usually arrested for public order or property offences, who pose considerable problems in management. They are rarely considered suitable for alcohol treatment programmes and there is a reluctance to send such men yet again to prison (although this is sometimes contemplated as a lifesaving or therapeutic measure). The immediate need is frequently for detoxification, but this can rarely be provided. Often these offenders are simply dismissed from court to the care of voluntary organisations or the probation service. The sterility of this cycle is evident, but with current attitudes to alcoholic offenders both inside and outside prison, there is no apparent remedy.

Pathological intoxication ('mania à potu') is a much debated entity. Anecdotal accounts of convincing cases have been described (Maletsky,

1976) but there has been criticism that it has not been possible to replicate in a clinical setting the reported spectacular effects caused by small amounts of alcohol. It has been suggested that in such a setting the necessary triggering situational factors are absent.

Drugs

Habitual criminality is an integral part of established drug dependence (Gordon, 1990). As with alcohol-misusing offenders, delinquent personality characteristics and non-drug related offending antedate drug misuse and drug-related offending. Drug misusers do not solely commit the specific offences of possession and supply of drugs, but a whole range of other offences to fund their habit. They may indulge in more organised serious criminal activities, including violence. In their pattern of offending, female addicts have much more in common with their male counterparts than non-addicted male and female offenders. They have even more disrupted and delinquent pre-addiction backgrounds, but do not commonly commit the more serious violent and organised drug-related offences. Successful treatment of the drug misuse does not necessarily abolish offending, and the beneficial maturational effects of ageing may take longer to appear than in non-addicted offenders.

Descriptions of clinical syndromes resulting from acute intoxication by, idiosyncratic reactions to, or chronic abuse of, drugs such as amphetamine, heroin, lysergic acid diethylamide (LSD) and solvents are not appropriate here. Cannabis, because of its wide use in psychiatric and offender populations, warrants some discussion. In an extensive review, Thornicroft (1990) concluded that there does not appear to be a separate clinical entity of cannabis psychosis. However, cannabis may produce an acute organic reaction and, in heavy users, may precipitate a schizophreniform psychosis. Prolonged heavy use is associated with an increased risk of developing schizophrenia in the subsequent 15 years. Drug-misusing defendants who appear psychotic require very careful evaluation to ensure that the correct diagnosis is made, especially when they are facing serious charges. The interplay of personality, illness and drug dependence needs proper consideration so that the correct disposal, to hospital or prison, is recommended. Such an assessment should usually be carried out in hospital.

Special syndromes

Morbid jealousy

Sexual jealousy is a powerful human emotion. The view taken of it has varied over culture and time, with a shift from a socially sanctioned response to infidelity, to a personal pathology which is the outward expression of unnatural possessiveness and insecurity (Mullen, 1993). The boundary between normal jealousy and morbid jealousy is indistinct. The strength of feeling and the results which flow from it are insufficient to make the distinction, as is the presence or absence of actual unfaithfulness by the sexual partner. Jealousy or a tendency to be jealous can be: a normal and relatively transient response in an otherwise well-adjusted individual to frank infidelity; a neurotic preoccupation of a vulnerable and insecure individual; one feature in an individual with a paranoid personality disorder; an overvalued idea with no additional features of psychosis; or a frankly delusional idea arising suddenly and unexpectedly either as a single delusional idea or one of a number of related delusional ideas in a typical psychosis. Over the years various authors have sought to classify morbid jealousy by particular psychopathological features, so far without complete success (Mullen, 1990). Box 3.5 summarises features of morbid jealousy.

The forensic importance of morbid jealousy is its association with violence, often repeated violence, usually towards the sexual partner. Morbid jealousy contributes significantly to wife battering and homicides of spouses, and in the latter, psychiatrists are regularly requested to offer an opinion on whether the jealousy is normal or morbid, and whether it amounts to an abnormality of mind sufficient for a finding of diminished responsibility. This is often difficult. The severity of distress of the jealous individual, and the presence or absence of the common features of depression, anxiety and anger, often in association with alcohol consumption, do not easily distinguish between normal and morbid forms. Frankly bizarre features such as elaborate surveillance, delusional misperceptions, or typical features of an organic, schizophrenic or affective illness make the diagnosis very much easier.

When morbid jealousy is only one feature of well-recognised psychiatric illness, the treatment is that of the underlying condition. This is often surprisingly effective. Jealousy which is part of a neurotic picture, and often a neurotic relationship with sexual difficulties and possible provoc-

---

Box 3.5 Morbid jealousy

The boundary between normal and pathological jealousy is indistinct

Jealousy may be psychotic or neurotic in type, or associated with personality disorder or alcohol misuse

It carries a high risk of violence to the sexual partner

Psychotic cases show a better response to treatment than others

It is essential to inform victims of potential risks

ative behaviour by both parties, is much more difficult to treat. Patterns of action and reaction are often well established and are difficult to break by psychotherapeutic means. Treatment of a paranoid personality disorder and overvalued ideas is even more difficult. It may be that the most effective approach is a merely symptomatic one, treating depressive features with an antidepressant, and tension and anger with a neuroleptic. Once the circle of events is loosened some progress may be possible. However, the risk of continuing jealousy, and more importantly the risk of continuing violence, must be assessed. If this seems grave, because a repeat of previous violence would be serious, or there are features which indicate that the risk of violence is increasing, or that the violence is increasing in severity, or there are new and important situational factors, then this risk should be imparted to both parties, particularly the victim. It may be that the only effective advice is that the partners must separate, although this is often difficult to achieve and sustain.

Erotomania

De Clerambault's syndrome, or erotomania, is described by Enoch & Trethowan (1979). The patient, typically a woman, presents with the delusional belief that a man, usually of higher social status, or sometimes a public figure, is in love with her. The condition may exist as a mono-delusion but is usually associated with a paranoid psychosis or schizo-phrenic illness (Rudden *et al*, 1990). Such patients may cause distress to the victim and his family, for example, by sending numerous letters, making repeated telephone calls or following the victim. It is when the love is unrequited that it may be replaced by anger, resentment and hatred. Repeated rebuttals may lead to dangerous behaviour, such as assaults and even attempts on the life of the victim or members of his family (Mullen & Pathé, 1994). In some cases the treating psychiatrist can become the object of the patient's delusions.

Münchausen syndrome

Münchausen syndrome is characterised by the triad of dramatic present-ations of acute medical or surgical symptoms, pathological lying or pseudologia fantastica, and wandering the country repeatedly presenting to accident and emergency departments (Bursten, 1965). Münchausen syndrome is best understood as a special presentation of a hysterical personality disorder. Such disabled personalities rarely cooperate with treatment; indeed, they usually quit hospital when the opinion of a psychiatrist is mooted. To fund their peregrinations they may commit thefts and create disturbances. A more recently described variant of particular importance is Münchausen syndrome by proxy, described in Chapter 2.

Pathological gambling

Gambling is a common social activity, but the frequency of excessive or pathological gambling in the general population is not known. "Maladaptive gambling behaviour" as defined in DSM–IV (American Psychiatric Association, 1994) suggests that the disorder has much in common with addictive behaviour or a dependency disorder. Moran (1990) has described five subgroups of pathological gamblers: symptomatic (associated with illness, e.g. depression); neurotic (in response to stress); impulsive (with loss of control); subcultural (socially acceptable); and psychopathic. This last group includes those whose gambling is part of a general pattern of antisocial and criminal behaviour. There is evidence that gambling is more common in offenders than in the general population (Cornish, 1978). Gambling and excessive gambling is highest in young offenders. Maden *et al* (1992) found gamblers had greater records of criminality, custodial sentences, local authority care and psychiatric contact than non-gambling young offenders. In some cases, excessive gambling may lead to criminal behaviour in order to finance the habit, but in many cases pathological gambling is more generally associated with recidivism and other delinquent activity.

Minority groups

Ethnic minorities

Afro-Caribbeans, but not Asians or other ethnic groups, are overrepresented in both the psychiatric and criminal justice systems, compared with their proportion in the general population of the UK. A disproportionate number of Afro-Caribbeans, particularly British-born young men, are admitted to psychiatric hospitals with a diagnosis of schizophrenia. They are more likely to be admitted following contact with the police and social services and to be detained under a section of the Mental Health Act 1983. The highest admission rates are found for forensic sections under Part III of the Act. McGovern & Cope (1987) found that male Afro-Caribbeans aged between 16 and 29 years were 25 times more likely than 'whites' to be detained as offender patients under Part III. Lipsedge (1994) has cautioned that the perception that Afro-Caribbeans are prone to manifest a violent form of schizophrenia is an example of dangerous stereotyping.

Afro-Caribbeans are also overrepresented in special hospitals, medium secure units and in locked wards in psychiatric hospitals. In a national survey of secure units, 20% of admitted patients were of Afro-Caribbean origin (Jones & Berry, 1986). An even higher proportion (38%) was found in the West Midlands in a survey of ethnic differences upon admission to a regional secure unit (Cope & Ndegwa, 1990). In this study, Afro-Caribbeans were significantly more likely to be admitted from prisons, especially while on remand. The majority of patients were considered to have a psychotic illness, almost invariably schizophrenia. Reasons for these findings are complex, but suggested factors include a more disturbed presentation of the illness, differential decision-making by psychiatrists, the police and courts, and a perception of the psychiatric services by patients as racist, coercive and inappropriate to the needs of Afro-Caribbean patients.

Afro-Caribbeans are also overrepresented among arrest rates and in the prison population. There are approximately 5% of Afro-Caribbeans in the general population, compared with 11% of men and 25% of women in the sentenced prison population (Home Office, 1993). The latter figure includes large numbers of women, normally resident in West Africa, serving sentences for drug smuggling. There is debate about whether these findings reflect disproportionate criminality in Afro-Caribbeans, whether it is a feature of social disadvantage, or whether it is an artefact caused by a discriminatory criminal justice system. Studies have repeatedly discounted systematic discrimination, but there is a widespread perception of racial bias. The literature on the subject is summarised by Fitzgerald (1993).

In the assessment of offenders and others from ethnic minorities who either do not speak English or easily communicate in English, specialist interpreters should be obtained. It is not good practice to use relatives or friends, who may unwittingly substitute their own interpretations in response to questions. Specialist interpreters are also available to the police and courts.

The deaf

Approximately 10% of referrals to specialist psychiatric units for the deaf come from the police, courts or solicitors. The majority have committed minor property or acquisitive offences, but a surprisingly high proportion have been charged with sexual offences. Deaf people do not commit disproportionately more sexual crimes than hearing people; their increased referral rate for court reports is more likely to be a reflection of a lower threshold for referral by magistrates.

Deaf offender patients, particularly those who have significant problems in communication, may be found unfit to plead (see Chapter 5). Grubin (1991) found that seven out of a series of 295 cases found unfit to plead were deaf. Psychiatric assessment of deaf offenders presents special problems, particularly if there is profound hearing loss, or coexisting mental illness or learning disability. In all cases, it is essential to obtain the services of a registered interpreter for the deaf. It is inappropriate to use a relative or social worker as interpreter, although it is often helpful to involve a specialist social worker for the deaf to aid assessment and evaluation. In all but the most straightforward cases, it is good practice to seek an expert opinion from a psychiatrist from one of the three specialist psychiatric units for the deaf, based in Birmingham, London and Manchester.

Elderly offenders

The offending rate of those over 60 years of age is very low, but physical and psychiatric illness is far more common than in younger offenders. Their profile of crime appears broadly similar to that of younger groups, although crimes of "disinhibition" (e.g. sexual exhibitionism) and violence as consequences of organic brain disease may be relatively more common. In a sample of over 1000 male remand prisoners, half of those over 55 years of age were recognised to be suffering from active psychiatric symptoms on admission. Alcoholism was common, and affective psychoses made up a substantial minority (Taylor & Parrott, 1988). Of those in this series who were convicted, a third were sentenced to prison, which is only a little lower than the figures for younger age groups. Most elderly offenders are socially isolated with broken marital and family ties, and they are frequently of no fixed abode (Goetting, 1983). It has been pointed out that prisons provide an even less suitable environment for the detention of the elderly than they do for the rehabilitation of younger offenders.

References

American Psychiatric Association (1994) *Diagnostic and Statistical Manual of Mental Disorders* (4th edn)(DSM–IV). Washington, DC: APA.

Bursten, B. (1965) On Münchausen's syndrome. *Archives of General Psychiatry,* **13**, 261.

Coid, J. (1986) Alcohol, rape and sexual assault: (b) socioculture factors in alcohol-related aggression. In *Alcohol and Aggression* (ed. P.F. Brain). London: Croom Helm.

—— (1988) Mentally abnormal remands. I: Rejected or accepted by the National Health Service. *British Medical Journal,* **296**, 1779–1782.

—— (1992) DSM–III diagnosis in criminal psychopaths: a way forward. *Criminal Behaviour and Mental Health,* **2**, 78–94.

Confidential Inquiry into Homicides & Suicides by Mentally Ill People (1994) *A Preliminary Report on Homicides.* London: Steering Committee to the Inquiry.

Cope, R. (1993) A survey of forensic psychiatrists' views on psychopathic disorder. *Journal of Forensic Psychiatry,* **4**, 215–235.

—— & Ndegwa, D. (1990) Ethnic differences in admission to a regional secure unit. *Journal of Forensic Psychiatry,* **1**, 365–378.

Cornish, D. B. (1978) *Gambling: a Review of the Literature and its Implications for Policy and Research.* Home Office Research Study No 42. London: HMSO.

Day, K. (1988) Hospital based treatment programme for mentally handicapped offenders. *British Journal of Psychiatry,* **153**, 635–644.

—— (1990) Mental retardation: clinical aspects and management. In *Principles and Practice of Forensic Psychiatry* (eds R. Bluglass & P. Bowden), pp. 399–418. Edinburgh: Churchill Livingstone.

—— (1994) Male mentally handicapped sex offenders. *British Journal of Psychiatry,* **165**, 630–639.

Dell, S. & Smith, A. (1983) Changes in the sentencing of diminished responsibility homicides. *British Journal of Psychiatry,* **142**, 20–35.

Dolan, B. & Coid, J. (1993) *Psychopathic and Antisocial Personality Disorders: Treatment and Research Issues.* London: Gaskell.

D'Orban, P. T. (1979) Women who kill their children. *British Journal of Psychiatry,* **134,** 560–571.

Enoch, M. B. & Trethowan, W. H. (1979) *Some Uncommon Psychiatric Syndromes* (2nd edn). Bristol: Wright.

Fenwick, P. B. C. (1990) Automatism. In *Principles and Practice of Forensic Psychiatry* (eds R. Bluglass & P. Bowden), pp. 271–285. Edinburgh: Churchill Livingstone.

Fitzgerald, M. (1993) *Ethnic Minorities and the Criminal Justice System.* Royal Commission on Criminal Justice Research Study No 20. London: HMSO.

Freeman, C. P. L. (1993) Personality disorders. In *Companion to Psychiatric Studies* (5th edn)(eds R. E. Kendell & A. K. Zealley), pp. 587–615. Edinburgh: Churchill Livingstone.

Gibbens, T. C. N., Palmer, C. & Prince, J. (1971) Mental health aspects of shoplifting. *British Medical Journal,* iii, 612–615.

Gillies, H. (1976) Homicide in the west of Scotland. *British Journal of Psychiatry,* **128,** 105–127.

Goetting, A. (1983) The elderly in prison: issues and perspectives. *Journal of Research in Crime and Delinquency,* **20,** 291–309.

Gordon, A. M. (1990) Drugs and criminal behaviour. In *Principles and Practice of Forensic Psychiatry* (eds R. Bluglass & P. Bowden), pp. 897–901. Edinburgh: Churchill Livingstone.

Grubin, D. H. (1991) Unfit to plead in England and Wales, 1976–1988. A survey. *British Journal of Psychiatry,* **158,** 540–548.

Gudjonsson, G. H. (1990) Psychological and psychiatric aspects of shoplifting. *Medicine, Science and the Law,* **30,** 45–51.

Gunn, J. (1977a) Criminal behaviour and mental disorder. *British Journal of Psychiatry,* **130,** 317–329.

—— (1977b) *Epileptics in Prison.* London: Academic Press.

——, Maden, A. & Swinton, M. (1991) Treatment needs of prisoners with psychiatric disorders. *British Medical Journal,* **303,** 338–341.

Guze, S. B., Woodruff, R. A. & Clayton, P. S. (1974) Psychiatric disorders and criminality. *Journal of the American Medical Association,* **227,** 641–642.

Hafner, H. & Boker, W. (1982) *Crimes of Violence by Mentally Abnormal Offenders. The Psychiatric Epidemiology in the Federal German Republic.* Cambridge: Cambridge University Press.

Hindler, C. G. (1989) Epilepsy and violence. *British Journal of Psychiatry,* **155,** 246–249.

Home Office (1993) *The Prison Population in 1992.* London: HMSO.

—— & Department of Health & Social Security (1975) *Report of the Committee on Mentally Abnormal Offenders* (Butler report) Cmnd no 6244. London: HMSO.

Humphreys, M. S., Johnstone, E. C., MacMillan, J. F., *et al* (1992) Dangerous behaviour preceding first admissions for schizophrenia. *British Journal of Psychiatry,* **161,** 501–505.

Jackson, H. F., Glass, C. & Hope, S. (1987) A functional analysis of recidivistic arson. *British Journal of Clinical Psychology,* **26,** 175–185.

Jackson, M. & Tarnopolsky, A. (1990) Borderline personality. In *Principles and Practice of Forensic Psychiatry* (eds R. Bluglass & P. Bowden), pp. 427–435. Edinburgh: Churchill Livingstone.

Joneś, G. & Berry, M. (1986) Regional secure units: the emerging picture. In *Current Issues in Clinical Psychology IV* (ed. G. Edwards), pp. 24–42. London: Plenum.

Langton, J., Krishnan, V., Cumella, S., *et al* (1993) Detentions in a mental handicap hospital: a ten-year retrospective study. *Journal of Forensic Psychiatry*, 4, 85–95.

Lewis, N. D. C. & Yarnell, H. (1951) *Pathological Fire-setting (Pyromania)*. Nervous and Mental Disease Monographs, No. 82. New York: Coolidge Foundation.

Lindqvist, P. & Allebeck, P. (1990) Schizophrenia and crime: a longitudinal follow-up of 644 schizophrenics in Stockholm. *British Journal of Psychiatry*, 157, 345–350.

Lipsedge, M. (1994) Dangerous stereotypes. *Journal of Forensic Psychiatry*, 5, 14–19.

Lund, J. (1990) Mentally retarded criminal offenders in Denmark. *British Journal of Psychiatry*, 156, 726–731.

Maden, T., Swinton, M. & Gunn, J. (1992) Gambling in young offenders. *Criminal Behaviour and Mental Health*, 2, 300–308.

Maletsky, B. M. (1976) The diagnosis of pathological intoxication. *Journal of Studies on Alcohol*, 37, 1215–1228.

Mathers, D. C. & Ghodse, A. H. (1992) Cannabis and psychotic illness. *British Journal of Psychiatry*, 161, 648–653.

Mawson, D. (1985) Delusions of poisoning. *Medicine, Science and the Law*, 25, 279–287.

Mayor, J., Bhate, M., Firth, M., *et al* (1990) Facilities for mentally impaired patients: three years' experience of a semisecure unit. *Psychiatric Bulletin*, 14, 333–335.

McGovern, D. & Cope, R. (1987) The compulsory detention of males of different ethnic groups with special reference to offender patients. *British Journal of Psychiatry*, 150, 505–512.

Moran, E. (1990) Pathological gambling. In *Principles and Practice of Forensic Psychiatry* (eds R. Bluglass & P. Bowden), pp. 841–847. Edinburgh: Churchill Livingstone.

Mowat, R. R. (1966) *Morbid Jealousy and Murder*. International Library of Criminology Delinquency and Deviant Social Behaviour No. II. London: Tavistock.

Mullen, P. E. (1990) Morbid jealousy and the delusion infidelity. In *Principles and Practice of Forensic Psychiatry* (eds R. Bluglass & P. Bowden), pp. 823–834. Edinburgh: Churchill Livingstone.

—— (1993) The crime of passion and the changing cultural construction of jealousy. *Criminal Behaviour and Mental Health*, 3, 1–11.

—— & Pathé, M. (1994) The pathological extensions of love. *British Journal of Psychiatry*, 165, 614–623.

Noble, P. & Rodger, S. (1989) Violence by psychiatric inpatients. *British Journal of Psychiatry*, 155, 384–390.

Oliver, J. E. (1970) Huntington's chorea in Northamptonshire. *British Journal of Psychiatry*, 116, 241–253.

Parker, N. (1979) Murderers: a personal series. *Medical Journal of Australia*, i, 36–39.

Persilia, J., Greenwood, P. W. & Lavin, M. (1978) *Criminal Careers of Habitual Felons*. National Institute of Law Enforcement and Criminal Justice. Washington, DC: US Government Printing Office.

Powell, G., Caan, W. & Crowe, M. (1994) What events precede violent incidents in psychiatric hospitals? *British Journal of Psychiatry*, 165, 107–112.

Rada, R. T. (1976) Alcohol and the child molester. *Annals of the New York Academy of Sciences*, 273, 492–496.

Robertson, G. (1981) The extent and pattern of crime amongst mentally handicapped offenders. *Apex, Journal of British Institute of Mental Handicap*, **9**, 100–103.

—— (1988) Arrest patterns among mentally disordered offenders. *British Journal of Psychiatry*, **153**, 313–316.

Rollin, H. R. (1969) *The Mentally Abnormal Offender and the Law*. Oxford: Pergamon Press.

Rudden, M., Sweeney, J. & Allen, F. (1990) Diagnosis and clinical course of erotomanic and other delusional patients. *American Journal of Psychiatry*, **147**, 625–628.

Smith, J. (1988) An open forensic unit for the borderline mentally impaired offender. *Psychiatric Bulletin*, **12**, 13–15.

—— & Hucker, S. (1994) Schizophrenia and substance abuse. *British Journal of Psychiatry*, **165**, 13–21.

Swanson, J. W., Holzer, C. E., Ganju, V. K., *et al* (1990) Violence and psychiatric disorder in the community: evidence from the epidemiological catchment area surveys. *Hospital and Community Psychiatry*, **41**, 761–770.

Tantam, D. & Whittaker, J. (1992) Personality disorder and self-wounding. *British Journal of Psychiatry*, **161**, 451–464.

Taylor, P. J. (1985) Motives for offending among violent and psychotic men. *British Journal of Psychiatry*, **147**, 491–498.

—— & Gunn, J. (1984) Violence and psychosis. I: Risk of violence among psychotic men. *British Medical Journal*, **288**, 1945–1949.

—— & Parrott, J. (1988) Elderly offenders: a study of age-related factors among custodially remanded prisoners. *British Journal of Psychiatry*, **152**, 340–346.

Tennent, G., McQuaid, A. & Loughane, T. (1971) Female arsonists. *British Journal of Psychiatry*, **119**, 497–502.

Thornicroft, G. (1990) Cannabis and psychosis: is there epidemiological evidence for an association? *British Journal of Psychiatry*, **157**, 25–33.

Tyrer, P. & Stein, G. (1993) *Personality Disorder Reviewed*. London: Gaskell.

Vize, C. & Tyrer, P. (1994) The relationship between personality and other psychiatric disorders. *Current Opinion in Psychiatry*, **7**, 123–128.

Walker, N. & McCabe, S. (1973) *Crime and Insanity in England II. New Solutions and New Problems*. Edinburgh: Edinburgh University Press.

Wessely, S., Buchanan, A., Reed, A., *et al* (1993) Acting on delusions, I: Prevalence. *British Journal of Psychiatry*, **163**, 69–76.

West, D. J. (1965) *Murder Followed by Suicide*. London: Heinemann.

—— (1988) Psychological contributions to criminology. *British Journal of Criminology*, **28**, 77–92.

Whitman, S., Coleman, T. E., Patmon, C., *et al* (1984) Epilepsy in prisons: elevated prevalence and no relationship to violence. *Neurology (Cleveland)*, **34**, 775–782.

Wilkins, J. & Coid, J. (1991) Self-mutilation in female remanded prisoners. *Criminal Behaviour and Mental Health*, **1**, 247–267.

Wolfgang, M. E. & Strohm, R. B. (1956) The relationship between alcohol and criminal homicide. *Journal of Studies on Alcohol*, **17**, 411–425.

Wulach, J. S. (1983) Mania and crime: a study of 100 manic defendants. *Bulletin of AAPL*, **11**, 69–75.

Zitrin, A., Hardesty, A. S., Burdock, E. I., *et al* (1976) Crime and violence among mental patients. *American Journal of Psychiatry*, **133**, 142–149.

4 The criminal justice system
Adrian Grounds

Criminal justice agencies • The criminal justice process • Addenda for Northern Ireland, Scotland and the Republic of Ireland

---

The purpose of this chapter is to give a brief description of the criminal justice system in England and Wales. Addenda at the end of the chapter refer to Northern Ireland, Scotland and the Republic of Ireland. The roles of the various criminal justice agencies, and the procedures of the police, the Crown Prosecution Service, and the courts in dealing with suspected offenders need to be understood, since they provide the context of much of forensic psychiatry practice. Psychiatric reports on people involved in criminal proceedings need to be based on an understanding of the legal questions that arise at different stages of the criminal justice process, and on an appreciation of the concerns and expectations of the other professions that are involved in responding to crime. Ideally, general psychiatry services should establish close links with local criminal justice agencies, and have arrangements in place that enable referrals from the police, probation officers and local magistrates' courts to be dealt with as promptly as emergency referrals from general practitioners.

The government is primarily responsible for defining contemporary criminal justice policy, and this sets the framework of goals within which the criminal justice system should operate. This chapter will briefly summarise the roles of the main agencies, the nature of criminal proceedings, and some of the main recent developments in policy and legislation. Particular reference will be made to the issues affecting mentally disordered offenders. An excellent guide to mental health legislation in this area is given by Hoggett (1990).

Criminal justice agencies

At central government level the Home Office is responsible for matters concerning the police, prisons, probation service and magistrates' courts. The Lord Chancellor's Department is responsible for issues relating to the judiciary, the higher courts and the administration of legal aid.

The police

The police in England and Wales are organised into 43 police forces headed by Chief Constables. Most constabularies are based on county boundaries, but in London the Metropolitan Police is responsible for most of the capital, excluding the City of London which has its own small force. Apart from the Metropolitan Police which reports to the Home Secretary, police constabularies report to local police authorities.

Crown Prosecution Service

The decision about whether an individual should be prosecuted for a criminal offence is generally taken by the Crown Prosecution Service, which is headed by the Director of Public Prosecutions. The Crown Prosecution Service is divided into areas, often covering one or two counties, and areas are divided into branches, each headed by a Chief Crown Prosecutor.

Courts

There are criminal courts and courts of appeal. These are summarised in Box 4.1.

Magistrates' courts

If the decision is made to prosecute, defendants are dealt with in criminal courts. Adult defendants will appear first in local magistrates' courts, which deal with 98% of criminal cases. It often takes some time for the prosecution and defence cases to be prepared, and so the first task of the magistrates' court may be to decide whether the defendant should be remanded on bail or in custody (i.e. prison) while awaiting trial. The magistrates' courts deal with minor offences themselves, and have limited sentencing powers. For example, a magistrates' court may not impose more than six months imprisonment for any offence. The Home Office regularly issues an updated handbook summarising the powers available to magistrates' courts (e.g. Home Office, 1990*a*). In the magistrates' courts the sentencers are lay 'justices of the peace', that is, members of the community drawn from a variety of occupations and backgrounds who are appointed to sit as magistrates on a part-time basis. Their training is limited, and most are not legally qualified. In some urban areas, particularly London, the courts have stipendiary magistrates, who are legally qualified and paid. Magistrates' courts are administered by justices' clerks, who are qualified lawyers. They provide guidance and legal advice to lay magistrates, and in some areas, one justices' clerk may be responsible for several local courts. Magistrates receive most of their training from their clerks, but journals such as *The Magistrate* also carry reviews of contemporary developments in the criminal law and criminal justice matters.

The Crown Court

There are three broad groups of criminal offences:

(1) minor or "summary" offences are dealt with in the magistrates' courts
(2) "indictable" offences (the most serious) are dealt with in the Crown Court
(3) an intermediate group, "triable either way" offences, may be dealt with in either.

Cases going to the Crown Court have to go through an initial procedure of being committed to Crown Court by the magistrates. Thus people charged with serious offences are likely to be committed by the magistrates' court to the Crown Courts for trial and sentencing. In addition, some people charged with minor offences may be committed to the Crown Court for sentencing because the Crown Court has wider sentencing powers than magistrates. The purpose of committal should be to ensure that the evidence is strong enough to justify proceeding to the Crown Court for trial, but in practice it is usually a formality that takes place when the written statements and papers comprising the prosecution case have been prepared. These papers are known as the "depositions".

In the Crown Court the defendant may plead guilty to the criminal charge, and then sentencing takes place. If the defendant pleads not guilty, the case is tried by a jury. Juries consist of 12 adults between the ages of 18 and 65 drawn from the electoral roll. People in the medical professions tend to be exempted from jury service. After hearing the prosecution and defence arguments and the judge's summing up, the jury's task is to decide on the evidence whether to convict the defendant. If they find the defendant guilty, sentencing by the judge follows.

The Crown Court has about 90 courts in England and Wales grouped into six regions, known as 'circuits'. Judges are responsible for sentencing in Crown Courts, and Crown Courts also deal with appeals from lower courts. However, Crown Courts consider only a tiny minority of criminal cases; the great majority are dealt with in magistrates' courts.

Youth Courts

Juvenile offenders (aged 10–17) are dealt with in the Youth Courts, which were established by the Criminal Justice Act 1991. The Youth Courts have been in operation since 1992, replacing the Juvenile Courts. The Children Act 1989 introduced a separation between criminal and civil proceedings. Youth Courts deal with criminal cases and the Family Proceedings Court deals with civil matters. The Youth Court has magistrates with specialist training and deals with the majority of cases. As with adults, juveniles charged with grave offences may be dealt with in the Crown Court.

Box 4.1 Criminal courts in England and Wales

Magistrates' court
- court of first instance for all crimes
- deal with 98% of crime
- hear all summary cases and some indictable cases
  cases heard by three lay magistrates advised by a legally
    qualified justices' clerk
- approximately 50 stipendiary magistrates, who hear cases on
    their own
- maximum sentence is six months imprisonment
- responsible for the bulk of hospital orders

Crown Court
- England and Wales is divided into six circuits
- presiding judges are of varying seniority according to the
    complexity of the case
- cases are heard by judge and jury
- hears appeals from magistrates' courts

Youth Court
- established by the Children Act 1989
- only deals with criminal matters
- cases heard by magistrates with special training
- serious cases are committed to Crown Court

Court of Appeal (Criminal Division)
- granting of leave to appeal is a necessary preliminary
- normally sits with three judges
- hears appeals by the defendant against conviction or sentence
- since 1989, can hear appeals by the Crown against sentence
- has power to increase (as well as reduce) a sentence

Queen's Bench Division (Divisional Court)
- hears appeals on technical points of law only

House of Lords
- hears appeals against decisions of the Queen's Bench Division
    and the Court of Appeal
- opinions are delivered by Law Lords
- must involve a point of law of general public importance

Courts of appeal

In addition to the magistrates' courts and the Crown Court, there are three
higher courts that deal with appeals (Box 4.1). Appeals on points of law
and procedure are dealt with by the Divisional Court of the Queen's Bench

Division of the High Court; appeals against conviction and sentence in the Crown Court are dealt with in the Criminal Division of the Court of Appeal; and appeals against the decisions of these two courts can be heard by the House of Lords.

Lawyers

The legal profession essentially consists of two kinds of lawyer. *Solicitors*, who constitute the majority, carry out a variety of work, and for defendants in criminal proceedings they provide initial legal advice and representation: for example, accompanying the defendant when he or she is interviewed by the police, and making representations to the magistrates in court. *Barristers* have a more specialist role and only become involved if requested by a solicitor. Barristers provide specialist advice on aspects of the law, and in the Crown Court and other higher courts they act as advocates: it is barristers who present the case for each side, question and cross-examine witnesses and put the arguments for their side to the judge. In this context, barristers are referred to as "counsel" , for example counsel for the prosecution and counsel for the defence. Judges are mostly drawn from the ranks of senior barristers and are appointed by the Lord Chancellor. There are five categories of judges, namely (in order of seniority):

(1) Law Lords (who sit in the House of Lords)
(2) Appeal Court judges (who sit in the Court of Appeal)
(3) High Court judges (who sit in the High Court, but may also preside in the most serious Crown Court cases)
(4) Circuit judges (who are full-time and sit in the Crown and County Courts)
(5) Recorders (who are part-time and sit in the Crown Court).

The probation service

The probation service is divided into 56 areas, mostly based on county boundaries, with each service being led by a chief probation officer. The tasks of the probation service include the provision of information and pre-sentence reports on offenders for courts, the supervision of non-custodial sentences and court orders, and the supervision and aftercare of released prisoners. Some probation officers are based in prisons and play an important role in liaison between prisoners and their families. Most probation officers, however, work in the community, and there are additional duties in magistrates' courts. Traditionally, probation officers have had social work training, and the probation service is facing new challenges in being expected to administer community-based sentences.

There are two other important areas of work in which the service is becoming involved. The first is bail information schemes, which provide information to courts about the personal circumstances of defendants, so that better decisions can be made about remanding in bail or custody. If a history of psychiatric disorder is elicited, this may highlight a need for medical assessment. Secondly, probation services are becoming increasingly involved in developing group-based programmes for offenders with alcohol problems and sexual offenders. The probation service deals with many individuals whose difficulties have a psychiatric component, and there are rewarding opportunities for joint working and liaison between probation officers and psychiatrists (Bowden, 1978).

The prison service

The prison service is managed centrally by a Director General and Prison Board at the Home Office. There is also an area level of organisation, and individual establishments are run by prison governors. Establishments for sentenced prisoners are categorised according to security status. In addition there are "local" prisons, which predominantly take people remanded in custody before trial or before sentence. The Health Care Service for Prisoners is part of the Prison Department and is administratively independent of the National Health Service. Its work is discussed in detail in Chapter 9.

The criminal justice process

Police action

The diagram below illustrates in a simplified form some of the main steps that may occur prior to and during criminal proceedings (Fig. 4.1). As the flow diagram illustrates, a criminal conviction and sentence are the outcome of a long and complex sequence of decisions. Offences first have to come to the attention of the police. Victims or witnesses may or may not decide to inform the police, and in only a proportion of these cases will an alleged offender be apprehended. The proportion of cases resulting in a criminal conviction will be smaller still. The 1988 British Crime Survey estimated that, of all offences committed, only about 41% are reported to the police, 26% are recorded, and 3% result in a criminal conviction (Home Office, 1991).

Police and mentally disordered offenders: Section 136, Mental Health Act 1983

When the police apprehend an alleged offender they may decide to take no further action as far as criminal proceedings are concerned. In the case of mentally disordered people, the police may make efforts to obtain psychiatric assessment and treatment as an alternative to prosecution. If an individual in a public place appears to a police officer to be mentally disordered and in need of care and control, he or she may be taken to a place of safety (which may include a psychiatric hospital) under Section 136 of the Mental Health Act 1983. This empowers the person's detention for up to 72 hours for the purpose of obtaining a medical and social work assessment of the need for compulsory admission. The Mental Health Act 1983 *Code of Practice* (Department of Health & Welsh Office, 1993) notes that a person who has been arrested by the police under Section 136 is entitled to have someone notified of his or her arrest and whereabouts, and the right of access to legal advice if he or she is in police detention. Efforts should always be made to ensure that the medical and social work assessments are carried out as rapidly as possible. The police are unlikely to "over-diagnose" mental illness, but Dunn & Fahy's (1990) research in London indicated that a disproportionate number of men from black ethnic minority groups were likely to be admitted to hospital under Section 136. The use of the power needs to be carefully audited.

Other action by the police

When an offender admits guilt and the police do not wish to proceed to court, the individual concerned may be given a formal caution by the police. Proceeding to a court appearance, however, requires that the person is charged. This process usually involves obtaining a statement in interview with the suspected offender. Awareness that an arrested person may be mentally disordered may not arise until the person is in police custody. Under these circumstances the police may call in a police surgeon (forensic medical advisor), who may in turn request a psychiatric assessment from the local psychiatric services. This could result in a voluntary hospital admission, other aftercare arrangements, or a compulsory admission under a civil section of the Mental Health Act 1983. The police are often reluctant to initiate criminal proceedings against someone that they recognise to be obviously mentally disordered, particularly if the alleged offending is minor.

Police interviews

Interviewing of suspects in police custody has to conform with the codes of practice issued under the Police and Criminal Evidence Act 1984 (Section 66). Suspects have the right to have a solicitor present and this is particularly advisable for vulnerable or mentally disordered suspects. In addition, under the *Code of Practice for the Detention, Treatment and Questioning of Persons by Police Officers* (Home Office, 1992), the custody officer must immediately call the police surgeon (or arrange alternative medical assistance in urgent cases) if the person appears to be suffering from mental disorder. The use of "oppression" in questioning of any suspect is prohibited, and a person who is mentally ill or has a learning disability should not be interviewed

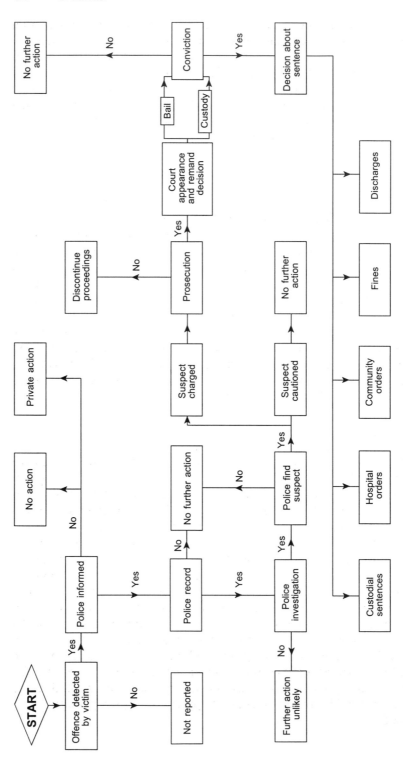

Fig. 4.1 A simplified flow chart of the criminal justice process.

or be asked to provide or sign a written statement in the absence of an appropriate adult. The appropriate adult may be a relative or guardian, someone with experience or training in work with the mentally disordered, or some other adult (who is not a police officer or police employee), such as the solicitor or a trained professional in psychiatric work. The role of the appropriate adult is not to observe passively but to supervise the person being interviewed, to see whether the interview is being conducted properly and fairly, and to assist in communication with the interviewee.

Unreliable confessions

There has been considerable concern in recent years about the possibility of unreliable, self-incriminating confessions being made under police interrogation (see Gudjonsson, 1992; *Lancet*, 1994), and the *Code of Practice* advises police officers that this risk may particularly apply to some mentally ill and handicapped defendants, and special care must be taken in conducting interviews with them. In overturning the convictions of the "Tottenham Three" in 1991, for example, the Court of Appeal accepted evidence that the testimony under police interrogation of one of the accused, Engin Raghip, could not be relied upon because of his low intelligence and abnormal degree of suggestibility (Rozenberg, 1992). The possibility of unreliable confessions is not confined to people with mental illness or a learning disability, but may also apply to other people in states of acute emotional distress following arrest.

Prosecution

The decision to proceed with prosecution is the responsibility of the Crown Prosecution Service, and guidelines for their decisions are laid down in the Code for Crown Prosecutors issued under Section 10 of the Prosecution of Offences Act 1985 (House of Commons, 1991). Government policy is that mentally disordered people should not be prosecuted unless it is clearly in the public interest (Home Office, 1990*b*). In their decision-making, Crown Prosecutors have to evaluate whether the evidence is sufficient, and in doing so they should have regard to whether the requirements of the Police and Criminal Evidence Act 1984 and its codes of practice, discussed above, have been met. In particular, have the individuals in police custody been properly treated and are there doubts about the reliability of any confessions or other statements made by the accused, bearing in mind his/her intelligence and apparent understanding? The Code for Crown Prosecutors also suggests that they consider whether the accused has any mental disability which may affect his credibility, and whether the public would consider it oppressive to proceed against the accused.

Secondly, having considered whether the evidence is sufficient the Crown Prosecutor should then decide whether a prosecution is required in the public interest. In particular, the Code specifies:

> "Whenever the Crown Prosecutor is provided with a medical report to the effect that an accused or a person under investigation is suffering from some form of mental illness or psychiatric illness and the strain of criminal proceedings may lead to a considerable worsening of his condition, such reports should receive anxious consideration . . .
> Where . . . the Crown Prosecutor is satisfied that the probable effect upon the defendant's mental health outweighs the interests of justice in that particular case he should not hesitate to discontinue proceedings" (para. 8 V(a)).

In appropriate cases, the provision of psychiatric reports at an early stage may have a useful role in influencing the prosecution decision.

Court proceedings

After being charged, a defendant's first court appearance will be at the magistrates' court. Cases are then usually remanded for trial, and the defendant may be remanded on bail or in custody. A remand on bail would be the normal course of events, and remands in custody require substantial grounds for believing that the defendant, if released, would commit further offences, abscond or interfere with witnesses. Remands on bail for very grave offences are unusual. Defendants with limited financial means can have legal representation paid for by Legal Aid, and solicitors acting for such clients can seek approval from the Legal Aid authorities to cover fees for medical and other reports that may be necessary.

Remands to hospital for report and treatment

In the case of the mentally disordered defendant, magistrates' courts have powers to remand to hospital for a report (Section 35, Mental Health Act 1983). This order initially lasts for 28 days and can then be renewed if necessary for two further 28-day periods. The court requires one medical recommendation which should confirm that the person may suffer from mental disorder, and that a hospital bed is available. If the defendant has not yet been convicted, the remand to hospital requires either that the court is satisfied that the person committed the offence, or alternatively that the defendant consents to hospital admission. Thus, at an early stage of criminal proceedings, before the prosecution evidence is fully prepared, it may not be possible to remand unwilling defendants to hospital for assessment. In addition, those detained solely under Section 35 of the

Mental Health Act 1983 cannot be given compulsory psychiatric treatment. The power to remand to hospital for the purposes of treatment (Section 36, Mental Health Act 1983) is only available to Crown Courts, and this power is rarely used. It requires two medical recommendations that the person is suffering from mental illness or severe mental impairment; the other categories of mental disorder are not included.

Remand on bail

Many psychiatric assessments for magistrates' courts are carried out while defendants are remanded on bail. Indeed, a remand to hospital for assessment should not be carried out unless the court thinks that it would be impracticable to obtain such a report by means of a remand on bail. These defendants are normally assessed in an out-patient clinic.

Remand in custody

Courts also have powers to remand to prison for psychiatric reports, and these custodial remands tend to be more common than remands to hospital (in recent years remands to hospital for assessment have numbered approximately 300 per year, and remands in custody for medical reports approximately 6000 per year). A remand in custody for a medical report does not require the availability of a psychiatrist to make a medical recommendation and advise on the availability of a bed, and it is therefore a simpler and less time-consuming procedure for busy courts. However, in consequence, mentally disordered people charged with minor offences can spend lengthy periods of time in the inappropriate conditions of remand prisons while awaiting psychiatric assessment (see Chapter 9).

Court diversion schemes

In September 1990 the Home Office issued a circular on provision for mentally disordered offenders (Home Office, 1990b) which emphasised the government policy aim that mentally disordered people should receive care and treatment from health and social services rather than in the criminal justice system, and that they should not be prosecuted unless it is in the public interest. Since that time, a growing number of court-based psychiatric diversion schemes have become established (Joseph, 1994). These aim to make rapid psychiatric assessments available to magistrates' courts, with a view to arranging care and treatment for those who require it while avoiding unnecessary remands in custody. The availability of a psychiatrist, either "on call" or on a regular sessional basis, together with the availability of an approved social worker, enables courts to obtain rapid opinions. Arrangements can be made for voluntary psychiatric treatment or compulsory admission under a civil order of the Mental Health

Act, or a remand to hospital under Section 35 of the Mental Health Act 1983. When informal treatment or compulsory civil admissions are recommended, the Crown Prosecution Service may choose to discontinue criminal proceedings. A report by Blumenthal & Wessely (1992) indicated that by mid-1992, only a quarter of purchasing health authorities had a policy dealing with diversion, and the overall response in providing court diversion schemes nationally was fragmented and fragile. For further discussion of court diversion schemes, see Chapter 7.

Trial and sentencing

The specific issues that arise in the trial and sentencing of mentally disordered defendants are covered in detail in Chapter 5. The framework of sentencing for normal offenders has been subject to major revision in recent years. In 1990 a Government White Paper on criminal justice policy in England and Wales, *Crime, Justice and Protecting the Public* (Home Office, 1990c), sought to establish a coherent legislative framework for the sentencing of normal offenders based on "just deserts" principles. (Sentences for mentally disordered offenders are based on different principles, namely to achieve psychiatric treatment and public protection). The White Paper contained proposals to strengthen community-based punishments and to make a sharper distinction between violent and non-violent crimes, signified by new powers for Crown Courts to impose longer sentences for violent and sexual offences when this is necessary to protect the public from serious harm. Legislation followed in the shape of the Criminal Justice Act 1991 which came into force in 1992. Its implications for psychiatric practice have been reviewed by James (1993).

Criminal justice policy is always subject to review, and at the time of writing, revisions to the Criminal Justice Act 1991 are already being discussed. Nevertheless, it was a substantial recasting of sentencing provisions, and it is therefore important to summarise it.

Criminal Justice Act 1991. The sentencing framework introduced in the Act included a new unit fine system. This quickly fell into disrepute because of perceived unfairness in its operation and it was repealed in September 1993. Among the other non-custodial forms of disposal, there are six types of sentence designated as "community orders", namely the Probation Order, the Community Service Order, the Combination Order, the Curfew Order, the Supervision Order and the Attendance Centre Order. The Combination Order combines elements of probation and community service.

In all cases the restriction of liberty imposed by the order should be commensurate with the seriousness of the offence(s). This may affect the imposition of Probation Orders with a condition of medical treatment. It will no longer be sufficient to regard the Probation Order as suitable solely because of the rehabilitation needs of the offender; the court must also be satisfied that the order is justified by the seriousness of the offence and that the restrictions on liberty are commensurate with the seriousness of the offence.

Under the Criminal Justice Act 1991, custodial sentences (sentences of imprisonment) require one of three conditions to be met. Either:

(1) the defendant has refused consent to a community order, or
(2) the offender has been convicted of a violent or sexual offence and a custodial sentence is needed to protect the public from serious harm, or
(3) the offence is so serious that only a custodial sentence can be justified.

Where the offender has been previously convicted of a violent or sexual offence the court may pass a sentence which is longer than would be commensurate with the seriousness of the offence.

This new framework needs to be borne in mind by forensic psychiatrists for several reasons. Firstly, when recommendations for psychiatric disposals are made, courts may be conscious of what sentence might have been imposed had the individual not been mentally disordered. If reports are to have credibility with courts they must be perceived as realistic. Secondly, the potential for imposing longer sentences following conviction for violent and sexual offences, when this is necessary to protect the public from serious harm, could lead to pressure to introduce psychiatric evidence to assist courts on these points. While it is appropriate for psychiatric reports to consider whether or not there should be a medical disposal, it is not acceptable that reports should be used only for the purpose of assessing "dangerousness" and the length of prison sentences (see Chapter 8). Thirdly, Section 4 of the Criminal Justice Act 1991 specifies that in any case where an offender is, or appears to be, mentally disordered, the court should obtain a medical report before passing a custodial sentence. While this requirement could be beneficial in assisting with the identification and diversion of the mentally disordered, the new requirement also has the potential for two adverse effects: increasing remands in custody for reports; and psychiatric reports influencing sentence lengths, as noted above. This will need to be carefully monitored.

Life imprisonment. Sentences of life imprisonment are reserved for the most grave cases. Following conviction for murder a life sentence is mandatory (i.e. the court cannot choose an alternative). Following conviction for certain other serious offences (e.g. rape, attempted murder) a life sentence is one of a range of sentences that can be imposed, and thus is discretionary. The view that an offender is highly dangerous due to mental instability may be an important factor in imposing a discretionary life sentence.

The length of time spent in prison by a life-sentence prisoner is indeterminate, and subject to intermittent reviews by the Parole Board (see Chapter 9). Psychiatrists are always included in the panels reviewing individual cases. At present the procedures for review and release operate differently for mandatory and discretionary life sentences. At the time of sentencing the judge indicates to the Home Office the period of time that represents the "tariff" for the particular offence, that is, the requirements of retribution and deterrence. Mandatory life sentence prisoners have a first review by the Parole Board, normally three years before their tariff date, and then subsequent annual reviews. The prisoner is not present or represented. Recommendations are made to the Home Secretary, but the Home Secretary does not have to accept a recommendation for release.

In contrast, discretionary life sentence prisoners who have passed the tariff period are entitled to hearings of "discretionary lifer panels" of Parole Board members. The prisoner can attend the hearing, be legally represented, and have independent psychiatric reports prepared. The panel has to decide whether continued imprisonment is needed for reasons of public safety, and if release is directed, the Home Secretary is obliged to accept this. For a recent review and discussion of the background to this complex state of affairs, see Windlesham (1993).

Addendum for Northern Ireland

By Fred Browne

In Northern Ireland, efforts to combat the "Troubles" have brought about significant differences in the criminal justice system compared with the rest of the UK. The most important pieces of legislation are the Northern Ireland (Emergency Provisions) Acts 1978 and 1987, and the Criminal Evidence (Northern Ireland) Order 1988. In addition, most of the Prevention of Terrorism (Temporary Provisions) Act 1989 which applies to the rest of the UK also applies to Northern Ireland.

The Northern Ireland (Emergency Provisions) Act 1987 states that terrorism means "the use of violence for political ends and includes any use of violence for the purpose of putting the public or any section of the public in fear". Schedule 4 of this act lists certain offences commonly associated with terrorism, including both hybrid offences and indictable offences. For these scheduled offences there are different regulations relating to powers of arrest and detention, photographing and fingerprinting of suspects, the granting of bail and committal proceedings. Because of fears that juries may be biased or intimidated, indictable offences are tried before Diplock Courts – a single judge sitting without a jury. Different criteria for the admissibility of a confession are used during the trial of a scheduled offence. Unlike a jury, the judge must give his reasons for his decisions. Because of the absence of a jury, people convicted on indictment of scheduled offences have greater rights of appeal. With the exception of the Diplock Courts, Northern Ireland has magistrates' and Crown Courts as in England, together with its own Court of Appeal. Ultimate appeal is to the House of Lords.

Some of the offences listed on Schedule 4 may be "descheduled" by the Attorney General if no element of terrorism is apparent, for example, in the case of a domestic murder.

The Criminal Evidence (NI) Order 1988 allows courts to attach whatever weight they think proper to the fact that someone remained silent in circumstances where an innocent person might reasonably have been expected to protest his innocence and draw attention to facts which were to establish it. This Order applies to the general criminal law and not specifically to terrorist-related offences.

The Police and Criminal Evidence (Northern Ireland) Order 1989 is similar to the Police and Criminal Evidence Act 1984, but again with differences in detail. Dickson (1989) summarises the legal system in Northern Ireland.

Addendum for Scotland

By Derek Chiswick

The criminal law of Scotland, its procedures and agencies, are different from those of England. Prosecution of serious crimes is the responsibility of the Lord Advocate, the Queen's senior law officer in Scotland. Much of the work is conducted by "advocates-depute" (lawyers seconded to this work) who, together with a staff of civil servants, constitute the Crown Office in Edinburgh. Less serious crime (in practice, the majority) is prosecuted locally by "procurators fiscal". A good working relationship between the local psychiatric service and the procurator fiscal is beneficial.

Prosecution may be under "summary" or "solemn" procedure. There are no committal proceedings comparable to those in England. On solemn procedure an accused may undergo judicial examination, that is, be questioned by a procurator fiscal before a sheriff, and given an opportunity to provide a disincriminating explanation. He is legally represented, and his answers or failure to answer may be subsequently referred to at trial. A person remanded in custody (prison or hospital) must come to trial within 40 days (under summary procedure) or 110 days (solemn), or be liberated with immunity from further prosecution for that alleged offence.

Courts

Box 4.2 shows the courts in Scotland. Trials take place in district courts (before one or more justices of the peace), in sheriff courts (before a sheriff), and in the High Court of Justiciary (before a High Court judge).

Box 4.2 Criminal courts in Scotland

District Courts
- cases heard by one or more lay justices of the peace
- maximum sentence is 60 days imprisonment
- stipendiary magistrates (currently only in Glasgow) have powers similar to the sheriff

Sheriff Court
- 49 courts organised into six sheriffdoms, each headed by a sheriff principal
- tries cases under summary procedure (sheriff sitting alone), or under solemn procedure (sheriff and jury of 15 people)
- maximum sentence is three months imprisonment (summary) or three years (solemn)
- remit to High Court for heavier sentence

High Court of Justiciary
Functions as court of:

Criminal Trial
- highest criminal trial court
- sits in Edinburgh, Glasgow and on circuit in other cities and major towns
- exclusive jurisdiction for serious crimes
- judge and jury of 15 people
- unlimited sentencing powers

Scottish Court of Criminal Appeal
- sole court of appeal from High Court and lower courts
- cases heard by three or more judges
- no appeal to the House of Lords

The bulk of the work is carried out in the sheriff courts. Sheriffs are legally qualified judges. Under summary procedure sheriffs sit alone (without a jury) deciding matters of law and fact. The maximum sentence under summary procedure is three months imprisonment on first offence, and six months in certain other circumstances. Under solemn procedure a sheriff sits with a jury, the latter deciding guilt. The maximum sentence under solemn procedure in the sheriff court is three years imprisonment; cases which may merit a longer sentence are remitted after conviction to the High Court. Major crimes are tried in the High Court where the sentences are unlimited. There are no youth courts in Scotland, and prosecution of children under 16 is only by leave of the Lord Advocate. Instead, the non-judicial children's hearings deal with all children in trouble (see Chapter 11).

At a trial there is no preliminary outlining of the case; the trial starts with the calling of the first Crown witness. Evidence in Scotland must be corroborated, that is, provided from at least two sources. Contrary to popular belief, conviction in Scotland can occur on precious little more evidence than a "confession" (Griffiths, 1992). A jury in Scotland consists of 15 people. In addition to verdicts of "guilty" and "not guilty", there is a third, "not proven", which results in acquittal. Decisions are by simple majority except that a guilty verdict requires at least eight jury members to be in favour of it. Scotland has its own Court of Criminal Appeal; there is no appeal to the House of Lords.

The Criminal Procedure (Scotland) Act 1975 governs procedural matters. Pre-trial remand to hospital is available (Sections 25 or 330) but after conviction it can only be provided by a remand on bail with a condition of residence in hospital (i.e. the patient is informal). A full range of post-conviction disposals is available. The Criminal Justice (Scotland) Bill, currently before Parliament, contains a proposal for a post-conviction remand to hospital. Transfer to hospital of an untried or sentenced prisoner is currently provided for under Sections 70 and 71 of the Mental Health (Scotland) Act 1984.

Addendum for the Republic of Ireland

By Enda Dooley

The Irish criminal justice system consists of the police (Garda Siochana), the courts, the prisons and places of detention, the Department of Justice, the Probation and Welfare Service, the office of the Director of Public Prosecutions, and the office of the Chief State Solicitor. This system inherited a bulk of British statute and common law at the time of Independence in 1922. Subsequently, a written Constitution was superimposed in 1937. The Constitution provides for the rigid separation of executive, judicial and legislative powers. All laws, including those of arrest, detention, and so on, are subject to the provisions of the Constitution. Where decisions are considered to be repugnant to the Constitution they may be referred for final arbitration before the Supreme Court. Various decisions of the Supreme Court have led to the introduction of significant changes in criminal justice procedures. Box 4.3 shows the criminal courts in the Republic of Ireland.

Following arrest, the decision to charge rests with the police. In serious cases such as murder, decisions regarding procedure involve the office of the Director of Public Prosecutions. Prosecution occurs in the courts and sentence is imposed by a judge following conviction by a jury (in indictable cases). Summary cases will be decided by a judge alone.

Box 4.3   Criminal courts in the Republic of Ireland

District court
- President and 39 legally qualified justices
- hears summary cases (maximum sentence six months imprisonment) and some indictable cases (maximum sentence 12 months)
- conducts preliminary hearing of serious cases

Circuit court
- President and ten judges
- cases are heard by judge and jury
- hears indictable cases only
- functions as a court of appeal for cases from district courts

Central Criminal Court (or High Court)
- President and 14 High Court judges
- cases are heard by High Court judge and jury
- only hears major crimes (treason, murder, attempted murder)

Special Criminal Court
- deals only with scheduled offences laid down by the government, usually terrorist cases
- cases are heard by three judges (majority decision)

Court of Criminal Appeal
- one justice of the Supreme Court and two High Court justices
- hears appeals from the Central Criminal Court, the Circuit Court and the Special Criminal Court
- majority decision

Supreme Court
- Chief Justice and other High Court justices
- hears appeals from the Court of Criminal Appeal
- exceptionally hears appeals from the Central Criminal Court

---

Once arrested and charged there is no provision in current Irish law to divert someone away from the criminal justice system. This includes the cases of those who are considered mentally ill or disordered at the time of arrest.

Section 165 of the currently applicable Irish mental health legislation (Mental Treatment Act 1945) allows a policeman to remove a person "believed to be of unsound mind" from a public place to a police station when it is believed that this is required for the safety of the public or the mentally ill person. It would be expected that in these cases, urgent psychiatric assessment would be arranged. In practice this provision is rarely used. More commonly, following arrest and charge a person is remanded in custody for the preparation of psychiatric and probation reports. There are no legislative provisions to allow the transfer of an individual on remand to a district psychiatric hospital for assessment or treatment. The only option available following remand in custody is for the accused to be transferred to the Central Mental Hospital in Dundrum (the only specific forensic psychiatry resource in the country) for assessment.

References

Blumenthal, S. & Wessely, S. (1992) *The Extent of Local Arrangements for the Diversion of the Mentally Abnormal Offender from Custody*. London: Institute of Psychiatry and King's College Hospital Medical School.

Bowden, P. (1978) A psychiatric clinic in a probation office. *British Journal of Psychiatry*, **133**, 448–451.

Department of Health & Welsh Office (1993) *Code of Practice, Mental Health Act 1983*. London: HMSO.

Dickson, B. (1989) *The Legal System of Northern Ireland*. Belfast: SLS Publications.

Dunn, J. & Fahy, T. A. (1990) Police admissions to a psychiatric hospital: demographic and clinical differences between ethnic groups. *British Journal of Psychiatry*, **156**, 373–378.

Griffiths, D. B. (1992) Confessions to the police in Scottish criminal law. *Journal of Forensic Psychiatry*, **3**, 215–218.

Gudjonsson, G. (1992) *The Psychology of Interrogations, Confessions and Testimony*. Chichester: John Wiley.

Hoggett, B. (1990) *Mental Health Law*. London: Sweet & Maxwell.

Home Office (1990*a*) *The Sentence of the Court*. London: HMSO.

—— (1990*b*) *Provision for Mentally Disordered Offenders*. Home Office Circular No. 66/90. London: Home Office.

—— (1990*c*) *Crime, Justice and Protecting the Public*. Cm 965. London: HMSO.

—— (1991) *A Digest of Information on the Criminal Justice System*. London: Home Office Research and Statistics Department.

—— (1992) *Code of Practice for the Detention, Treatment and Questioning of Persons by Police Officers*. London: HMSO.

House of Commons (1991) *Annual Report: Crown Prosecution Service April 1990– March 1991*. London: HMSO.

James, A. (1993) The Criminal Justice Act 1991. Principal provisions and their effect on psychiatric practice. *Journal of Forensic Psychiatry*, **4**, 285–294.

Joseph, P. L. A. (1994) Psychiatric assessment at the magistrates' court. *British Journal of Psychiatry*, **164**, 722–724.

Lancet (1994) Guilty innocents: the road to false confessions. Editorial. *Lancet*, **344**, 1447–1450.

Rozenburg, J. (1992) Miscarriages of justice. In *Criminal Justice under Stress* (eds E. Stockdale & S. Casale), pp. 91–117. London: Blackstone Press.

Windlesham, Lord (1993) Life sentences: law, practice and release decisions, 1989– 93. *Criminal Law Review* [1993], 644–659.

5 Psychiatry and criminal proceedings
Paul Bowden

Psychiatric issues before or during a trial • Psychiatric disposals after conviction • Addenda for Northern Ireland, Scotland and the Republic of Ireland

---

This chapter is concerned with the ways in which a psychiatric disorder might affect the trial, conviction and disposal of an accused person. In practice, most psychiatric disposals take place after conviction when guilt has been established. However, the psychiatric issues relating to the procedure of trial and determining guilt are of great importance, although they are rarely raised. Three of the subjects – muteness, fitness to plead, and amnesia – relate to circumstances where courts have evolved modifications of the criminal justice process to deal with defendants who may be mentally disordered. The other subjects – insanity, automatism, diminished responsibility, suicide pacts and infanticide – are essentially legal concepts whose central concern is criminal responsibility or blameworthiness.

Criminal acts are defined by two characteristics: the act is proscribed, and transgression carries a penalty. Where mental disorder is present, a person's responsibility to pay the penalty may be lessened.

Fitness to plead is theoretically an issue at all trials, but for reasons which will be explained later, it is only raised in a very small number. Similarly, the effects of alcohol could be an issue in many cases, but the law has evolved so that its effect on the criminal justice process is extremely limited. Where a trial does take place, and it concerns one of the esoteric matters dealt with below, the level of proof is different for the prosecution and the defence. For the prosecution the case must be proved beyond reasonable doubt, whereas for the defence the burden of proof is on the balance of probability.

In some circumstances the presence of mental disorder may mean that offending behaviour is more likely to be detected, or that the perpetrator may draw attention to himself or be less able to talk his way out of a difficult situation. In other cases a mentally disordered person may not be charged with an offence, for example, when the Crown Prosecution Service may be reluctant to prosecute a hospital in-patient. For some mentally disordered offenders, treatment as an out-patient or in-patient may be arranged informally or formally without recourse to the courts (see Chapter 4).

Where numerical information appears in this chapter it has been taken from *Criminal Statistics*, a volume produced annually by the Home Office.

The reader is also referred to Walker (1968) for an authoritative account of the history of the legal issues discussed, and to Archbold (1985) for a description of legal procedure. Where the Butler Report appears in the text it refers to the *Committee on Mentally Abnormal Offenders* (Home Office & Department of Health and Social Security, 1975). Chapter 6 provides a detailed description of the way in which defendants should be assessed for providing court reports.

Psychiatric issues before or during a trial

Muteness

It is not uncommon for the police to be faced with individuals who do not speak. If they are suspected of a criminal offence they may be charged and be remanded in custody as "male (or female) anon". The great majority have a severe mental illness, usually schizophrenia; for a minority who are not mentally ill their silence may be a protest or a political gesture.

From medieval times courts have had to deal with defendants who have failed to answer "guilty" or "not guilty" on arraignment, which is that stage in the criminal proceedings where the charge is put. In these circumstances the court may simply remand the case until a later date. Alternatively, where a magistrates' court is satisfied that a person is mentally ill or severely mentally impaired, and that he did the act charged, it can make a hospital order (described later in this chapter) without convicting the defendant (Section 37(3), Mental Health Act 1983).

If the case reaches the Crown Court the question is raised: "is he mute of malice or by visitation of God?" The origins of these quaint phrases are to be found in the 18th century, when the court's remedy was to order the man to be subjected to *piene forte et dure* which consisted of slowly pressing him to death unless he spoke, which halted the process and allowed the trial to continue.

Nowadays the issue is decided by a jury. Where a verdict of mute of malice is returned, a plea of not guilty is entered and the trial proceeds. If the verdict is "mute by visitation of God" the jury must then decide the separate issue of fitness to plead (see below).

Assessing the mental state of a mute defendant calls for particular skills: in obtaining descriptions of behaviour from the arresting police officer and others charged with the person's care; and in patiently observing behaviour and interpreting its meaning. Malingering is hardly ever an issue and the most urgent task is often simply to find out the identity of the accused person. In the unlikely event of the matter reaching a Crown Court, a deaf and dumb individual may be found mute by visitation of God, but he or she would usually be fit to plead with the help of a lip-reader or sign-language interpreter.

Case example 1

A man charged with theft was remanded in custody for a psychiatric report. On interview he was mute and sat with a serene smile on his face. He obeyed instructions, for example to close the door, and cooperated with physical examination, which was normal. Prison officers reported that he had shown odd behaviour, in that he would talk to himself in his cell, he would lie prostrate on the ground with his arms outstretched and he frequently made the sign of the cross. He was admitted to hospital on a transfer direction, and soon began to talk, stating he was Jesus Christ, and that he had the gift of healing. With treatment, his mental state improved, and by the time of trial he was fit to plead.

Fitness to plead

Legal aspects

Like muteness, but unlike the other issues dealt with in this chapter, fitness to plead is concerned with a defendant's mental state *at the time of trial*. The principal of being unfit to plead, which is also known as being *under disability,* was first established in statute in Section 2 of the Criminal Lunatics Act 1800.

> "Persons indicted for any offence, and upon arraignment . . . found to be insane . . . the court shall order them to be kept in custody till His Majesty's Pleasure be known."

The tests of disability are from the case of a deaf mute (*R v Pritchard,* 1836).

> "Whether he can plead to the indictment . . . [and] . . . whether he is of sufficient intellect to comprehend the course of proceedings on trial, so as to make a proper defence – to know that he might challenge any of you [the jury] to whom he might object – and to comprehend the details of evidence . . ."

Box 5.1 shows how this judgement is interpreted today.

Box 5.1 Fitness to plead

The defendant must have the capacity to:
- understand the charge
- instruct a lawyer
- challenge a juror
- plead to the charge
- understand the evidence

The phrase "unfit to plead" is the marginal note alongside the text of Section 4 (i), Criminal Procedure (Insanity) Act 1964. The Act prescribes that fitness is tried by a jury whose members take a special oath. If the issue is decided at the beginning of the trial, and the defendant is found fit to plead, a separate jury decides the criminal case. Fitness to plead should not be confused with fitness to appear in court, although some defendants unable to appear in court will also be unfit to plead. Those unable to appear in court will include the physically ill and some very psychotic defendants whose appearance in court might lead to public scandal. It does not follow that a defendant who is highly abnormal or who does not act in his best interests is automatically unfit to plead. The test is his capacity to meet the criteria described above.

Case example 2
An 87-year-old woman was found with her elderly sister who had been battered to death. Evidence pointed unequivocally to the woman as having been responsible for the killing. She was in a state of gross dementia and was found unfit to plead by a jury on the basis that she could not fulfil any of the five tests of fitness. She was detained on a psychogeriatric ward subject notionally to Sections 37 and 41, Mental Health Act 1983. She died some months later.

A person found unfit to plead might improve after treatment and return to court for trial.

Case example 3
A solicitor became depressed after being charged with fraud involving a large amount of money. His trial was delayed on several occasions but he was found unfit to plead on the basis that his illness prevented him from adequately instructing his legal advisors in matters involving the examination of schedules and complex financial transactions. He remained a patient in a psychiatric unit and 18 months later he had improved to the extent that he was able to stand trial.

Before 1991 a person found under disability in terms of the 1964 Act was admitted to a hospital specified by the Secretary of State. Such patients were subject notionally to a hospital order with a restriction on discharge (Sections 37 and 41, Mental Health Act 1983). The inescapable imposition of the restriction order meant that, other than unwittingly, the defence was only used in grave circumstances. The Criminal Procedure (Insanity and Unfitness to Plead) Act 1991 has made two essential changes. Firstly, there is now a trial of 'facts' after a finding of unfitness to plead, and secondly, disposal is at the discretion of the judge and not limited to mandatory hospital and restriction orders. If the facts are not found then the accused is released. If the facts are found, the range of flexible disposals is described below. Patients who recover their fitness can be returned to court for trial at the discretion of the Home Secretary. There is a right of appeal against a finding of unfitness to plead.

Fitness to plead in practice

Despite the steep rise in recorded crime, from 750 000 offences in 1959 to more than 3 million in 1989, the number of unfitness findings has fallen (see Table 5.1).

Mackay (1990) has provided a profile of the 300 persons found to be under disability between 1976 and 1988 under the 1964 Act. Reflecting the sex distribution of those charged with criminal offences, the majority were male. Schizophrenia and learning disability were the most common diagnostic groups. The typical person found under disability had previous convictions and a history of psychiatric treatment. Most crimes were of a moderate or severe nature, and violent and sexual offences were over-represented. There was usually strong evidence to link the accused with the offence charged.

Grubin (1991) has also reviewed persons found to be under disability between 1976 and 1988. About a third were detained in special hospitals, the remainder in local hospitals and regional secure units. While only 12% of those found unfit to plead before 1983 were remitted to court for trial, the proportion from that date was 45%. After 1982, three-quarters of those returned to court did so within one year of the unfitness finding. Secure hospital containment, a diagnosis of mental illness and a history of previous convictions for violence were the best predictors of an early return to court.

Table 5.1 Numbers of defendants in England and Wales found unfit to plead, expressed as averages for 9-year periods

Decade	Average annual unfitness findings	In murder cases only
1948–1957	46	15
1958–1967	43	6
1979–1988	22	2

Clinical assessment of fitness to plead

Fitness to plead is only likely to be an issue in relation to severe psychiatric disorder, and therefore abnormality is likely to manifest itself early in the criminal trial process. The prison medical officer or the defendant's solicitor may have raised the issue even before assessment by a psychiatrist. Assessment of fitness to plead requires time, patience and a suitable location for the examination(s). Usually the case is one of severe functional psychosis or learning disability. In practice, the issue of fitness to plead

---

Box 5.2 Clinical assessment of fitness to plead

The following questions may be asked:
- Do you know what the police say you have done?
- Do you know the difference between saying "guilty" and "not guilty"?
- Can you tell your solicitor your side of things?
- If you think a witness in court is not right in what they say, who would you tell?
- Do you know what it means if they say you can object to some of the people on the jury in your case?

---

is rarely raised, as many of these defendants, often psychotic, are admitted to hospital from prison under Section 48 of the Mental Health Act 1983 for urgent psychiatric treatment (see Chapter 7). By the time they go to trial they are fit to plead.

Relevant questions (Box 5.2) based on the criteria which have been described must be put to the defendant in simple, clear language (Chiswick, 1990). In practice the psychiatrist is looking for a global view of whether or not the accused knows what's going on and can give instructions of some form to his lawyer. It is important to re-examine the defendant on the morning of the trial if it is some time since he was last seen. The most severe problems in determining fitness to plead usually concern people with a learning disability.

The insanity defence

Legal aspects

The importance of the insanity defence does not lie in the frequency with which it has been used, but in the position it holds in the history of medical jurisprudence throughout the world. The marginal note alongside the text of Section 1 of the Criminal Procedure (Insanity) Act 1964 states "Acquittal on grounds of insanity" and the section reads:

> "The special verdict required by Section 2 of the Trial of Lunatics Act 1883 (hereinafter referred to as the *"special verdict"*) shall be that the accused is not guilty by reason of insanity."

An appeal against acquittal on the grounds of insanity is available. Until recently, when the special verdict was returned the court made an order such that the accused be admitted to a hospital specified by the Secretary of State. As with unfitness, those found legally insane were subject notionally to orders under Sections 37 and 41 of the Mental Health Act 1983. Hence it was only prudent to raise the defence where the charge was serious. The Criminal Procedure (Insanity and Unfitness to Plead) Act 1991 now gives the judge discretion in sentencing after an insanity finding, and does not limit the disposal to mandatory committal to hospital (see below). The defence of insanity is based on the absence of *mens rea*, or guilty mind. It depends on the mental state of the accused at the time of committing the act; it therefore requires a retrospective diagnosis. The legal test of insanity is to be found in the Law Lords' answers to questions put to them after the trial of Daniel McNaughton in 1843 (see West & Walk, 1977) where part of the judgement was:

> "to establish a defence on the grounds of insanity, it must be clearly proved that at the time of the committing of the act, the party accused was labouring under such a defect of reason, from disease of the mind, as not to know the nature and quality of the act he was doing, or if he did know it, that he did not know that what he was doing was wrong."

While the presence of mental disorder may lessen criminal responsibility, or negate it completely as in the case of legal insanity, the law is nothing if not practical: "The purpose of legislation relating to the defence of insanity, ever since its origin in 1800, has been to protect society against recurrence of dangerous conduct" (Lord Diplock in *R v Sullivan*, 1984).

The defining criterion of legal insanity is impaired reasoning due to disease of the mind. What is disease of the mind? It will be clear from what follows that the law defines medical terms by the end it wishes to achieve.

> "The major mental diseases which doctors call psychoses, such as schizophrenia are clearly diseases of the mind . . . any mental disorder which has manifested itself in violence and is prone to recur is a disease of the mind. At any rate it is the sort of disease for which a person should be detained in hospital . . " *(Bratty v Attorney General for Northern Ireland*, 1963).

And what is the mind?

> "The law is not concerned with the brain but with the mind, in the sense that 'mind' is ordinarily used, the mental faculties of reason, memory and understanding *(R v Kemp*, 1957).

The nature and quality of the act refers to its physical characteristics. Knowledge that the act was wrong, meaning against the law, is a legal criterion rather than a moral one.

Case example 4
A middle-aged man killed and beheaded a neighbour. For some time he entertained a system of delusional beliefs, supported by auditory

hallucinations, that he was God. While he knew the nature and quality of the act of killing, the court accepted that he did not know that it was wrong in that his godly status, and belief that the neighbour was the devil, justified his behaviour. He was found not guilty by reason of insanity and was detained in a maximum security hospital.

The insanity defence in practice

Before the 1957 Homicide Act, which introduced the defence of diminished responsibility in murder cases, in about half the trials where a medical defence succeeded it was on the basis of legal insanity. In contrast, since 1957 there have only been about three insanity findings each year (range 1–6). Half were diagnosed as suffering with schizophrenia and a quarter with depression, epilepsy, or substance abuse (Mackay, 1990). In the decade from 1978, only seven individuals charged with homicide were found legally insane.

Criticisms of the insanity defence

The Butler Committee (1975) suggested that the concept of legal insanity should be broadened and, as with unfitness to plead, that discretionary sentencing should be available. The latter proposal was accepted and is one of the provisions of the Criminal Procedure (Insanity and Unfitness to Plead) Act 1991. The Committee's criterion of insanity was to be "severe mental illness", which was defined as being of such severity that the link between the offence and the defendant's mental condition could be safely presumed. It was this last suggestion which has been a major hurdle in gaining support for the recommendations.

Clinical assessment

This defence, and that of diminished responsibility (see below), depend on the examiner making a retrospective diagnosis; he needs to "reconstruct" the mental state of the accused at the time the alleged offence was committed. The first task is to come to a clinical view of his former mental state based on examination, listening to tape-recorded interviews (see Chapter 6) and usually interviewing witnesses or other people who knew the accused. Having reached a clinical conclusion that there was a disease of the mind present, it is then necessary to consider whether the defendant's reasoning was defective as a result of the disease. Thus far the tasks are not dissimilar from ordinary clinical practice (except that we do not normally talk about "diseases of the mind"). There then comes the imposs-ible part, namely making a judgement about what the accused did, or did not, know – psychiatrists are much more used to saying what they think their patients "think" rather than what they "know". The examiner must come to a view based on a global consideration of the defendant's former mental state and all other information available to him. It is rarely easy.

Criminal Procedure (Insanity and Unfitness to Plead) Act 1991

The issue of fitness to plead is normally determined by a jury as soon as it arises. The jury bases its decision on the written or oral evidence of two or more medical practitioners, at least one of whom is approved under Section 12 of the Mental Health Act 1983 (see Chapter 10). If the jury then decides that the accused is unfit to plead, the court is required to conduct "a trial of the facts". The burden of proof is the same as in other criminal proceedings, that is, beyond reasonable doubt. If the jury is satisfied on the evidence that the accused did not commit the offence, he must be acquitted. Those found under disability receive one of the disposal options described below (Box 5.3)(Kellam, 1992).

The 1991 Act and its provisions for discretionary sentencing in insanity and unfitness cases (and a trial of facts with unfitness) might lead to an increase in the use of these legal provisions.

Box 5.3 Disposal options for defendants found either unfit to plead or acquitted on grounds of insanity

Admission order: equivalent to a hospital order (Section 37) with or without restriction under Section 41 of the Mental Health Act. Where the offence is unlawful killing, there is a mandatory hospital order with restriction without limit of time

Guardianship order: equivalent to Section 37 of the Mental Health Act

Supervision and treatment order: equivalent to a probation order with a condition of psychiatric treatment (Section 9(3), Criminal Justice Act 1991)

Absolute discharge: where the offence was trivial and the person clearly does not require treatment and supervision in the community

---

Diminished responsibility

The doctrine of diminished responsibility applies only to murder. It reduces the category of crime from murder to manslaughter. Murder is the killing of a human being with malice aforethought, and conviction for it carries a mandatory and indeterminate sentence of life imprisonment. On conviction for manslaughter the judge can impose any sentence. Many authorities have argued that if the sentence on conviction for murder was at the discretion of the judge, diminished responsibility would be unnecessary.

Furthermore, in most circumstances psychiatric evidence would be given after conviction rather than being tailored to suit the adversarial process of a trial.

Legal aspects

Diminished responsibility is often referred to as "Section 2 manslaughter" and can be raised only by the defence. It is not an illness from which defendants suffer but a marginal note to the text of Section 2 of the Homicide Act 1957, which introduced the concept into English law. The same Act also introduced provocation as grounds for the lesser charge of manslaughter.

Section 2 reads:

> "Where a person kills . . . he shall not be convicted of murder if he was suffering from such an abnormality of mind (whether arising from a condition of arrested or retarded development of mind or any inherent cause or induced by disease or injury) as substantially impaired his mental responsibility for his acts . . ."

Again we are dealing with legal concepts, the terms being defined by case law rather than medical opinion. For example, 'abnormality of mind' is a broader concept than that of mental disorder, and is defined as:

> "A state of mind so different from that of ordinary human beings that the reasonable man, earlier defined as "a man with a normal mind", would term it abnormal. It appears to us to be wide enough to cover the mind's activities in all its aspects, not only the perception of physical acts and matters, and the ability to form a rational judgement as to whether the act was right or wrong, but also the ability to exercise will-power to control physical acts in accordance with that rational judgement." (Lord Chief Justice in *R v Byrne*, 1960)

The phrase "whether arising from a condition of arrested or retarded development of mind or any inherent cause or induced by disease or injury" was borrowed from the definition of mental defectiveness in the Mental Deficiency Act 1927. The whole bracketed part of Section 2 appears to be a limiting clause which was intended to confine the application of the Act to causes which are recognisably pathological and not merely transient.

Although psychiatrists are supposed to pronounce on the matter, mental responsibility belongs solely to law and morality. There is no such faculty as mental responsibility which means liability to punishment. And what constitutes substantial impairment? "Substantial does not mean total . . . At the other end [it] does not mean minimal or trivial. It is something in between" *(R v Lloyd, 1966)*.

Case example 5

A 25-year-old man killed his father. For some weeks he had experienced a variety of abnormal perceptions and unsystematised delusional ideas. Shortly after the killing he was noted to be in a state of acute fear with a pronounced delusional mood. When he came to court the Crown accepted the defence plea of manslaughter on the grounds of diminished responsibility. There was no trial, the judge made hospital and restriction orders (Sections 37 and 41, Mental Health Act 1983) and the man was admitted to a regional secure unit.

Case example 6

A middle-aged man was charged with the murder of his wife. He had a long history of dependant and aggressive behaviour and she left him having formed a new relationship. The defence plea of guilty to manslaughter on the grounds of diminished responsibility was not accepted by the prosecution and there was a trial. Disagreement between expert witnesses centred on both the degree of personality disorder and depressive reaction (and therefore the nature of the abnormality of mind) and also on their effect on his judgement and will power (which related to impairment of mental responsibility). The jury found him guilty of murder and he was sentenced to life imprisonment.

Diminished responsibility in practice

Since the 1957 Homicide Act, the previously used medical defences of legal insanity and unfitness to plead have been almost completely replaced by diminished responsibility. It was anticipated that the introduction of the concept would result in more of those charged with murder being found guilty of a lesser offence. In fact, as the homicide rate has risen, the proportion of assailants whom courts deem to be mentally abnormal has fallen (see Table 5.2). This trend reflects Schipkowenski's rule that there is an inverse relationship between the murder rate and the proportion of

Table 5.2 Number of people in England and Wales indicted for murder expressed as averages in three 4-year periods, and the percentage convicted of Section 2 manslaughter (diminished responsibility)

Years	Annual average no. indicted for murder	Section 2 manslaughter (%)
1978–1982	453	21
1983–1987	469	16
1988–1992	474	15

both mentally abnormal murders and murder/suicides (West, 1965; Schipkowenski, 1973).

When a defendant who is charged with murder pleads guilty to manslaughter on the grounds of diminished responsibility the Crown accepts the plea in about 80% of cases (Dell, 1984). The judge then proceeds to sentencing. Where the prosecution challenges the defence there is a trial and the usual verdict is murder. These contested cases can involve psychiatrists giving conflicting evidence and their judgements being subjected to critical scrutiny. Even when unchallenged expert evidence that a defendant is mentally disordered is put to a jury, they can convict of murder if there is other evidence before them which throws doubt on the psychiatric testimony.

The Privy Council has ruled:

> "Whether the accused was at the time of the killing suffering from an abnormality of mind in the broad sense . . . is a question for the jury. On this question medical evidence is no doubt of importance, but the jury are entitled to take account of all the evidence. They are not bound to accept the medical evidence if there is other material before them which, in their good judgement conflicts with it and outweighs it." (Elliott & Wood, 1974)

Sentencing

For the years 1983–1992 there was an annual average of 58 findings of Section 2 manslaughter. Their sentences are shown in Table 5.3. There is evidence that an increasing proportion are sentenced to imprisonment. Those sentenced to life imprisonment on conviction for Section 2 manslaughter tend to be the personality disordered, and they may spend longer in prison than others found guilty of murder. This is because the spectre of dangerousness, which is often raised in establishing their defence of diminished responsibility, can count against them later when the decision to release them from prison is considered.

Table 5.3 Sentencing of diminished responsibility cases in England and Wales 1983–1992

Sentence	%
Life imprisonment	10
Other imprisonment	28
Restriction order (S. 37/41)	36
Hospital order (S. 37)	11
Probation order	12

Psychiatric aspects

The assessment of the defendant is of his mental state at the time of the homicide. There is no criterion of abnormality of mind other than the judgement of the reasonable man (being defined legally as the man with the normal mind). Each case is decided on the basis of the evidence presented: pre-menstrual tension, transient situational disturbance and homosexual panic have all succeeded where frank psychosis has failed. Where a person is not psychotic the diagnosis is usually of personality disorder or depression.

Criticism of diminished responsibility

The Butler Committee (1975) recommended the abolition of the mandatory life sentence for murder, thereby rendering the provisions of Section 2 Homicide Act superfluous. This suggestion has received the support of the Criminal Law Revision Committee, but the mandatory life sentence seems likely to remain because its repeal would be politically unacceptable.

Suicide pacts

Suicide and its attempt ceased to be offences in the Suicide Act 1961. Hamilton (1990) stated that suicide pacts are very uncommon, accounting for only 1% of suicides. Rosen (1981) showed that most involved married couples and young lovers and there was a high incidence of physical and mental disorder. Section 4 of the Homicide Act 1957 altered the category of crime for homicide by the survivor of a suicide pact from murder to manslaughter. Section 4(i) reads: "It shall be manslaughter, and shall not be murder, for a person acting in pursuance of a suicide pact between him and another to kill the other or be party to . . . being killed by a third person".

> **Case example 6**
> A man was charged with the murder of his partner. She was found strangled and he took a non-fatal overdose of a tranquilliser. The man was an alcoholic and sexually deviant; the woman was said to have a neurotic personality. In court he pleaded manslaughter on the grounds that it was a suicide pact. The Crown did not accept the plea and a jury found him guilty of murder because of the lack of evidence of both a common agreement and of his settled intention of dying.

It is for the defence to prove that a suicide pact existed and the phrase is defined in Section 4(3):

> ". . . a common agreement between two or more persons having as its object the death of all of them whether or not each is to take his own life, but nothing done by a person who enters into a suicide

pact shall be treated as done by him in pursuance of the pact unless it is done while he has the settled intention of dying in pursuance of the pact".

Infanticide

Legal aspects

No woman has been executed in England for the killing of her child under the age of one year since 1889. Until the Infanticide Act 1922, judges went through the ritual of pronouncing the death sentence in such cases, knowing full well that it would never be carried out (Morris & Blom-Cooper, 1964). The 1922 Act provided that if a woman wilfully caused the death of her newly born child, but at the time the balance of her mind had been disturbed by the effects of childbirth, she committed the crime of infanticide and not murder. The existence of infanticide has several advantages: it allows a prosecution other than for murder; it concedes the presence of mental disorder; and it allows the court to pass any sentence.

"Newly born" was not defined in the 1922 Act, whereas the Infanticide Act 1938 specified the period after childbirth in which disturbance of the mind can be claimed. Section 1(i) reads:

> "Where a woman by any wilful act or omission causes the death of her child under the age of twelve months, but at the time of the act or omission the balance of her mind was disturbed by reason of not having fully recovered from the effect of giving birth to the child or by reason of the effect of lactation consequent on the birth . . . she shall be guilty of [an offence], to wit of infanticide . . ."

Psychiatric aspects

The degree of mental disorder which amounts to a disturbance of the balance of a woman's mind is much less than that required to fulfil the criterion of abnormality of mind as is contained in the Homicide Act 1957. Once again, the issue is the mother's mental state at the time of the killing. The wider aspects of the killing of children are described in Chapter 2.

Case example 7
A woman asphyxiated her 4-month-old child after a succession of sleepless nights caused by the infant's miserable crying. She felt overwhelmed by the child's demands, unsupported as a mother, and that the child was selfish and gave her nothing. She was found guilty of infanticide even though there was little evidence that she was mentally disordered. She was put on a probation order.

Case example 8
After the birth of her third child a woman became depressed and psychotic. She killed her three children to save them from what she

believed to be a worse fate. She was found guilty of infanticide in killing the baby and of manslaughter on the grounds of diminished responsibility with regard to the two older children. She was made subject to Sections 37 and 41 of the Mental Health Act 1983 and was admitted to a regional secure unit.

D'Orban (1979) has examined infanticide in the context of 89 maternal filicides where 44% of the victims were under one year. Offenders who killed or attempted to kill children within 24 hours of birth (neonaticide) were very likely to be found guilty of infanticide, although most had no demonstrable psychiatric abnormality. Two-thirds of battering women who killed children under one year were also found guilty of infanticide. Mentally ill mothers were likely to be found guilty of manslaughter on the grounds of diminished responsibility rather than infanticide.

Sentencing in infanticide

In the decade from 1978 there was an average of five findings of infanticide each year (range 1–7). The usual sentence on conviction for infanticide is a probation order but a few hospital orders are also made. The Butler Committee (1975) recommended the abolition of infanticide and that the defence should be subsumed under the doctrine of diminished responsibility.

Legal automatism

Almost every criminal offence requires *mens rea* or guilty mind. If the mind does not have the potential to control physical acts, there is an absence of *mens rea* and this forms the basis of the defence of automatism. The legal definition of automatism was given by the Lord Chancellor, Viscount Kilmuir in the case of *Bratty v Attorney General for Northern Ireland* (1963).

> "The state of a person who, though capable of action is not conscious of what he is doing . . . it means unconscious involuntary action and it is a defence because the mind does not go with what is being done"

Legal automatism has no relationship to the clinical concept of automatic behaviour.

In law there are two types of automatism: sane (automatism simpliciter) and insane. The distinction is based on the defendant's dangerousness as measured by the prospect of the behaviour recurring. If the behaviour can recur it is labelled insane automatism and is said both to be due to the disease of the mind and, illogically, to have an internal cause. A finding of insane automatism formerly resulted in the accused's admission to hospital subject notionally to hospital and restriction orders (Sections 37 and 41, Mental Health Act 1983). Under the Criminal Procedure (Insanity and Unfitness to Plead) Act 1991, sentencing is now left to the discretion of the judge. Insane automatism includes behaviours caused by brain diseases, tumours and epilepsy. A recent judgement ruled that sleepwalking was also an example of insane automatism (*R v Burgess*, 1991).

Case example 9

A known epileptic was admitted to hospital after two grand mal fits. He was confused, paranoid and hallucinating. Following a minor seizure he assaulted a fellow patient inflicting serious injuries. At his trial for attempted murder the jury found him legally insane and he was admitted to a regional secure unit subject notionally to a hospital order and restriction order.

In contrast, sane automatisms are once-only events and are said, again illogically, to be due to external causes. A finding of sane automatism results in an acquittal and the defendant is free to leave court. Sane automatisms include confusional states and concussion, reflex actions following, for example, a bee sting, dissociative states, night terrors, and hypoglycaemia.

Case example 10

A man strangled his wife during a dream in which he believed he was being pursued by soldiers. It was accepted at his trial that he experienced a night terror and he was acquitted.

The legal distinction between internal and external causes has no physical basis. Similarly the ascription of disease of the mind only to insane automatisms, on the basis that they may recur, is difficult to understand when night terrors, which are said to be sane automatisms, are excluded (Fenwick, 1990).

It is likely that as the provisions of the Criminal Procedure (Insanity and Unfitness to Plead) Act 1991 take effect, the distinction between insane and non-insane automatisms will cease to exist; its only purpose was to secure the prospect of indeterminate detention of the insane group on the grounds that they were dangerous.

Alcohol and drugs

The extent to which voluntarily taking alcohol or drugs (here called intoxication) affects criminal liability is a controversial subject. In essence the purpose of legal judgements in the area is restrictive, limiting greatly the circumstances in which intoxication can be used as a defence. Almost all offences require two elements: *actus reus* and *mens rea*. The *actus reus* is the prohibited act, and the *mens rea* the intention or recklessness; the latter may be affected by alcohol or drugs.

The law regarding the defence of intoxication in crimes of specific intent (see below) was stated by Lord Birkenhead in *Director of Public Prosecutions v Beard* (1920). The law can be summarised thus:

(1) If intoxication causes insanity, for example, *delirium tremens* or drug-induced psychosis, the McNaughton rules apply, and a defence of insanity may be possible.
(2) Intoxication is a defence if it prevents the accused forming specific intent. The latter applies only to certain crimes (see below).
(3) Intoxication not negating *mens rea* but merely making a defendant more likely to behave as he did is no defence.

In general, voluntary intoxication is considered a defence only with crimes of specific intent: murder, wounding with intent, burglary with intent to steal, handling stolen goods. In contrast, manslaughter, malicious wounding, assault occasioning actual bodily harm, common assault, and rape are held to be offences of basic intent and therefore intoxication is no defence. It follows that where voluntary intoxication is insufficient either to constitute legal insanity or to negate specific intent, then it is assumed that a person intends the consequence of his acts. The House of Lords recently ruled that involuntary intoxication was not a defence where a person was shown to have the necessary criminal intent (*R v Kingston, The Times* law report, 22 July 1994).

The neuropsychiatric sequelae of alcohol abuse (e.g. Korsakov's syndrome or alcoholic dementia) may provide grounds for a defence of diminished responsibility.

Amnesia

Amnesia for all or part of the thoughts, feelings and behaviours which accompany criminal acts is not uncommon. As with other dramatic events, little may be remembered of chaotic and emotionally charged situations. A variety of emotional and physical factors can operate simultaneously, and over a period of time different factors may produce amnesia. Thus what begins as an alcohol-induced amnesia may be reinforced voluntarily and later maintained by hysterical mechanisms. Box 5.4 summarises the conditions with which amnesia may be associated.

Courts have resisted attempts to make amnesia a bar to trial, not least because of the difficulty of distinguishing between real and faked forgetfulness. In addition, amnesia can often be recognised as self-serving and the fact that a person claims not to remember what he did, or why, does not mean that at the time he did not intend his actions. Being amnesic often makes the long wait to the trial bearable, and it may allow a defendant to face himself, his family, and fellow prisoners. Being amnesic could handicap a defendant in providing a defence, such as an alibi, but courts

---

Box 5.4 Amnesia

Amnesia may be associated with:
- periods of impaired consciousness or acute intoxication
- hysterical dissociation
- unconscious denial

Alternatively, the subject may be lying

---

have decided unequivocally that it does not form the basis for a successful defence of unfitness to plead.

Case example 11
A man charged with shooting and killing a policeman sustained a head injury during his arrest. His defence that amnesia made him unfit to plead was not accepted by a jury and a second jury found him guilty of murder. *(R v Podola, 1960)*

Case example 12
A police inspector was charged with theft by shoplifting. Examination revealed him to be suffering from a mixed affective disorder associated with constitutional factors and stress at work and at home. He was amnesic for the period when he was shopping and the charge against him was dismissed when expert evidence suggested that his preoccupation with morbid thoughts led to inattentiveness and lack of criminal intent.

Clearly, if amnesia is associated with an identifiable psychiatric disorder such as a head injury or florid psychosis, then the primary condition may form the basis of a medical defence, such as automatism. Alternatively it may result in mitigation, with reduction to a less serious charge, or the imposition of treatment rather than punishment.

Psychiatric disposals after conviction

The most frequent route to treatment for a mentally disordered offender is provided after conviction. The main psychiatric consideration becomes the requirement for treatment. At this stage, insanity and responsibility are redundant issues. Box 5.5 summarises the way in which the courts link in with the mental health system.

Further information will be found in *A Guide to the Mental Health Act 1983* (Bluglass, 1983), and the four official publications on which the section is based: *The Mental Health Act 1983* (HMSO, 1983); *The Sentence*

Box 5.5 Psychiatric disposals after conviction

Hospital order (Section 37(2), Mental Health Act 1983)
Interim hospital order (Section 38)
Guardianship order (Section 37(1))
Restriction order (Section 41)
Probation with a condition of treatment (Section 9(3), Criminal
    Justice Act 1991)

---

of the Court (Home Office, 1986); *Provision for Mentally Disordered Offenders*
(Home Office, 1990); *Code of Practice* (Department of Health & Welsh
Office, 1993).

Hospital orders

This is the most important psychiatric disposal available to the court. Where
a mentally disordered person is convicted of an offence the court may
well wish to consider the appropriateness of psychiatric treatment. This
may be obtained by imposing a hospital order under Section 37(2) of the
Mental Health Act 1983. The offence must be one which is punishable on
conviction by imprisonment, and not one for which the sentence is fixed,
such as murder.

The grounds for making the order are that the court must be satisfied
on the evidence of *two registered medical practitioners, one of whom is
approved* under Section 12(2) of the Act as having special experience in
the diagnosis and treatment of mental disorder, that *the offender is suffering
from mental disorder of a nature or degree which makes it appropriate for
him to be detained in hospital for treatment, and in the case of psychopathic
disorder or mental impairment that the treatment is likely to alleviate or
prevent a deterioration of the condition.*

Treatment is defined in very broad terms by Section 145(1), Mental
Health Act 1983: "'medical treatment' includes nursing, and also includes
care, habilitation and rehabilitation under medical supervision".

*The court must be satisfied that arrangements have been made for the
offender's admission to hospital within 28 days* on the basis of either written
or oral evidence from the doctor who is to be in charge of the treatment,
or some person representing the managers of the hospital. Courts have no
power to order a hospital to take a particular patient.

The person on whom a hospital order is made can be detained in a
place of safety, usually a prison hospital, for up to 28 days if a bed is not
immediately available. *Hospital orders last for six months and are renewable.*
Patients can be discharged at any time by the responsible medical officer

(RMO). An application can be made to a mental health review tribunal after a period of six months in hospital.

> **Case example 13**
> A 26-year-old man with a history of schizophrenia was arrested following a disturbance at his home. Unable to secure his immediate admission to hospital, the police charged him with assault and he was remanded in custody for medical reports when he appeared in a magistrates' court the next day. In prison he was seen by his catchment area consultant and a member of a nursing team and the necessary reports were completed. When he returned to court two weeks after his first appearance a hospital order was made and he went back to prison awaiting availability of a bed in hospital.

The provisions of Section 37(3) allow a magistrates' court to make a hospital order without convicting the defendant provided it is satisfied that the accused did the act and that the requirements of Sections 37(1) and (2) (see above) are fulfilled.

Hospital orders in practice

The process of remands into custody for medical reports is grossly inefficient and the importance of diverting people from the criminal justice system at the earliest possible stage cannot be overemphasised (Joseph, 1990, and see Chapter 9). The *Code of Practice* (Department of Health & Welsh Office, 1993) makes it clear that the purpose of legislation is to ensure that those subject to criminal proceedings who are both in custody and in need of treatment for mental disorder should receive such treatment. Mentally disordered individuals are particularly vulnerable in custody; there is a high incidence of suicide, and treatment with medication without consent is difficult other than in urgent and grave situations.

Those in custody should have the same quality of service which other citizens enjoy, and where there is difficulty in obtaining an assessment or treatment, Section 39(1) requires regional health authorities to furnish courts with information with respect to the hospital(s) at which arrangements could be made for admission of the person. Regional health authorities usually appoint a person to respond to these requests but it does not mean that the authority must find the offender a place.

Problems sometimes arise with persons who have *no fixed abode*. In such cases the responsible district services are identified according to the following generally accepted criteria:

(1) If the patient has relatives known to take an interest in his welfare, the health authority where the nearest caring relative resides is responsible for placement.

(2) Even if the nearest relative is not interested in the patient's welfare, the health authority where the relative resides will be responsible unless the relative is hostile to the placement and the patient has no contact with the area.
(3) If there is no relative available but the patient has some long association with an area, then the authority for the area concerned is responsible.
(4) In cases where the above do not apply, the authority for the area where the patient committed the offence is responsible.

Interim hospital orders

Section 38 of the Mental Health Act 1983 introduced interim hospital orders. They are imposed after conviction by both magistrates' courts (where the offence must be imprisonable) and Crown Courts (but not for murder). The circumstances in which the order can be made are broadly similar to those which apply to hospital orders under Section 37. Section 38 orders are for 12 weeks, renewable for 28 days at a time for up to six months.

The orders were designed to be used to test individuals' cooperation with, and response to, treatment. They have been used little, almost exclusively with persons designated legally as having a psychopathic disorder.

Guardianship orders

Section 37(1) of the Mental Health Act 1983 allows a court to place a convicted person under guardianship. The procedure is identical to that for making a hospital order except that the purpose is not to provide treatment but to ensure that the offender receives care and attention. The offender must have reached the age of 16, and the order places him under the care of the local authority social services or an approved person. A court can only make a guardianship order if the authority or approved person is prepared to receive the offender.

> **Case example 14**
> A 19-year-old man with a learning disability was found to have been interfering sexually with a niece. He had attended special schools and was unemployed. He lived with his mother and a sister who had a 3-year-old daughter. He had no friends or social outlets. He was deemed fit to plead and found guilty of indecent assault. Assessment suggested that he lacked social skills and needed help to direct his sexual feelings appropriately. Medical reports stated that he was mentally impaired and he was received into guardianship with the specific purpose of controlling access to the niece and other young children.

The effect of the order is described in Chapter 10. The goal is to enable an offender to manage in his own home or hostel. No sanction is available in the event of non-compliance with the order. In the five years from 1983, only eight guardianship orders were made on offenders who had been remanded in prison.

Restriction orders

A restriction order imposes control on both the offender and his RMO (see Chapter 7). In any case, where a hospital order under section 37(2), Mental Health Act 1983 is made, a Crown Court may add a restriction order under Section 41 of the same Act. Magistrates' courts cannot make restriction orders. The decision is for the judge and rests on *the necessity to protect the public from serious harm*. To make a restriction order the Crown Court must hear the *oral evidence of one of the doctors* who recommended the hospital order.

The imposition of restriction orders is based on consideration of the *nature* of the offence, the *antecedents* of the offender, and the *risk of his committing further offences* if at liberty. Restriction orders can be made for a specific period of time, which is very unusual; generally they are unlimited in duration. The latter is known as *"without limit of time"*. The effect of the restriction order is that the patient may not be granted leave of absence or transferred to another hospital without the consent of the Home Secretary. Only the Home Secretary or a mental health review tribunal can discharge a restricted patient (see Chapter 10).

Discharge can be *absolute* or *conditional*. Conditionally discharged patients remain liable to recall to hospital, and are subject to conditions relating to residence and supervision by a doctor and social worker or probation officer. They are monitored by the C3 Department of the Home Office to whom supervisors are required to report regularly. The overriding concern is for public safety (see Chapter 7).

> **Case example 15**
> A young man with schizophrenia killed his father. He had a history of non-compliance with treatment, lacked insight and had often behaved violently in response to his abnormal thoughts and perceptions. He was admitted to a special hospital subject to a hospital order and a restriction order. Six years later he was transferred to a regional secure unit and after 18 months was conditionally discharged to a hostel. Four years later he remains conditionally discharged and subject to psychiatric and social work supervision. Although the restriction order does not sanction his compulsory treatment in the community, the prospect of a recall to hospital ensures that he continues to receive depot neuroleptic medication.

Robertson (1989) has described the restriction order in practice. Up to 1985, between 100 and 120 orders were made each year. The majority of patients were admitted to special hospitals. Since 1986, the numbers have been increasing, and between 150 and 170 restricted hospital orders are now made annually (Home Office, 1994). The numbers admitted to special hospitals have remained relatively constant over the years, but increasing numbers are now admitted to regional secure units. About 65% of restricted patients are diagnosed mentally ill, and the remainder as psychopathic or mentally impaired. Ninety per cent are male, and a similar proportion are convicted of offences of violence. Each year about 50 conditionally discharged patients are recalled to hospital for reasons such as reconviction, non-compliance with treatment, and perceived dangerousness.

Probation order with a condition of treatment

While it is only a minor aspect of its work, the probation service contributes to the network of agencies which provide accommodation, care and treatment for mentally disordered offenders in the community. A probation order can be imposed only if the offender has reached the age of 17 and has agreed to comply with its requirements. The declared purpose of a probation order is to help an offender to strengthen his resources to cope with the problems which led to his offending. The word "breach" is used to describe a failure to comply with the conditions of the probation order.

Courts have the power to include in a probation order any requirements that it considers necessary, and this may include a requirement that the offender should undertake treatment. This can be as an out-patient, day patient or in-patient. If it is the latter, it should be remembered that the admission is a voluntary one. Section 9(3) and Schedule 1A of the Criminal Justice Act 1991 make statutory provision for a probation order with a condition of treatment. This is a probation order adapted to meet the needs of the offender who does not need to be detained in hospital but is suffering from a mental condition which can be treated and needs treatment.

It is important to note that making a probation order requires the consent of the offender. The reporting doctor, who must be approved under Section 12(2), Mental Health Act 1983 (Chapter 10), should confirm that the offender requires treatment for his mental condition but does not need to be detained. The length of treatment, which is usually as an out-patient, may be for part or all of the order's duration. Failure to comply with the treatment can result in the offender being in breach of probation; any sentence for breach will take into account the offence for which the order was initially imposed. In practice, it is rare for people who fail to comply with a treatment condition to be returned to court.

Case example 15

A young woman was charged with her third offence of theft by shoplifting. There was some evidence that the thefts were associated with a breakdown in her marital relationship. With her consent and the agreement of a psychotherapist she was placed on a probation order with a condition of treatment for two years during which period she attended an out-patient psychotherapy group.

The use of probation orders with treatment conditions has declined over the years: there were 2000 in 1973 and only 750 a decade later. In 1983, 78 orders were made on offenders remanded into custody and the equivalent figure for 1988 was ten. These orders are used mainly for substance abusers, non-violent sex offenders and those who can broadly be described as personality disordered.

Addendum for Northern Ireland

By Fred Browne

In Northern Ireland the procedures in relation to unfitness to be tried and the finding of insanity are covered under Articles 49 and 50 of the Mental Health (Northern Ireland) Order 1986. The criteria for being found unfit to plead or unfit to be tried are the same as in England and Wales. The McNaughton rules are obsolete in Northern Ireland and the defence of insanity comes under the Criminal Justice Act (Northern Ireland) 1966, which states that an insane person shall not be convicted. "Insane person" means a person who suffers from mental abnormality which prevents him from (a) appreciating what he is doing; (b) appreciating that what he is doing is either wrong or contrary to law; or (c) controlling his own conduct. The term "mental abnormality" is defined as "an abnormality of mind which arises from a condition of arrested or retarded development of mind or any inherent causes or is induced by disease or injury". When a person is found unfit to be tried or not guilty on the grounds of insanity he is admitted to hospital under an order which has the same effect as a hospital order together with a restriction order made without limitation of time.

The Criminal Justice Act (NI) 1966 also provides for the defence of impaired mental responsibility:

> "Where a person charged with murder has killed or was a party to the killing of another, and it appears to the jury that he was suffering from mental abnormality which substantially impaired his mental responsibility for his acts and omissions in doing or being a party to the killing, the jury shall find him not guilty of murder but shall find him guilty (whether as principal or accessory) of manslaughter".

As in England and Wales the finding of manslaughter permits flexibility in sentencing.

Further details of the criminal law in Northern Ireland are given in Stannard (1984). Boyle & Allen (1983) provide a guide to sentencing law and practice. Psychiatric disposals in Northern Ireland are similar to those in England and Wales, but with some differences in detail – for example, in Northern Ireland a condition of medical treatment attached to a probation order may not exceed 12 months, whereas in England and Wales it may last up to three years.

Addendum for Scotland

By Derek Chiswick

Fitness to plead (also known as insanity in bar of trial), the special defence of insanity and diminished responsibility all apply in Scotland. Their criteria are based on a combination of common and case law. Procedural matters only are governed by the Criminal Procedure (Scotland) Act 1975.

A finding of insanity in bar of trial is returnable under summary and solemn procedure (see Chapter 4). The criteria (see *HMA v Brown,* 1907) are broader than those of England, but in recent years practical application has been based on understanding the charge and proceedings, and giving instructions. The disposal is by mandatory hospital order; in solemn proceedings there is a mandatory restriction order and disposal is to the State Hospital except in special circumstances. The insanity defence depends on the judge's charge to the jury in the case of *HMA v Kidd* (1960). The disposal is the same as for insanity in bar of trial. It is disputed whether or not the plea is possible under summary procedure (Nicholson, 1981). The Criminal Justice (Scotland) Bill now before Parliament contains proposals for a trial of the facts in unfit to plead cases, and for flexible disposals for these and insane acquittal cases.

Diminished responsibility was a Scottish creation in 1867 which results in reduction of murder to culpable homicide. Ironically its interpretation is wider elsewhere than in its country of birth (Walker, 1968). It is governed by case law, currently *HMA v Savage* (1923), and not statute. Psychopathic disorder is excluded from its ambit, as is an absence of intent to murder resulting from voluntary intoxication. Successful pleas are usually accepted pre-trial by the Crown; the few that are contested have a high failure rate. Judges have complete flexibility in sentencing in culpable homicide. Infanticide has never existed in Scotland; it is normally indicted by the Crown as culpable homicide.

Scotland has historical and contemporary interest in automatism. It was the home of one of the earliest trials concerning sleepwalking (*HMA v Simon Fraser,* 1878). For many years Scotland has not recognised automatism simpliciter and all cases have been regarded as insane automatism. However, in a recent case (*Ross v HMA,* 1991) the Scottish Court of Criminal Appeal ruled that the involuntary ingestion of drugs could cause an absence of *mens rea* leading to complete acquittal.

At the post-conviction stage judges have available the complete range of psychiatric disposals described for England (hospital and restriction orders, interim hospital order, guardianship order, and psychiatric probation order). In addition they can defer a case for sentence with almost unlimited conditions, which could include voluntary psychiatric treatment. Treatment by a chartered clinical psychologist, as a condition of probation, is proposed in the Criminal Justice (Scotland) Bill. Offender patients detained in hospital have broadly the same rights of appeal as civil patients.

Addendum for the Republic of Ireland

By Enda Dooley

In the Republic of Ireland the issue of fitness to plead before the courts is still decided on the basis of early 19th century laws. The same stipulations as in the UK apply to the issue of fitness to plead in Ireland. The issue is decided by a jury separate from that which tries the case in question. There is no defence of diminished responsibility currently available under Irish law. In situations where psychiatric disorder is considered relevant, the only psychiatric defence available is that of insanity, based on the McNaughton rules. In raising this defence (which, if successful, leads to a special verdict of "guilty but insane") it is open to the accused to plead that he did not know the nature of the act, did not know that it was wrong, or "was debarred from refraining from committing the damage because of a defect of reason due to his mental illness" (*Doyle v Wicklow County Council* ,1974). A finding of insanity results in detention in the Central Mental Hospital, Dundrum for treatment. A recent Supreme Court decision (*Director of Public Prosecutions v Gallagher,* 1991) has established definitively that decisions regarding discharge lie with the Minister for Justice and not the courts. Due to concern regarding the apparent deficiencies in the present law regarding insanity, which have been highlighted in a number of recent cases (*People [DPP] v Ellis,* 1991; *DPP v Gallagher,* 1991), it is likely that the present legislation will be updated in the near future to include provisions in relation to fitness to plead, insanity, and diminished responsibility.

Under Irish law the crime of infanticide is dealt with under the Infanticide Act 1949. This states that where a woman by any wilful act or omission causes the death of her child under 12 months old, but at the time of the offence it is accepted by the court that her mind was disturbed due to the effects of giving birth, then she should be convicted of infanticide.

There is currently no form of hospital order available under Irish law where, following conviction, a psychiatrically disturbed person may be committed to hospital for treatment. The only way to provide access to hospital following appearance in court is to arrange for the charge to be dropped (if the offence is relatively minor and this course is agreeable to the arresting police officer and the court) and to arrange for subsequent admission to psychiatric hospital for treatment. It is hoped that a review of civil mental health legislation currently being undertaken by the Department of Health (see Chapter 10) will include provisions for the diversion to hospital of mentally disordered persons appearing before the courts.

Law reports

Bratty v Attorney General for Northern Ireland (1963) AC 386
Director of Public Prosecutions v Beard (1920) AC 479
Director of Public Prosecutions v Gallagher (1991) ILRM 339.
Doyle v Wicklow County Council (1974) IR 55.
HMA v Brown (1907) Session Cases (Justiciary) 67.
HMA v Simon Fraser (1878) Couper 78.
HMA v Kidd (1960) Justiciary Cases 61.
HMA v Savage (1923) Session Cases (Justiciary) 49.
People (DPP) v Ellis (1991) ILRM 225.
R v Burgess (1991) 2 WLR 120
R v Byrne (1960) 44 Cr App R 246
R v Kemp (1957) 1 QB 339
R v Lloyd (1966) 2 WLR 13
R v McNaughton (1843) 4 St T 847
R v Podola (1960) 1 QB 325
R v Pritchard (1836) 7 C & P 303
R v Sullivan (1984) AC 156
Ross v HMA (1991) Scots Law Times 564.

References

Archbold (1985) *Pleading, Evidence and Practice in Criminal Cases* (eds S. Mitchell, P. Richardson & J. Huxley Buzard). London: Sweet & Maxwell.
Bluglass, R. (1978) Infanticide. *Bulletin of the Royal College of Psychiatrists*, 139–141.
—— (1983) *A Guide to the Mental Health Act 1983*. Edinburgh: Churchill Livingstone.
Boyle, C. K. & Allen, M. J. (1983) *Sentencing Law and Practice in Northern Ireland*. Belfast: SLS Legal Publications.
Chiswick, D. (1990) Fitness to stand trial and plead, mutism and deafness. In *Principles and Practice of Forensic Psychiatry* (eds R. Bluglass & P. Bowden), pp. 171–177. Edinburgh: Churchill Livingstone.

Dell, S. (1984) *Murder into Manslaughter.* Oxford: Oxford University Press.

Department of Health & Welsh Office (1993) *Code of Practice.* London: HMSO.

D'Orban, P. (1979) Women who kill their children. *British Journal of Psychiatry,* **134**, 560–571.

Elliott, D. & Wood, J. (1974) *A Casebook of Criminal Law.* London: Sweet & Maxwell.

Fenwick, P. (1990) Automatism. In *Principles and Practice of Forensic Psychiatry* (eds. R. Bluglass & P. Bowden). London: Churchill Livingstone.

Grubin, D. (1991) Regaining fitness: patients found unfit to plead who return for trial. *Journal of Forensic Psychiatry,* **2**, 139–152.

Hamilton, J. (1990) Manslaughter: assessment for court. In *Principles and Practice of Forensic Psychiatry* (eds. R. Bluglass & P. Bowden). London: Churchill Livingstone.

Home Office (1986) *The Sentence of the Court.* London: HMSO.

—— (1989) *Criminal Statistics in England and Wales 1988.* Cmnd 847. London: HMSO.

—— (1990) *Provision for Mentally Disordered Offenders.* London: HMSO.

—— (1994) *Statistics of Mentally Disordered Offenders, England and Wales 1992.* Home Office Statistical Bulletin. London: HMSO.

—— & Department of Health and Social Security (1975) *Report of the Committee on Mentally Abnormal Offenders.* Cmnd. 6244. London: HMSO.

Joseph, P. (1990) Insanity and fitness to stand trial. *Journal of Forensic Psychiatry,* **1**, 277–304.

Kellam, A. (1992) The Criminal Procedure (Insanity and Unfitness to Plead) Act 1991. *Psychiatric Bulletin,* **16**, 201–202.

Mackay, R. (1990) Insanity and fitness to stand trial. *Journal of Forensic Psychiatry,* **1**, 277–304.

Morris, T. & Blom-Cooper, L. (1964) *A Calendar of Murder.* London: Joseph.

Nicholson, C. G. B. (1981) *The Law and Practice of Sentencing in Scotland.* Edinburgh: Green.

Robertson, G. (1989) The restricted hospital order. *Psychiatric Bulletin,* 4–11.

Rosen, B. (1981) Suicide pacts: a review. *Psychological Medicine,* **11**, 525–533.

Schipkowenski, N. (1973) *Epidemiological Aspects of Homicide.* World Biennial of Psychiatry and Psychotherapy (ed. S. Arieti). New York: Basic Books.

Stannard, J. E. (1984) *Northern Ireland Supplement to Smith and Hogan, Criminal Law.* Belfast: SLS Legal Publications.

Walker, N. (1968) *Crime and Insanity in England, I. The Historical Perspective.* Edinburgh: Edinburgh University Press.

West, D. (1965) *Murder Followed by Suicide.* London: Heinemann.

—— & Walk, A. (1977) *Daniel McNaughton.* London: Gaskell.

6 Writing reports and giving evidence

Robert Bluglass

Structure of the report • Reports in criminal proceedings • Reports in civil proceedings • Appendices

---

Court reports display one aspect of the public face of psychiatry. A well crafted report demonstrates objectivity, detachment, humanity and professionalism. A carelessly constructed report reveals much about the author, does little for the patient, and does less for the credibility and image of the profession of psychiatry. Although initially psychiatrists may find an encounter with the legal process daunting, and even intimidating, for the patient it may be crucial. The role of the doctor in providing a medicolegal opinion on the patient's behalf can be just as important as a diagnostic decision or treatment recommendation.

Psychiatrists are increasingly requested to provide a report in connection with the legal process (see Table 6.1), and few will avoid doing so on occasion during a career. Many psychiatrists, from all specialities, find that report-writing eventually forms an important part of their professional work. In this chapter, reference is made to the law in England and Wales, but the principles of report-writing are of universal application.

Structure of the report

The report should always be based upon a comprehensive assessment. It is important to have clear instructions about the issues in question and to understand the problems before conducting the interview. The approach to the case and the report will depend upon the purpose for which it is requested, which must be kept in mind throughout the assessment.

The subject of the report will not usually be in a therapeutic relationship with the reporting doctor and he will not have been referred by another medical practitioner. As several authors have pointed out (e.g. Chiswick, 1985), in these circumstances the subject of assessment finds himself in unfamiliar circumstances; he is in the position of client rather than patient. Confidentiality will almost certainly not apply as the report will inevitably pass to a third party, such as a lawyer, and it will often be seen by many others. It is important, therefore, that the purpose of the interview on which the report will be based is clearly understood from the outset and that the patient/client is reminded who requested the examination (his lawyer or

Table 6.1 Psychiatric reports: source of request and matter under consideration

Requests made by:	Matter under consideration:
Court (youth, magistrates', Crown or appeal) or solicitor	Criminal proceedings
Solicitors or (rarely) courts	Civil proceedings (e.g. compensation for mental injury, child custody or access dispute, divorce, contested will, capacity to manage affairs)
Mental health review tribunals, solicitors, hospital managers	Applications for discharge from hospital
Home Office	Treatment of restricted patients, transfer of prisoners to hospital, review of long-term prisoners
Special Hospitals Service Authority	Admission and discharge of special hospital patients
Parole boards and discretionary lifer panels	Early release from prison
Prison medical officers, other consultants, probation officers and social workers	Management and dangerousness
Driver and Vehicle Licensing Agency	Fitness to hold a driving licence
Health authority (or trust), medical defence organisation or solicitor	Allegation of medical negligence
Professional body (e.g. General Medical Council)	Professional competence (and perhaps mental health) of a psychiatrist, or mental health of any doctor
Employing authority	Mental health of employee and fitness for employment, or for a particular task

the other side). In civil proceedings the individual may have been referred to a variety of specialists and may well not know why he is seeing yet another one. It is always important for the doctor to introduce himself, explain his position, the nature of his specialty, ensure that the purpose of the interview is understood and that the subject recognises that the information he imparts will be included in the report. He should have the opportunity of giving or refusing consent to be interviewed once the explanation has been given. If he chooses not to proceed, his right to do so should be accepted. Ethical aspects of confidentiality are discussed in Chapter 12.

In preparing a report it is important to remember that the psychiatrist is addressing a lay recipient (when this is the case) such as a court, judge or lawyer, or professionals from other specialities. This is often forgotten and many reports are peppered with complex jargon familiar to colleagues, but misunderstood or perceived as nonsense by others. All information can be imparted or explained in clear and understandable language.

Reports in criminal proceedings

A report may be requested on behalf of the prosecuting authorities by the Crown Prosecution Service (see Chapter 4), the Clerk of a court, the Probation Service on behalf of the prosecution, or, more rarely, by the police. For individuals remanded in custody the request will usually be to the prison medical officer who will be responsible for preparing the report himself, or he will pass it to a visiting psychiatrist. In bailed cases the request will be made to a psychiatrist directly, although sometimes the Crown Prosecution Service consults the prison medical authorities, and in some cases prison medical officers assess individuals on bail. More rarely a judge or magistrate will initiate the request.

Defence solicitors are entitled to obtain an independent psychiatric opinion on behalf of their clients and will make the request directly to a psychiatrist of their choice. In controversial cases, or if the defence has doubts about the authority or opinion presented in the report, a second opinion may be obtained.

Background information

It is important to ensure that comprehensive information is provided by those requesting a report as early as possible in the investigation and, as further sources of information are identified, that other papers and reports are requested. For Crown Court cases this will include all the papers which form the basis of the case for the prosecution, once the accused has been committed for trial by a magistrates' court. These will comprise:

(1) A letter of request for a report briefly summarising the background to the case.
(2) Formal documents specifying the charge(s).
(3) Typed statements of witnesses taken at police interview.

(4) Typed records of interviews between the investigating police officers and the accused. These are now usually transcripts taken from taped recordings, but are frequently edited and are then not complete. For this reason, they may sometimes be unreliable.
(5) Signed statement(s) made by the accused if one has been made.
(6) Copies of documents to be submitted as exhibits, such as room plans, birth certificate, school reports, cash receipts, letters or medical records.
(7) Record of previous offences, prosecutions and their outcome.
(8) A recent pre-sentence report and sometimes copies of previous reports.
(9) Possibly photographs of the scene of the crime.
(10) Sometimes a copy of the investigating officer's summary of the investigation. This is essential for a full understanding of the case, even though much of the content may be irrelevant to the psychiatric assessment. It may include important observations by witnesses which describe the mood or behaviour of the accused prior to, or at the time of, the alleged offence. These independent comments can be helpful in attempting to reconstruct the state of mind of the accused at the material time.
(11) Often, tape recordings of interviews by the police with the accused. In serious cases the psychiatrist may be given as many as ten or more such tapes and time must be found to listen to them.
(12) Rarely, video tapes which may be a visual record of the police interrogation, or of the scene of the crime.

A request from defence solicitors will usually be accompanied by similar material, sometimes with copies of reports from psychiatrists instructed by the prosecution and other reports obtained by the defence.

Requests to assist proceedings in magistrates' courts will usually be supported by more limited information, and practices vary from one court to another. At best, there may be details of the charge, a summary of the circumstances and background and probation reports. If the psychiatrist considers that information is lacking he should insist that more is provided by the solicitor, probation officer or court office, before completing the assessment. Where typed witness statements are available they should be provided.

As the psychiatric investigation progresses, the psychiatrist will often be made aware of other sources of information that can be helpful (e.g. hospital records, previous psychiatric reports, school reports, work records, probation reports and social services reports).

Interviewing the defendant

The psychiatrist can expect (but will not always receive) reasonable time to gather information, carry out interviews and any necessary investigations before submitting a considered report. When the accused is remanded in custody the prison hospital should be contacted to check the periods during which he is available for interview. There is a need to fit in with staff shifts and meal times. Many prisons are becoming more flexible in their arrangements. Several visits may be necessary to complete the assessment.

When the accused is on bail he can be seen at an out-patient clinic; sufficient time must be provided for a relaxed and extensive interview. It is good practice to request that close relatives, or friends who know the defendant well, also attend so that they can be interviewed independently.

The interview

Whether the defendant is in custody or on bail it is very rarely necessary to have a protective escort present for the interview. It is always preferable to see the person alone, although it is a wise precaution to know how to obtain assistance should it be required. The interview should otherwise be conducted as for any other patient.

Forensic patients presenting for assessment may be coping with not only with the problems engendered by a psychiatric illness, but also apprehension about a forthcoming trial, compounded perhaps by guilt, or even grief, if they have been responsible for an offence. The person should be put at ease and treated courteously. He or she is entitled to be addressed according to his or her choice.

At the outset the psychiatrist should check the defendant's correct name and other personal details. Particularly in a busy remand prison it is not uncommon for the wrong prisoner to be produced for interview. The psychiatrist should introduce himself and establish the basis of the interview with the accused, who will often wrongly presume that the encounter is on a confidential basis.

> "I am Dr — and I have been asked by the prosecution to interview you to provide a report. I would like you to understand that what you tell me will be used in my report which will be seen by other people. This interview is not confidential as it normally is when you go to see your own doctor. Do you understand?"

If the report is requested by the defendant's solicitor, it should be explained that it may be passed to others.

The interview then proceeds in the way that seems most appropriate for the individual person and the circumstances of the case. Many defendants will wish to talk about the circumstances of the offence, which is clearly their prime concern, at the earliest opportunity. A psychiatric interview is usually the first opportunity for them to talk to a sympathetic and understanding listener. For others, the psychiatrist will gain a better understanding by first taking a personal history, allowing the offence to be placed in the context of a chronological narrative.

The interview should be comprehensive and may require more than one session. It should include the features of the standard psychiatric interview: a developmental history from infancy, through childhood and adolescence; family background and environment; school performance; further education; family relationships; sexual history; employment history; marital history and relationships; drinking patterns; substance abuse; history of offending; medical and psychiatric history; and any family history of illness or offending behaviour. The defendant should be invited to provide his account of his involvement in the alleged offence in the way that he chooses to give it.

The psychiatrist should note the person's appearance, demeanour, behaviour and changes of mood throughout the interview, recording evidence of hostility, anger, resentment, depression, or signs of psychotic behaviour, impulsivity, irritability or inappropriate behaviour or use of language, and cognitive functioning.

A physical examination should be performed if it is indicated. Other clinical investigations may be necessary such as an electroencephalogram (EEG), neurological assessment, psychological investigation, x-rays, a computerised axial tomography (CAT) scan, biochemical tests or chromosome analysis. These may have to be arranged with the cooperation of the prison medical officer or hospital departments. If investigations will take time, a further period of remand may have to be requested, but if the authorities insist on proceeding before the psychiatrist is ready he should make it clear that the value of any report is qualified.

Occasionally the defendant will refuse to be interviewed or will fail to attend, and this must be reported. The psychiatrist should not give an opinion on the papers alone. A defendant on bail may be remanded in custody for non-attendance to provide a further opportunity for interview.

Purpose of the report

Frequently the request is simply for "a psychiatric report" but sometimes the psychiatrist is asked to give an opinion on a specific matter. In most cases the issues shown in Box 6.1 should be addressed.

The report

The psychiatrist should always remember that the report is written to assist laymen who are not trained in medicine or psychiatry. Although experienced lawyers often learn to interpret complex reports remarkably well, terms that are familiar to the psychiatrist are easily misunderstood or misinterpreted and no assumptions should be made. The report should always be written in standard English and should be jargon-free. If it is

---

Box 6.1 Psychiatric issues in reports for the criminal courts

Fitness to plead
Fitness to stand trial
Mental state at the time of the alleged offence
Any psychiatric factors that might assist in understanding or
    explaining behaviour, or have a bearing on forming an intent,
    or on criminal responsibility
Mental state at the time of examination
Recommendations for disposal or treatment
Prognosis where this seems relevant

---

essential to use a technical word such as schizophrenia, epilepsy, or affective disorder, then its meaning should always be given, in parenthesis, in simple English. The author should not write anything that he would regret were it to be quoted to him in court. It is important to exercise caution in reporting as fact what the accused says. While it seems reasonable to write "he was an only child raised by his parents in Warcester" (if that is what the person says), it would be unwise to state as fact "his wife is irresponsible in handling money", unless this is verifiable from independent sources. Psychiatric reports therefore make frequent use of phrases such as "he says that . . ." or "he reports that . . ." or "he describes his wife as . . ."

Before compiling the report it is essential that the psychiatrist is confident that he understands the legal issues that may be relevant in the particular case, such as fitness to plead, diminished responsibility, or the criteria for recommending a hospital order disposal (see Chapter 5). Vagueness, inaccuracies or omissions on these crucial matters cause confusion. The form of the report is to some extent a matter of individual style and preference, but the following format is suggested and encompasses the important headings which should be used as a basis for the report (see Box 6.2). A sample report is provided in Appendix I. Fact should be clearly separated from opinion. The following is a summary of the information that should be contained in the report.

(1) Name and charge or indictment.
(2) A brief introduction indicating on whose behalf the report is prepared, where the interview took place, dates of interviews and who else was interviewed (together or separately).
(3) A list of documents received and studied.
(4) Full name, age and recent occupation of the accused.
(5) A brief statement indicating whether the accused understood the nature of the charge against him and its possible implications.

(6) Personal history: childhood (including emotional and physical development in infancy, childhood and adolescence), family environment and structure, schools attended and educational performance, behaviour, hobbies and interests. Employment record and performance, sexual and marital history, interests and activities.

(7) Dependency on alcohol or other substances.

(8) Medical and psychiatric history (including details of hospitalisations and out-patient referrals).

(9) Family history of relevance (including psychiatric history).

(10) History of offending behaviour (if any).

(11) The present offence: the accused's account of the circumstances, of his state of mind at the time and his explanation for his behaviour.

(12) Findings on examination. This should include a description of the accused's state and behaviour at the time of interview; features suggestive of mental illness, such as his descriptions of delusional beliefs or of experiencing hallucinations, of depressed mood or of bizarre or inappropriate activity. The report should be structured indicating the presence or significant absence of the standard elements of mental state examination. The psychiatrist should also describe any significant features of the defendant's personality and intellectual functioning.

(13) Reports of any interviews with close relatives or partners.

(14) Discussion. This may not always be necessary, but in complex cases it may be helpful to explain the relevance of findings in this section.

(15) *Opinion.* The lawyers will find this the most important part of the report and it is helpful to the reader to deal with the opinion in stages. Remember that opinions should be supported by material in the body of the report.

    (a) Fitness to plead. Although this is rarely at issue, it is a useful discipline to mention it to indicate that it has been considered.

    (b) Conclusions regarding the defendant's mental state at the time of the offence with appropriate supporting references to the body of the report, to other papers and to interviews with relatives.

    (c) Any appropriate comments if psychiatric factors have affected the ability to form an intent. This is particularly important in cases of murder, manslaughter, automatism, provocation, where the misuse of alcohol or drugs is in question, and when the defendant is assessed as severely mentally impaired.

    (d) An opinion as to the presence and nature or absence of mental illness or other disorder at the present time with supporting evidence.

    (e) Recommendations as to the need for treatment and whether or not this should be on a compulsory basis in hospital (and if so whether in a secure hospital), or as an out-patient as a

---

Box 6.2 Psychiatric report in a criminal case

Name of defendant and charge
Introduction
- at whose request? Place and date(s) of examination? For how long?
- documents studied, other information obtained, other informants interviewed
- description of defendant: age, occupational and social situation, and capacity to understand purpose of interview

Personal history
- developmental, educational and social history; family relationships; psychosexual and marital history; hobbies, interests and activities; use of alcohol, drugs or illicit substances

Medical and psychiatric history
- all previous contacts with medical and psychiatric services

Family history
- medical, psychiatric or other relevant factors

Previous offending behaviour
- nature and court disposals

Present offence(s)
- defendant's own account of his actions and state of mind at time of offence(s)

Findings on clinical examination
- the salient features (positive and negative) of the examination upon which your opinions will be based

Information from other sources
- relevant information summarised from other documents or from informants

Discussion
- required only in cases of unusual complexity

Opinion
- the most important section for the reader; opinion concerning particular issues of relevance; must be supported by findings in body of report; treatment recommendations (if any) should be clear and unambiguous

Mental Health Act approval status
Name, qualifications, designation, signature and date

---

requirement of a probation order, or in any other circumstances.
(f) An opinion may be given about the medical prognosis and the risk to others of dangerous behaviour in the future.
(g) If a hospital order is recommended, an opinion should also be given as to the need for a restriction order (with or without a time limit). Arrangements should have been made for admission

to a named hospital and the report should specify whether a bed is immediately available. It is bad practice to make a recommendation for a hospital order without finding a bed, although there are sometimes circumstances which might make this necessary (e.g. a grave shortage of beds).

(h) Any other comments.

(16) The author should state whether he is approved by the Secretary of State for the purposes of Section 12(2) of the Mental Health Act 1983.

(17) The qualifications and principal appointment should follow the signature and name of the author.

(18) The date of the report.

Psychiatric reports provided in jurisdictions other than England and Wales are prepared on the same principles described above, but there are important differences in legislation and procedure. In Scotland, for example, depositions by the prosecution do not exist by that term. Psychiatrists preparing reports do not normally have sight of the statements, or precognitions, of Crown witnesses. It is advisable to ask the procurator fiscal for necessary information and to indicate if the report is based solely on information provided by the defendant. It is also customary in Scotland to include a statement that a report is given "on soul and conscience" (i.e. that it is a true report).

The use of psychiatric reports to court

Psychiatric reports in Crown Courts are used to provide advice about disposal and in mitigation after a plea of guilty (Mackay, 986). Reports are requested on about 5% of cases committed for trial and the majority originate as a result of requests from solicitors. Evidence is offered in mitigation in the hope that it will reduce the punishment imposed on a convicted person. Only mitigating factors of a psychiatric nature should be addressed in a report, for example, the stress caused by a recent bereavement. In practice, many psychiatrists seem to stray from their remit in relation to mitigating factors.

A report for the defence becomes the property of the solicitor who may decide not to use it if in his view it is not helpful to his client. Psychiatrists may feel wounded by the thought that their hard work has ended up on file or in the waste paper basket; however, our system of justice is adversarial and partisan and the lawyers have little interest in the doctor's conflicting wish to be independent, objective and detached from the contest.

The defence is not obliged to reveal the psychiatric report unless it is to be used. The Crown, on the other hand, must reveal reports they commission to the defence. It is now good practice for psychiatrists to discuss their findings with each other, although some defence solicitors will wish to give their endorsement first.

The destiny of psychiatric reports

It should be remembered that although requested originally by one agency, the psychiatric report may have a long life. It will be included in case records and becomes an important reference against which to assess future progress. It may also be useful in future legal proceedings. It may be requested by others, be copied, and be passed between lawyers, prison or probation authorities. It can be an important document even years later in the event of an appeal or a review of a long-term prisoner or patient. It is therefore all the more important to be comprehensive, crystal-clear and non-judgmental. The report may be valuable in future research (e.g. Dell's (1984) review of diminished responsibility cases). If a copy of a report is requested, the permission of the author and, where appropriate, the patient or his agent should be obtained if it is possible to do so.

Giving evidence in criminal proceedings

The majority of psychiatric reports prepared for court proceedings are not followed by a request to give oral evidence; the report is used by the lawyers and judge without a need for challenge or clarification. The judiciary invariably take careful note of psychiatric reports and are prepared to act without hesitation on definite medical recommendations.

The psychiatrist will be requested to be further involved in the following instances:

(1) If the report is unclear, ambiguous, or equivocal and clarification is needed.
(2) If the court finds it difficult to accept the opinion and requires persuasion.
(3) If the court has several reports with conflicting opinions, each of which needs to be evaluated.
(4) In specific cases where oral evidence is sometimes requested or may be obligatory, for example:
    (a) in support of a defence of diminished responsibility
    (b) in infanticide cases
    (c) where a restriction order is under consideration
    (d) when a probation order with a requirement of psychiatric treatment is under consideration
    (e) when a court is evaluating the future risk to the public
    (f) in consideration of fitness to plead.

In criminal proceedings the trial date is fixed in advance, and although most courts and solicitors will try to accommodate psychiatric witnesses, there is less flexibility than in the civil courts.

The psychiatrist is involved as an expert witness rather than as a witness to fact, or as a professional witness (when the accused may have been his patient). He is there because of the expertise he can provide to assist the court in understanding matters which are outside the court's competence or experience (in practice, to comment on abnormality rather than normal behaviour, which the court and jury are assumed to understand). He must understand from the outset that his involvement, initially to provide a report, may result in a request to give oral evidence, and he should not resent it as an intrusion on his time or be intimidated by the prospect.

In advance, the psychiatrist may be requested to attend a conference in chambers with the barrister ('counsel') who is acting as advocate in court and the solicitor for the Crown Prosecution Service, or the defence, as the case may be. In major cases the case will be taken by a senior barrister, a Queen's Counsel (or "silk" because he wears a silk gown in court), who will often be accompanied by a junior barrister. Other experts for the side may also be present. The term 'chambers' refers to the barristers' offices, usually in one of the Inns of Court in London or in similar premises in the provinces. The conference reviews the issues in the case and assists the advocates in understanding the points made in the expert's report.

The Crown Prosecution Service or solicitor will usually notify the expert of the date of trial and whether or not he will be required throughout the hearing or only to give his evidence. The attendance of witnesses can be assured by serving upon them in person a witness summons ('subpoena') which means that the expert will be in contempt of court and liable to a penalty for non-attendance. Alternatively, a judge can issue a bench warrant summoning attendance. These steps are unusual because expert witnesses are professionals who know the importance of attending court, as agreed, and they may reasonably resent their legal colleagues doubting their integrity. However, some lawyers rarely deal with experts or believe that they are being helpful in assisting the doctor in obtaining release from other duties in hospital (and this may be so) by serving a summons.

Attendance at court

The psychiatrist should prepare in advance for his attendance at court by reviewing the papers and re-reading his report. He should consult any appropriate references or legal authorities and try to anticipate any issues that may arise. He will be required to substantiate the opinions that he has given in his report when confronted with them in court.

He should try to present himself in a smart, confident and professional way, dressing appropriately and arriving in good time. If the court is a considerable distance from base it may be wise to spend the night before in a local hotel rather than rely on a train or a long, early drive. At Crown Courts the judge will usually sit at 10.00 or 10.30 am, break for an hour for lunch at 1.00 pm and rise at 4.00 or 4.30 pm.

Counsel may request a conference in a room in the court building to review last minute issues before the court sits. It is usually wise to have a brief interview with the accused in the cells below the court beforehand, particularly if he has not been seen for some time. This will be necessary if the issue is fitness to plead, as the decision is determined on the accused's mental state at the time of his court appearance.

At court, as an expert, the psychiatrist is entitled to expect to be present in court to hear witnesses if he wishes, as the evidence that he hears may affect his opinion (the reason why witnesses as to fact are excluded). Indeed, he may subsequently be asked if he has listened to a witness, particularly another doctor. He should request a seat in the well of the court rather than accept exclusion.

Court proceedings

Crown Court proceedings are held before a judge of the High Court (addressed as "My Lord" or "My Lady"), or a local judge ("Your Honour"). Magistrates' courts are presided over by three lay magistrates or a single stipendiary (paid) magistrate (all addressed as Sir or Madam).

When the presiding judge or magistrate enters the court, all those present stand and the judge bows to the court. The Clerk will then call the defendant who enters the dock and the charge or indictment is read out. In jury trials, a jury is then called and sworn; a defence lawyer may raise an objection to a potential juror.

The lawyer representing the Crown will outline the background of the case against the accused and proceed to call witnesses. They are examined by way of questions, cross-examined by the defence, then re-examined by the Crown. When the case for the Crown is completed, the Defence will proceed in a similar manner, with the Crown counsel cross-examining.

In the witness box

When the doctor is called to give evidence he should walk calmly to the witness box where he will be required to take the oath by swearing on the Bible (or other religious book) to tell the truth (or he may choose to affirm without a religious book). He will then be questioned by the barrister or solicitor who called him, be cross-examined and re-examined. When there is a difference in medical opinion between the two sides the doctor for the prosecution side may be called out of sequence, after the defence doctor, in 'rebuttal' (to say why he takes a different view to the defence).

For the inexperienced, an appearance in the witness box can seem a frightening ordeal. In ordinary medical practice the doctor is not used to having his opinion challenged, or to explain or justify what he has written in the way that is customary in court, where cross-examination can feel threatening, hostile or even offensive. Judges should (and usually do) protect witnesses from unacceptable bullying or from counsel who insist on "yes/no" answers and prevent the witness from explaining himself, but there are unfortunate exceptions.

In the witness box the psychiatrist may have his notes and papers in front of him and will be allowed to refer to them (it is perhaps polite to ask the judge formally if he may do so); he is not expected to remember every detail of the case or his examination. He must restrict himself to giving his opinion within the rules of evidence (see May, 1990) although it is for the lawyers to ensure that this is so.

The expert should speak up clearly and audibly so that he can be heard by the jury, lawyers and the bench. It is best to speak more slowly than one would in normal conversation. The witness should try to appear confident and remember that he is the expert and knows more about the technical issues than the non-psychiatrists present. During his evidence the judge or clerk will be making notes; he should keep an eye on the judge's pen, pausing from time to time to give the judge time to allow his evidence to be written down.

It is important for the expert to stick to his own opinion. But he should be prepared to accept an argument that convinces him to move in another direction and, admit the possibility that he can be wrong if that seems appropriate. However, he should sustain his opinion where he feels that the evidence justifies it. It is the barrister's job to 'test' the quality of his opinion if it differs from that of a colleague; convincing answers will add weight to his conclusions.

After giving evidence the expert may be asked to remain at the trial to hear other witnesses or to advise lawyers in the interpretation of the evidence of others.

As experience is gained, many psychiatrists become increasingly expert in giving evidence and as a result are a valuable asset to the criminal justice system. Many psychiatrists eventually enjoy the process, but should then try to avoid becoming a 'performer' or pseudo-advocate, or to become known as a professional defence or prosecution expert.

Reports in civil proceedings

Claims for compensation for personal injury or loss

Most psychiatric reports in civil courts relate to claims following accidents at work or road accidents associated with physical injury. A recent analysis of the files of one insurance company (Cornes & Aitken, 1992) indicates that 14% of claims were related to deaths and 45% were connected with severe or serious injuries. Orthopaedic surgeons are most frequently requested to provide reports but, increasingly for these cases, a psychiatric report is also requested to advise upon the element of claim made for psychological trauma or injury, mental illness, personality change or post-traumatic stress disorder which is said to have resulted from the injury.

The parties involved in civil claims are referred to as the plaintiff and defendant. The plaintiff is the claimant in an action in which damages are claimed on the basis of liability on the part of an employer or some other person or institution. Liability means that the defendant has a responsibility for health or safety of his employees (or for persons to whom a service is provided, or whose premises are used). In road accidents the defendant is the driver of another vehicle, an insurance company, or other liable individual.

Those claiming injury may be disabled to a variable degree and for varying lengths of time. Their livelihood, quality of life, family or marital relationships may suffer. If injury is successfully demonstrated, a financial settlement will often have a significant effect on future life.

Reports are requested on behalf of the plaintiff or defendant and by their solicitor in writing. Most claims (90%) are ultimately settled between the lawyers on behalf of the parties, but only after a long period of time since the accident, often years. Court hearings are expensive, and lawyers will seek to avoid their client having to bear these costs.

Psychiatrists are particularly involved in cases of head injury because of the increased likelihood of psychiatric symptoms such as depression, anxiety or brain damage.

Background information

As in criminal proceedings, it is essential to have full information and this is usually provided. The papers will include:

(1) A letter requesting a report from the referring solicitor with a full summary of the circumstances of the case.
(2) Sometimes a verbatim account of the accident and its consequences for him as given by the plaintiff to his solicitor.
(3) Hospital and consultant reports, representing other specialities, general practitioner records and reports.
(4) Expert reports obtained from other specialists.
(5) Defendants sometimes include covert video recordings obtained by private investigators, attempting to demonstrate that disability is less than claimed.

If any information is missing it should be requested.

Interviewing the plaintiff

The plaintiff can be seen at the out-patient clinic or rooms and it is usually essential for a close relative or friend to attend, who can give an independent account of the person's previous personality and demeanour and the extent of any change since the accident. This information, together with evidence of previous symptoms gained from the general practitioner or hospital records, will be very important in the assessment.

At the beginning of the interview the personal details of the client should be checked with him. This is important information, but also allows a period of time for the person to relax and accustom himself to the situation. The psychiatrist should make plain the basis of the interview, including on whose behalf he is carrying out the assessment, and it should be made clear that the report will go to the lawyer concerned and may then be passed elsewhere. Even though the interview may have been requested by the "other side", it should be made clear that the doctor is providing his independent expert view which will not favour one side or the other.

The interview will then proceed in the usual way, the psychiatrist noting the way in which the person relates to him, his mood, attitude, demeanour and evidence of any abnormal behaviour or symptoms.

The interview should always be comprehensive and include the usual features: a developmental history through infancy, childhood and adolescence; family background and environment; school performance; further education; sexual history; marital history; family history; employment history; drinking pattern; history of substance abuse; previous medical and psychiatric history; previous accidents and claims for personal injury; and the plaintiff's recollections of the circumstances of the accident. He should describe his subsequent physical and mental disabilities, treatment and progress. He must describe his state of mind, prevailing mood, and complaints at the present time.

Purpose of the report

In such cases the purpose of a psychiatric report is:

(1) to assist the parties in establishing what mental damage has been sustained and whether the defendant is liable
(2) to assist the parties to decide on 'quantum' or the amount of damages appropriate in the case, to compensate for the direct mental consequences of the accident and the indirect consequences, including the effects on employment, family life, the need for nursing care or medical treatment and future earning potential
(3) to provide a prognosis and estimate the likelihood of improvement or recovery
(4) to indicate any need for treatment and recommend what form it should take.

The report

As for other reports, the recipients will be laymen, although as legal specialists in compensation claims they are often well versed in medical technicalities. It is best to assume no specialised knowledge on the part of the reader, but to explain carefully any technical terminology. Fact and opinion should be clearly differentiated in the report. A sample report is provided in Appendix II.

The general structure of the report should be as follows:

(1) Heading indicating the names of the parties in the action for damages, for example, "Mrs Helen Smith v Midland and Stratford Railway Company".

(2) An introduction indicating who was examined, when, where, how often, for how long and who else was independently interviewed (e.g. accompanying relative).

(3) A list of documents received and studied, (name and status of author for each report, and the date it was prepared). Sometimes lawyers will request removal of this paragraph if they do not wish to reveal the existence of certain documents when the report is passed to others.

(4) Full name, age and recent occupation of subject.

(5) A brief statement indicating that the person understood the basis of the interview and that a report would be sent to the commissioning lawyer (i.e. that the person consents to the interview with understanding).

(6) Personal history from childhood, including emotional and physical development in infancy, childhood and adolescence, family environment, background and structure, schools attended, educational performance, behaviour, hobbies and interests, employment record and performance, sexual and marital history, current interests, activities and hobbies.

(7) Dependency on alcohol or substance abuse.

(8) Previous medical and psychiatric history with details of accidents, hospitalisation, out-patient treatment, general practitioner history.

(9) Relevant family history.

(10) The plaintiff's own account of the accident, injury or loss suffered.

(11) Immediate consequences; physical and mental.

(12) Longer term consequences.

(13) Any treatment received.

(14) Present complaints.

(15) Findings on examination, including any specialised tests (EEG, biochemistry, neurology).

(16) *Opinion*
    (a) Description/summary of previous personality, relevant history, stability prior to the incident.
    (b) Consistency between accident, complaints and findings.
    (c) Cause of any psychiatric condition found.
    (d) Prognosis for disability or handicap.
    (e) Need for further treatment or rehabilitation.
    (f) Any other pertinent comments.

(17) The report should end with the author's signature, name, qualifications and appointment, and the date.

The lawyers may find it helpful to be provided with a separate sheet providing more details of the consultant's qualifications, appointments, experience and standing to establish his credentials as an expert. This is occasionally required in the report itself.

Paul (1981) provided a useful checklist of guidance to consultants on the essential 28 points that should be covered in a compensation report. Analysis of 602 reports by Cornes & Aitken (1992) indicated that some topics are generally poorly covered or omitted. They include no mention of consent, age, occupation, family circumstances or social history in many reports. Psychiatrists were especially bad in this respect. The analysis noted that recurrent themes in requests for compensation reports from psychiatrists were for advice regarding cognitive deficits, behavioural problems, traumatic neurosis and "functional overlay" (the rather dismissive generalised term used by non-psychiatric doctors to indicate the presence of emotional factors).

Civil reports on specific issues

Mental health and professional competence

Doctors: Reports are requested from the Registrar of the General Medical Council, usually following the criminal conviction of a medical practitioner or a complaint against him. Most reports are requested to assist the Health Committee to decide whether the doctor's health is such that he is unfit to practise, or that he should only be allowed to practise to a restricted extent, or with conditions that he receives treatment or supervision. Most cases relate to dependency on alcohol or drugs, but some to psychiatric illness.

The report should provide a full medical, psychiatric and social assessment after interviews with the practitioner, independent interviews with relatives and consultation with other doctors who have provided treatment or supervision. The General Medical Council will require the results of blood and urine tests where this is appropriate, in drug or alcohol cases. Some cases are concerned with sexual behaviour, violence or unacceptable behaviour towards patients or staff, which may result from psychiatric abnormality.

The report should give an opinion upon the doctor's mental health and his ability to practise, with a comment on any qualifications or restrictions that should be applied, for instance, regarding access to controlled drugs and authority to write prescriptions. The report should discuss any need for treatment and the prognosis. The report must take into account the need to protect the public and others. Reports are shown to the doctor. He is entitled to a report from a doctor of his choice. Periodic further reports may be required.

Psychiatrists are sometimes asked to provide reports about nurses, police officers, teachers and others by their professional body, regarding fitness to practise or in connection with the investigation of complaints.

Allegations of medical negligence

Reports are requested from lawyers for the plaintiff or respondent in cases alleging medical negligence or malpractice. If the allegation is sustained, damages will be claimed. In these cases the plaintiff is usually an aggrieved or injured patient and the respondent the doctor or doctors, together with the employing health authority or trust.

Medical negligence cases are broadly of two kinds:

(1) *Non-psychiatric cases:* The allegation is of damage through medical care, some other specialist involvement or general practitioner care. These may involve wrong or delayed diagnosis or surgical errors. Where a claim for additional psychological injury or trauma (or 'nervous shock' in legal parlance) is made then this aspect will require psychiatric assessment.

The psychiatrist must report after a full examination. It is necessary to assess personality and evidence of mental illness or symptoms (if any) present before the incident, and then to decide to what extent subsequent psychiatric complaints or disability clearly result from the negligent acts.

(2) *Psychiatric cases:* These are increasingly common. Here the allegation concerns psychiatric care and management. Examples are allegations of 'failure of duty of care' when a patient claims to have suffered through a failure of good practice. This may include attempted or successful suicide (when the relatives may make the allegation), or errors due to failure to observe the requirements of mental health legislation, such as consent to treatment. The psychiatrist may be asked to give an opinion on the documents alone. He will be asked to comment on the circumstance of the case and whether or not, in his opinion, the staff involved acted in accordance with accepted practice. The status and level of training of the practitioners is also relevant.

Medical negligence cases can be protracted and require a number of conferences with counsel. Many are eventually settled without proceeding to a hearing. Powers & Harris (1994) give a comprehensive account of the issues and valuable guidance.

Appendix I

Example of a report to a Crown Court in a case of criminal damage.

James Dee is to be tried at Midshires Crown Court charged with criminal damage. He had deliberately set fire to a neighbour's barn causing extensive destruction.

PSYCHIATRIC REPORT

Shires Clinic,
England Road,
Warcester,
Midshires.

Chief Crown Prosecutor,
Crown Prosecution Service,
Warcester,
Midshires.

James Dee (DOB: 17.02.65)
Charge of Criminal Damage
Midshires Crown Court 4th May 1993

I examined the above-named at HM Prison, Midshires on 2 February 1993, 23 February 1993 and on 1 March 1993. I interviewed his mother, Mrs Janet Dee, at my out-patient clinic at the Shires Clinic on 2 March 1993. I confirm that I have read the following:

(1) details of the indictment
(2) a comprehensive bundle of witness statements
(3) edited transcripts of interviews with accused taken from the audio-taped recordings and dated 10 and 11 December 1992
(4) a signed statement from Mr Dee
(5) four audio tapes of interviews with Mr Dee
(6) letters from previous employers.

I have also discussed the case with Dr P. Brown who has also examined him, and the prison medical officer, Dr Smith, and hospital officers at HM Prison, Warcester.

Mr James Dee is a single man of 28 years who was recently unemployed. At the time of each of my interviews he was aware of the charge against him and understood its possible implications. He understood that as a result of my interviews I would prepare a report which would be sent to you.

Personal history

I understand from my interviews and documentation that Mr Dee was born in Birmingham in 1965, an only child. He had a deprived and disrupted early life. He was brought up for the first ten years by both parents, but his father had suffered brain damage as a result of a road traffic accident in 1960 and was often violent, unpredictable, intoxicated and in trouble with the police. His mother had poor control over the defendant and was often absent from home when in employment.

Mr Dee's father is now aged 58; his whereabouts are unknown. He separated from his wife ten years ago. His mother is aged 55, suffers from chronic bronchitis and has a history of several admissions to a local psychiatric hospital suffering from depressive episodes.

Development: Mr Dee was a weak, underweight child who is reported to have had feeding difficulties as an infant and suffered from enuresis (bedwetting) until the age of 12. Until the age of five he exhibited severe temper tantrums.

Schools and educational progress: He attended Lower Warcester Infant and Junior Schools from 5 to 11 years where he was initially noted to be slow, withdrawn and a poor mixer with other children. By the age of six he was more outgoing, bright and was enjoying school life, although his progress in learning to read and write was slow.

From 11 to 16 he attended Warcester Comprehensive School. He was, from the start, easily influenced by other more dominant children, suffered some bullying and often truanted. His reports were indifferent. His home life was increasingly unstable at this time. He enjoyed football and showed an artistic talent which gave him some degree of self-confidence and status. He failed two CSE examinations and was considered for special education.

Employment: On leaving school at the age of 16 he had difficulty in obtaining a job and was accepted for a Youth Training Scheme in painting and decorating which he managed to complete successfully. He has since found difficulty obtaining any further work although he has had several casual jobs. A report from one employer (J. & C. Dobbs, Builders) in the case papers comments satisfactorily on the two months Mr Dee spent with them in 1985. However, during the past eight years he has been virtually continuously unemployed.

Sexual history and relationships

He began to show an interest in girlfriends during his last year in school and had two short-lived relationships. He has always felt shy and awkward in developing his contacts with girls. At the age of 20 he was attracted to a 16-year-old girl in his village with whom he had his only sexual experience, but the relationship ended after six weeks.

Alcohol and substance abuse

He began drinking at the age of 15 with others from school, and from 17 onwards would often drink excessively, and was arrested on several occasions. Drinking was sometimes associated with violence, particularly against property; he was involved in several burglaries but was not arrested. He has smoked cannabis infrequently.

Hobbies and interests

He tends to spend time on his own wandering aimlessly with his dog. He has had an interest for some years in collecting Second World War memorabilia, although this is more of an aspiration than a success. He has one or two items such as badges and bullets.

Previous medical and psychiatric history

(1) He was referred for an assessment to a school psychologist at the age of 12. His intelligence was assessed as below average and advice was provided to the school on his management.
(2) At the age of 17 he had an appendectomy.
(3) Aged 25 he was assessed by a consultant psychiatrist as an out-patient at Midshires County Hospital psychiatric department on the referral of his general practitioner. He presented with a history of withdrawal, hallucinations (hearing voices), delusions (he believed that neighbours were in a conspiracy to shoot him) and he demonstrated inappropriate sudden giggling. It was considered that he may be suffering from schizophrenia, and medication was recommended. He did not persist with this.

Family history

His father showed considerable instability (see above). His paternal uncle suffers from schizophrenia and is under the care of Midshires County Hospital.

Present offence

He could remember very little of the alleged offence but at the second interview recalled that he had experienced the voice of his next-door-neighbour, a man, telling him to set fire to the barn or he would be caught and shot. He tried to resist this, but felt that the instruction, which was repeated increasingly often, was insistent. It continued during a three-week period. He drank whisky at home in his room which suppressed the voice, but then it returned.

On the night concerned, after drinking, he left home at 2.00 am, walked to the barn and set fire to some papers. He stayed at a distance to watch the flames and the arrival of the fire brigade. He was seen and subsequently questioned and arrested. He was remanded in custody.

Examination

At my interview with him, Mr Dee presented as a thin, withdrawn young man who looked older than his age. He was initially uncommunicative but at the second and third interviews he was more forthcoming, cooperative and coherent. He was able to give me a reasonably relevant account of himself, but he showed little emotion. At times he stopped talking and I had the impression he was listening to inner voices. His account of his alleged offence was sometimes difficult to follow. He would occasionally move irrelevantly to an unrelated topic. During the interviews he giggled inappropriately several times.

I had the impression that he was of below average intelligence. His prevailing mood was depressed and he seemed perplexed. He still believed that he was hearing voices within his head which came from his neighbours at home. He did not consider that he was ill.

Interview with Mrs Janet Dee

Mr Dee's mother could not provide any helpful information. She was a depressed and inarticulate lady who was able to endorse some aspects of the childhood history.

Opinion

(1) James Dee is able to understand the nature of the charge against him, and can understand the meaning of a plea of guilty or not guilty. He is able to instruct his legal advisers and follow the proceedings in court. He is fit to plead and to stand trial.

(2) Mr Dee had an unhappy, disrupted and deprived childhood. His emotional development was retarded and his school performance was poor. He was drinking excessively from an early age, used cannabis and was in trouble. From his teens he was often withdrawn, isolated and sometimes hostile.

(3) Since the age of 20 he has shown deterioration of his personality with incipient signs of mental illness which led to his first referral to a psychiatrist when aged 25.

(4) In my opinion he now suffers from schizophrenia, a mental illness within the meaning of the Mental Health Act 1983, characterised by

hallucinatory experiences (voices), persecutory delusional beliefs (false beliefs which have no factual basis) and disruption of his thought processes. He has inappropriate mannerisms and moods. In my opinion the offence with which he is charged occurred as a result of his mental illness which influenced his behaviour although he knew that his actions were wrong. (5)   He has accepted treatment voluntarily while on remand in prison and he is now somewhat improved but still shows signs of active illness.

I believe that he requires further treatment and recommend that the court should consider a Hospital Order, should he be found guilty.

Furthermore, in view of the seriousness of the offence and the uncertain prognosis, I would recommend a restriction order (Section 41, Mental Health Act 1983) without limit of time. A bed in a medium secure hospital would be appropriate and I am willing to accept him at the Shires Clinic, a regional secure unit. On his return to the community he will eventually be supported by a community team from the clinic.

I am approved by the Secretary of State for the purposes of Section 12(2) of the Mental Health Act 1983.

Dr Malcolm Barchester, MB BS MRCPsych, Consultant Forensic
Psychiatrist, Shires Health Trust.
17th March 1993

Appendix II

Example of a report to the solicitor acting for a plaintiff in a compensation case.

Mr John Brown was a bus driver involved in a road traffic accident.

PSYCHIATRIC REPORT

Shires Clinic,
England Road,
Warcester,
Midshires.

Wisdom and Advice,
Solicitors,
20 High Street,
Warcester.

Brown v Allbash Insurance Company

At the request of Wisdom and Advice, Solicitors, acting for Mr John Brown (DOB 07.01.33) I provide the following psychiatric report. I examined Mr Brown at the Shires Clinic for one hour 30 minutes on 20

February 1993. I have been asked to give an opinion on the nature and degree of any mental injuries sustained by Mr Brown as a consequence of a road traffic accident in which he was involved on 8 November 1990. I confirm that I have read the following:

(1) A copy of the Statement of Claim in Brown v Allbash Insurance Company
(2) Medical records and a medical report dated 15 October 1992 from his general practitioner, Dr R. Ahmed, Medical Centre, Warcester.

I have also interviewed Mrs Jean Brown, his wife.

Mr Brown is a 61-year-old retired bus driver who lives with his wife at the above address. He was a cooperative informant who understood the purpose of the interview.

Personal history

He was born in Warcester the middle of three children. His father, who had been a serving soldier, deserted the family home leaving his wife to bring up the three children. He lived with his siblings and mother in Warcester and completed his schooling at Warcester County School. He left school at the age of 14 years and served an apprenticeship as a motor engineer. He was called up for National Service in the Royal Air Force and afterwards remained in the Force serving a total of 12 years in the motor transport division. After leaving the RAF he worked as a car mechanic. He was made redundant from this work and for the last 12 years of his working life was employed as a bus driver with the Midshire Omnibus Company. His work involved driving buses in central and southern England. He retired from work on health grounds in February 1992 (aged 60) having been on sick leave for approximately six months.

He has been married for 35 years. The couple have two grown-up children who live near Warcester. His wife works as a cashier in a butcher's shop. The couple own their own home. The marriage is happy and there have been no separations.

Mr Brown was a smoker until ten years ago. He drinks an occasional pint of beer but there is no history of any heavy alcohol intake. There is no history of any drug misuse.

Previous medical history

He has had a variety of physical conditions over the years including a left inguinal hernia, arthritis of his cervical spine, and kidney stones, for which he has had surgical treatment on five occasions.

There is no previous history of any psychiatric disorder.

Family medical history

There is none of any relevance.

Functioning prior to accident on 8 November 1990

Mr Brown said he had enjoyed his work and had always been an active man; he played football regularly until the age of 40. He anticipated working until he was 65 and his outside interests included fishing, gardening and home decorating. He always enjoyed family holidays. He said there were no personal problems in his life before the accident and he regarded himself as having a happy and contented disposition.

Plaintiff's account of accident on 8 November 1990

Mr Brown described how he was driving his bus on a rainy morning. He had done the journey many times before. He told me that he was taking a right-hand bend, when a car "bulleted round the corner" on the wrong side of the road and crashed head-on into his vehicle. He had 15 passengers on board including many elderly people, and he assisted them off the bus to safety. The other vehicle was badly damaged and he saw its female driver immobile in the driving seat. He remained at the scene of the accident while the woman was assisted by emergency services into an ambulance. He gave statements to the police at the time and recalls being told by them "he was blameless".

Physical symptoms following accident

Mr Brown experienced an exacerbation of his neck pain and was treated with analgesics and physiotherapy. He was off work for three weeks and then asked to return to work. The pain has, however, continued and he now attends privately for reflexology treatment.

Mental symptoms following accident

Mr Brown said he experienced increasing tension in the months after the accident. He was preoccupied by disturbing visual images of the accident. His sleep pattern was impaired and he often dreamed about the accident. He complained to his general practitioner. He recognised that he was increasingly short-tempered and irritable. He found no enjoyment in two holidays taken in 1991. He found it difficult to concentrate on his work, and was preoccupied about what shifts he would be working; previously he had taken shift work in his stride. In July 1991 he felt he was a liability at work and he proceeded on sick leave due to what he referred to as "depression" (see below). His public service vehicle driving licence was revoked in September 1991 on the grounds of ill health and he finally retired from work on health grounds in February 1992.

Over the following months there was some improvement but later in 1992 he was required to attend court in connection with a civil action against his employers by the driver of the other vehicle. His sleep pattern became worse and he was constantly preoccupied with the prospect of giving evidence in court. He duly appeared in court and gave evidence for approximately 90 minutes.

He has continued to experience significant mental symptoms in the last three months. He remains preoccupied with the accident and his sleep pattern is disturbed. He wonders whether he might have been able to rescue the driver and so prevent some of her injuries. He feels low in mood and has episodes of weeping. He has lost interest in gardening and home decorating. He no longer drives as he feels he does not have "the confidence" to do so.

He has very restricted interests, spending much of his time in the house apart from occasionally walking his dog. His appetite is poor and he lacks energy. He says he has lost his normal sex drive. He feels he has now taken "second place" to his wife who is in employment while he remains at home.

Treatment received

He is currently attending private therapists for reflexology and acupuncture for his neck pain. He finds both these treatments helpful. In addition he is receiving antidepressant medication (amitriptyline) from his general practitioner whom he has been consulting since the accident.

Information from Mrs Jean Brown (wife)

Mrs Brown said that prior to the accident her husband was "always full of life" though there had always been an "intolerant" edge to him. He had been extremely conscientious in his work. She said that since the accident he appeared to have "changed completely". He had lost interest in all his normal activities. Whereas he had previously dealt with problems in his stride, he had appeared completely preoccupied with the accident since it happened. She particularly mentioned his irregular sleeping, his agitation, his avoidance of social interactions and the fact that he is made anxious by trivial events. She confirmed that he appeared to have lost all interest in sexual activity. He tells his wife he is "useless".

Examination

Mr Brown is a tall man (6 feet in height) of medium build (12 stones 8 pounds). He was smartly dressed and was entirely cooperative. He appeared ill-at-ease, preoccupied and at times became tearful. He spoke spontaneously in a fluent and articulate fashion and gave no impression of seeking to exaggerate or dramatise his account. He continues to think daily about the accident and remains fearful when travelling by road.

He described feelings of poor self-image, guilt, depression of mood and anxiety. Subjectively he complained of poor concentration, but formal testing of his concentration and short-term memory showed no significant impairment.

Opinion

Nature and degree of mental symptoms: Mr John Brown describes no problems with his mental health prior to the accident in November 1990. His work record was stable and he had many leisure interests.

In the months immediately following the accident he developed significant mental symptoms of two types. Firstly, there was a preoccupation with thoughts of the accident, disturbing visual images, disturbed sleep, and increased irritability. These symptoms increased in intensity over the following 12 to 18 months and have continued but with less intensity since that time. In my opinion these symptoms are characteristic of a condition known as post-traumatic stress disorder. This was initially present at a moderate degree and is now mild to moderate in intensity.

Secondly, he has experienced persistent feelings of low mood, loss of self-confidence, social withdrawal, lack of energy and drive, a poor sense of self-worth and loss of libido. In my opinion these symptoms, taken together with your client's presentation at interview, indicate that he has developed a depressive disorder at a moderate degree of severity.

Taken together, the development of the post-traumatic stress disorder and the depressive disorder have produced what is now a significant degree of impaired mental health. His capacity to enjoy life and the quality of his interpersonal relationships have been seriously impaired.

Relationship of mental symptoms to accident on 8 November 1990: Mr Brown does not appear to have suffered from any psychiatric symptoms before November 1990 and does not appear to be predisposed to any psychiatric disorder. In my opinion the condition of post-traumatic stress disorder developed as a result of the accident. The subsequent development of the depressive disorder is commonly seen in combination with post-traumatic stress disorder. Other factors, in particular the persisting problem of neck pain, may have contributed to the development of depressive symptoms. The conditions of post-traumatic stress disorder and the depressive disorder are interrelated and on balance I think his current level of psychiatric disorder is largely attributable to the accident in November 1990.

Treatment required: Mr Brown finds treatment by reflexology and acupuncture helpful for his neck symptoms. I anticipate that he will continue to receive this treatment. He attends his general practitioner regularly and is receiving antidepressant medication at an appropriate dosage. However, the condition has remained fairly static and it may well be that your client will require extended treatment, either with alternative medication or by referral to a specialist service.

Prognosis: The prognosis for people who develop post-traumatic stress disorder is varied. In the case of Mr Brown there has been some improvement in the intensity of his symptoms with the passage of time. It is, however, notable that there was a deterioration following the court case in 1992. I would expect the symptoms of post-traumatic stress disorder to improve gradually over a prolonged period. In my opinion the outlook for his depressive disorder is less good. His symptoms are complicated by his changed social situation (he is no longer a breadwinner in the home) and he has suffered a loss of status since retirement. This is likely to aggravate his symptoms of low mood and poor self-worth. I doubt that there will be any significant improvement in his depressive disorder in the near or medium-term future.

Summary

(1) Mr Brown was involved in a head-on collision while driving his bus on 8 November 1990. He did not sustain any serious physical injuries, although there was an exacerbation of previous neck symptoms.
(2) Following the accident he has developed symptoms of post-traumatic stress disorder which were initially moderate in severity and are now mild to moderate in intensity. This condition was caused by the accident.
(3) He has also developed a depressive disorder which continues at moderate severity. In my opinion this condition is largely attributable to the accident.
(4) The psychiatric disorders have seriously reduced his quality of life.
(5) There will probably be continued improvement of the post-traumatic stress disorder but the depressive disorder is unlikely to improve in the medium-term future.

Dr Malcolm Barchester, MB BS MRCPsych, Consultant Forensic
Psychiatrist, Shires Health Trust.
26 February 1993

References

Chiswick, D. (1985) Use and abuse of psychiatric testimony. *British Medical Journal*, **290**, 975–977.

Cornes, P. & Aitken, R. C. (1992) Medical reports on persons claiming compensation for personal injury. *Journal of the Royal Society of Medicine*, **85**, 329–333.

Dell, S. (1984) *Murder into Manslaughter*. Oxford: Oxford University Press.

Mackay, R. D. (1986) Psychiatric reports in the crown court. *Criminal Law Review*, April, 217–225.

May, R. (1990) Rules of evidence. In *Principles and Practice of Forensic Psychiatry* (eds R. Bluglass & P. Bowden), pp. 35–41. Edinburgh: Churchill Livingstone.

Paul, D. M. (1981) Writing medico-legal reports. *British Medical Journal*, **282**, 2101–2102.

Powers, M. & Harris, N. (1994) *Medical Negligence* (2nd edn). London: Butterworths.

Further reading

Bluglass, R. (1979) The psychiatric court report. *Medicine, Science and the Law*, **19**, 121–129.

—— (1990) The psychiatrist as an expert witness. In *Principles and Practice of Forensic Psychiatry* (eds R. Bluglass & P. Bowden), pp. 161–166. Edinburgh: Churchill Livingstone.

Bowden, P. (1990) The written report and sentences. In *Principles and Practice of Forensic Psychiatry* (eds R. Bluglass & P. Bowden), pp. 183–197. Edinburgh: Churchill Livingstone.

Chiswick, D. (1990) The psychiatric report: Scotland. In *Principles and Practice of Forensic Psychiatry* (eds R. Bluglass & P. Bowden), pp. 199–203. Edinburgh: Churchill Livingstone.

Faulk, M. (1994) Writing a report. In *Basic Forensic Psychiatry* (ed. M. Faulk)(2nd edn), pp. 287–314. Oxford: Blackwell Scientific.

Storey, P. (1990) Reports for compensation after injury. In *Principles and Practice of Forensic Psychiatry* (eds R. Bluglass & P. Bowden), pp. 1117–1122. Edinburgh: Churchill Livingstone.

7 Facilities and treatment
Peter Snowden

Psychiatric services • Special hospitals • Regional forensic psychiatry services • General adult psychiatry services • The independent sector • Services for other groups of mentally disordered offenders • Treatment • Role of the Department of Health and the Home Office • Interrelationship of services • Appendix

---

In general psychiatry, after the assessment of a new case, the main focus is on treatment. Where this should take place (hospital, day hospital or in the community) is relatively easy to decide. In forensic psychiatry the issues are more complex. Determining the appropriate setting for treatment is necessary before the treatment approach can be considered. To do this one needs knowledge of the variety of psychiatric services available for mentally disordered offenders, the interrelationship of these health services with the criminal justice system, and the roles of the Department of Health and the Home Office.

Psychiatric services

The treatment of mentally disordered offenders is carried out by a range of psychiatric services (see Table 7.1):

(1) special hospitals
(2) regional forensic psychiatry services
(3) district-based general adult psychiatry services
(4) services provided by the independent sector.

Services for offenders with a learning disability and for juveniles are described separately.

Special hospitals

The role of the special hospital has been reviewed by Hamilton (1990) and more recently by the Department of Health (1994). In England and Wales the special hospitals, which form part of the NHS, provide an in-patient service under conditions of maximum security for mentally disordered offenders who are so dangerous that they would cause grave concern if managed elsewhere. There are three such hospitals in England

164

Table 7.1 Hospital services for mentally disordered adult offenders (MDOs)

	Security	Type of service
Special hospital	High	In-patient service, long-stay (on average 8–9 years
Regional forensic psychiatry services	Medium	(a) In-patient secure unit (RSU), most patients stay for less than two years (b) Out-patient community forensic psychiatry service (CFPS)
District psychiatric services	None/low	Variable interest in MDOs. Some provide an out-patient and in-patient service in open or locked wards. Variable length of stay
Independent sector	Low/medium	Various hospital units around the country offering in-patient services for patients who do not fit current health service facilities or who live in an area with inadequate resources. Variable length of stay

and Wales. Broadmoor Hospital in Berkshire was the first to be established in 1863 and serves most of the south of England. In 1914, Rampton Hospital in Nottinghamshire was opened and serves roughly the east of the country. Ashworth Hospital in Merseyside is an amalgamation of Park Lane and Moss Side Hospitals and provides a service for the rest of England and Wales, including the geographically distant North West Thames health region.

In Scotland, the State Hospital at Carstairs (see Fig. 7.1) is the sole provider of treatment in conditions of special security. It currently has approximately 230 patients, most of whom are mentally ill, but also some with a learning disability or personality disorder. It is responsible to the Secretary of State for Scotland, but will shortly be administered by the equivalent of a special health authority. There are no special hospital services in Northern Ireland – indeed, there is no dedicated facility for forensic psychiatry in the Province. Patients from Northern Ireland requiring special security are treated principally at Carstairs, although there is a small number in the English special hospitals. The only specified facility for forensic psychiatry in the Republic of Ireland is the Central Hospital, Dundrum. This is a secure psychiatric hospital, with approximately 80 beds, administered by the Eastern Health Board. Over 90% of its admissions are from prisons, with only a small number admitted from local facilities.

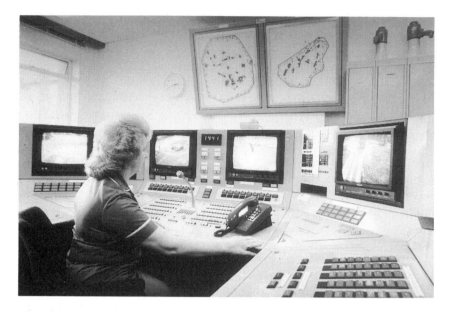

Fig 7.1 The control room of the State Hospital, Carstairs.

Management

In 1968 there was a total of 2200 special hospital beds in England. Rebuilding and other service developments have allowed the numbers to fall to 1676 beds by January 1993.

The Special Hospitals Service Authority (SHSA) is based in London and manages the special hospitals. There are signs of significant changes in the style and organisation of special hospital services. At the local level, each hospital has a stronger management team than under the old central DHSS management. The response to the Inquiry of Complaints at Ashworth Hospital (see below) by the SHSA has been positive and energetic.

Security

Maximum security is provided by the perimeter security, made up of high walls (similar to those found in prisons), and entry into the hospital is through a double (or in some cases triple) door airlock system under electronic control, with security cameras monitoring this weak point in the secure shell. Patients (without parole) and visitors are escorted throughout the hospital. Within the hospital are areas that remain highly secure, but in Ashworth Hospital there are some trusted patients who have a degree of parole within certain areas of the hospital campus. Security in special hospitals is mainly the responsibility of nursing staff. In each hospital there is a group of nurses who have primary responsibility for security, while the rest of the nurses need to balance their therapeutic and security tasks. Ward areas contain single bedrooms (usually locked at night), large day areas and, on certain wards, a seclusion room.

Admission criteria

In contrast with consultants in other hospital services, a special hospital consultant cannot admit patients directly. Each patient referred for admission is considered by a local special hospital admissions panel made up of medical, nursing, psychology, social work and administrative representatives. Patients are referred to the panel after examination in prison or in hospital by a forensic psychiatrist, prison medical officer or general psychiatrist. About half of referrals result in the offer of a bed, and although the special hospital psychiatrist's recommendations can be overturned by the admissions panel, there is agreement in the majority of cases (Close & Larkin, 1994).

> **Case example 1**
> A man in his early 30s left the Royal Navy after he developed schizophrenia, which led to a number of hospital admissions because of poor compliance with treatment after discharge. On two occasions he broke into dwelling houses, frightening female occupants, and on one occasion a Section 37 hospital order was imposed. These incidents occurred in the setting of a psychotic relapse, but were not easily attributable to any single psychopathological symptom. Before the index offence he sexually assaulted an elderly female patient in the grounds of a mental illness unit where he was an informal inpatient. After absconding, he tricked his way into an elderly woman's flat and subjected her to a violent and prolonged physical (using a knife and other implements) and sexual assault, ending in rape. At interview in a remand prison, the forensic psychiatrist found evidence of an acute relapse of his schizophrenia. He had been taking neuroleptic medication up to only a few days before the offence.

If a special hospital bed is considered necessary, the assessing psychiatrist must first contact a special hospital consultant (many of whom are trained forensic psychiatrists) from the hospital that serves the relevant geographical area. Both doctors must then agree that:

(1) the person is mentally disordered with the meaning of the Mental Health Act;
(2) there is evidence of violence of a severe nature to person or property (i.e. arson). The term "grave immediate danger to the public" is often used to separate these cases from others;
(3) maximum security is necessary.

Issues such as level of physical aggression, harm to the victim, whether weapons were used, response to treatment, compliance and history of absconding are relearnt in deciding why other hospital facilities are inappropriate.

In the case example above, both doctors agreed that the patient's poor cooperation with psychiatric services, his history of absconding, sexually assaulting a female patient when on appropriate treatment, the two unauthorised forced entries into dwellings some years before, and the recent serious sexual attack on an elderly female using a weapon, indicated the need for prolonged treatment in a maximum secure hospital, as he would have been an immediate risk to others if he absconded. All of the relevant reports and documents were sent to the local special hospital admission panel who made a place available. The judge followed medical advice and ordered a medical disposal.

Admission sources

There were 194 special hospital admissions in 1992 (see Table 7.2). The great majority (69%) were admitted from prisons and the courts. Most were subject to a restriction order. More than one in five admissions were from regional secure units and other psychiatric facilities. Among these are non-offender patients who have shown serious violence. Admissions from the community (5% of the total in 1992) are usually conditionally discharged restricted patients who are recalled by the Home Secretary. Overall, two-thirds of the special hospital population have restrictions on discharge.

Clinical services and facilities

Clinical teams made up of doctors, nurses, psychologists, and social workers provide the same treatment one would expect to find in any other psychiatric unit. Other professionals, such as teachers, may be involved in

Table 7.2 Special hospital admissions and departures in 1992 (Department of Health, 1994)

Sources	Admissions n (%)	Departures n (%)
Prisons	80 (41)	32 (15)
Courts	55 (28)	–
Medium secure units	37 (19)	57 (26)
Other special hospitals	6 (3)	–
Other NHS	6 (3)	44 (20)
Other (including community)	10 (5)	68 (31)
Deaths	–	16 (7)
Total	194	217

treatment. Patients are usually admitted first to the most secure (admission) wards, with the highest nursing staff numbers and physical security. Following assessment and as improvement occurs, patients are moved to less secure wards with less intensive nursing input.

There are at present very few occupational therapists. The large well-equipped occupation centres are staffed by occupational officers who are not clinically trained. The facilities within the special hospitals for sport, education and recreation are extremely good and necessary as patients may spend many years in a special hospital.

Psychologists have an important role in the assessment and treatment of patients with psychopathic disorder. The psychology departments are well staffed and have sophisticated equipment (e.g. for penile plethys-mography) that is rarely used in ordinary hospital practice. Recent developments within special hospitals include rehabilitation departments, which aim to break the institutional mould and prepare the patient for life away from the unavoidable routines of a special hospital.

Patient characteristics

The characteristics of patients in special hospitals are shown in Box 7.1.

Discharge

In 1992 the average length of stay for the 201 patients of all legal categories discharged from special hospital was 6.9 years, but for the Section 37/41

Box 7.1 Characteristics of special hospital patients

The total population is approximately 1700
84% are male and 16% are female
Nearly 18 % are from ethnic minorities
The average age is nearly 40 years
77% are detained under Part III of the Mental Health Act (i.e. under court orders or directions of the Home Secretary)
One in seven are non-offenders
The majority (60–70%) have a diagnosis of mental illness, of which schizophrenia is the most common diagnosis. A minority (3–10%) have other conditions (e.g. manic–depressive psychoses or organic states)
25% are detained under the legal category of psychopathic disorder
9% are detained under the legal categories of mental impairment or severe mental impairment
Each year there are approximately 200 admissions and departures, a turnover of 10%

patients the figure was 8.7 years (Department of Health, 1994). When appropriate, transfer to a lesser degree of security (such as a regional secure unit or catchment area hospital) is more common than direct discharge to the community (Table 7.2). The special hospital consultant contacts the relevant regional forensic psychiatry service, or catchment area consultant, who then assesses the patient with members of the multidisciplinary team. The assessment should be thorough, as there is often much detailed information to be assimilated (see Table 7.3). The

Table 7.3 Tasks in the assessment of a special hospital patient with a view to transfer to a less secure hospital unit

Source of information	Task	Reason
Clinical records	Read all clinical notes, reports, summary of offence. If possible, obtain photocopies of important documents	Gather enough information to make a decision
Patient	Interview on ward	Gather enough information to make a decision
Patient's room	Ask patient to show you his room (i.e. look at books, decor, etc)	Ascertain whether patient's interests are as described on interview
Nursing staff	Interview on ward	Nursing views are not always stated clearly in notes alone. Can relate all recent events involving patient. Ask about patient's daytime occupation
Medical staff	Speak with responsible medical officer	Can update information and clarify psychiatric opinion
Psychologist	Speak with psychologist	This is important if the psychologist is involved in patient care, particularly if no up-to-date reports are available
Relative	Note recorded views or arrange interview	Ascertain attitude of family

need for a careful assessment is paramount since an inadequate understanding of a case accepted for transfer may have extremely serious consequences.

Unrestricted special hospital patients, who are few in number, may be transferred to another hospital in the normal way, but restricted patients require the approval of C3 Division and sometimes support from a mental health review tribunal before transfer. Initially the Home Office usually agrees to a 6-month period of trial leave before full transfer. If there is a problem, the patient can be transferred back to special hospital without the necessity for a formal admission. Delays in finding a hospital willing to accept a special hospital patient may be due to inadequate services or disagreement over whether a patient is ready to move (Dell, 1980).

Clinical services in special hospitals

In 1991 the Secretary of State for Health ordered an inquiry into complaints about the death of a patient and mistreatment of others at Ashworth Hospital (Department of Health, 1992). Psychiatrists, nurses, and the general standard of patient care (including the use of seclusion) were criticised, as were the response to complaints by patients and the general management of the hospital. All security hospitals, but the maximum security special hospitals in particular, can lose contact with developments in mainstream psychiatry, and with appropriate standards of patient care. Physical security can readily become a psychological barrier. The report of the 1992 inquiry into Ashworth Hospital has had a considerable impact on the special hospital services. Ashworth Hospital has been reorganised into a hospital with geographical units (closely linked to the medium secure units that this hospital serves) to ease patient movement both up and down the security ladder. Specialist units, including those for the treatment of patients with psychopathic disorder and learning disability, are being developed.

Follow-up studies of patients discharged from the special hospitals are reviewed in Chapter 8. In general, poorer outcome, defined by reoffending, is associated with patients in the legal category of psychopathic disorder, with absolute discharge and discharge directly to the community rather than through a regional secure unit (RSU) or other hospital.

Regional forensic psychiatry services

Each regional health authority (RHA) in England and Wales has a forensic psychiatrist with responsibility for developing services for mentally disordered offenders throughout the region. The development of these services followed the Butler report in 1975, which recommended the development of RSUs and regional forensic psychiatry services. Those regions that appointed forensic psychiatrists early opened what were called temporary or interim secure units. These were usually converted wards, rarely with more sophisticated security than a singled locked door. These units were the service models for RSUs and the forensic community services (Snowden, 1990). They closed when definitive RSUs opened. There were a variety of reasons for the delays in opening RSUs from 1975 and throughout the early eighties (Snowden, 1985), but most RHAs now have forensic psychiatry services with an RSU.

The RSU serves three functions. Firstly, it is the administrative, teaching and research base for all staff. Secondly, it is the clinical base for those staff who are primarily involved with the community forensic psychiatry service. Thirdly, it is the in-patient resource. Forensic services have developed in a slightly different way from region to region, often depending on the interests and service philosophy of the forensic psychiatrist involved in planning. Some RSUs have their own out-patient area; at least two regional forensic psychiatry services have an additional community base in a city centre, with out-patient, administrative and treatment facilities. Factors such as regional geography, location of the RSU, and areas of population density have also influenced the different service patterns.

The situation in Scotland, where there are no RSUs, is different. The State Hospital at Carstairs has a more flexible role than an English special hospital. A small number of area forensic psychiatrists, most of whom have in-patient units, work in collaboration with colleagues in general psychiatry. It is easier to move patients through the system according to their need for security and specialist forensic services than it is south of the border.

In Northern Ireland, each large psychiatric hospital has a locked ward, and the Province has two consultants in forensic psychiatry. There is no equivalent of a RSU, although negotiations are currently taking place to provide one. In the Republic of Ireland, two consultant forensic psychiatrists are based at the Central Hospital, Dundrum; there is no other forensic facility in the country.

Regional secure units

Only a few regional forensic psychiatry services have access to open beds. Most have a RSU that provides what is termed medium security. This means the RSU is not escape-proof or as secure as a special hospital, but is more secure than a locked ward. There is no standard design, but all units are secure enough for the majority of patients who need secure in-patient care, and even the most dangerous patients should be manageable until another more secure placement can be found. Table 7.4 shows the locations of RSUs in England and Wales.

Table 7.4 Medium secure units in England and Wales, 1994

Region	Medium secure unit	Beds
Northern	Hutton Unit, St Luke's Hospital, Middlesborough	34
	Secure Unit, St Nicholas Hospital, Newcastle	10
Yorkshire	Newton Lodge, Pinderfields Hospital, Wakefield	44
Trent	Arnold Lodge, Towers Hospital, Leicester	58
East Anglia	Norvic Clinic, St Andrew's Hospital, Norwich	34
Wessex	Ravenswood House, Knowle Hospital, Fareham	28
South Western	Butler Clinic, Langdon Hospital, Dawlish	30
	Fromeside Clinic, Blackberry Hill, Bristol	30
South West Thames	Secure Unit, Springfield Hospital	10
South East Thames	Dennis Hill Unit, Bethlem Royal Hospital	30
	SASS Unit, Cane Hill Hospital, Coulsdon	15
	Trevor Gibbens Unit, Oakwood Hospital, Maidstone	15
	Bracton Clinic, Bexley Hospital	15
	Ashen Hill, Hellingly Hospital, East Sussex	15
North East Thames	Camlet Lodge, Chase Farm Hospital, Enfield	34
	Secure Unit, Runwell Hospital	14
	Secure Unit, Hackney Hospital	12
North West Thames	Three Bridges Secure Unit, Ealing Hospital	54
Oxford	Wallingford Clinic, Fairmile Hospital, Oxfordshire	13
West Midlands	Reaside Clinic, Rubery, Birmingham	77
North Western	Edenfield Centre, Prestwich Hospital, Manchester	65
	Langdale Unit, Whittingham Hospital, Preston	24
Mersey	Scott Clinic, Rainhill Hospital, Merseyside	42
Wales	Caswell Clinic, Glanrhyd Hospital, Bridgend	18

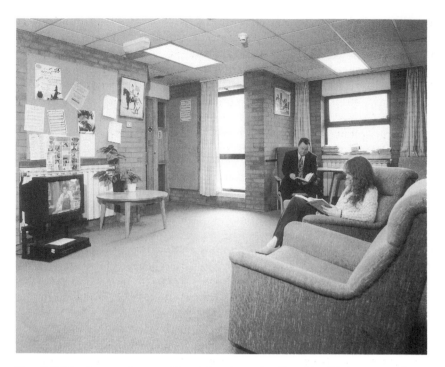

Fig. 7.2 The lounge in a residential unit of the Reaside Clinic regional secure unit, Birmingham.

Security provision and RSU design

RSUs have been built on hospital sites adjacent to other services. Each has been designed to fit in with the surrounding buildings and topography so that the security is not obvious. Most have a secure exercise area bounded by perimeter fencing, rather than a high wall as in special hospitals. Entry into the unit is invariably through an electronic double door airlock system. On entry, staff exchange an identity card for a key at the control centre where staff monitor entry, exit, patient movement and alarms. Sometimes office and administrative areas are situated outside the secure shell, but most of the clinical and administrative areas are located inside the secure shell. Within the unit, access to secure areas is through locked doors. Electronic door locks inside the building are not found in many units. Nursing staff are usually responsible for monitoring the security arrangements.

Most RSUs have opted for functional ward arrangements with more than one clinical team having access to an admission ward (often the most secure), treatment wards and rehabilitation/pre-discharge wards (sometimes at a lower level of security). Ward areas are designed to facilitate nursing observations, in order to reduce the likelihood of escape, damage to the ward, or use of furniture as weapons. A seclusion room is usually found in at least one ward area. Most RSUs have single bedrooms, and some of the larger units have facilities such as occupational therapy departments, a gymnasium, a patients' canteen and shop. Compared with special hospitals, RSUs are small, varying in size from 30–100 beds. As the length of stay is usually less than two years, patients have less need for the longer-term employment and leisure facilities available in the special hospitals. Those who cast an envious eye on the facilities in RSUs and special hospitals should remember that the patients they contain are potentially violent, locked up, and detained on a Mental Health Act order for long periods.

Staffing

Multidisciplinary teams consisting of forensic psychiatrists, nurses, psychologists, social workers and occupational therapists all bring their expertise to the assessment, treatment and rehabilitation of in-patients. Nursing numbers may at first seem more generous than in an ordinary psychiatric in-patient unit. However, the real number of staff available for clinical duties may be much lower than staff numbers suggest, because of other duties such as specialling (see below), escorting patients to and from court and the community, and the need to make assessments in other institutions. Nevertheless, it is the nursing staff who provide the first line of security through their skills and expertise in planning nursing strategies, setting limits, anticipating incidents, and dealing with problems when they occur. There are now special nursing courses for forensic nurses in order to develop these skills. Although there is a national shortage of clinical psychologists and occupational therapists, forensic specialisation is now a recognised career development for these professions.

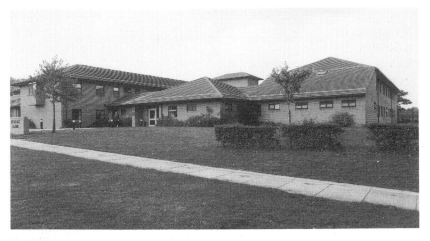

Fig. 7.3 External view of the Reaside Clinic regional secure unit, Birmingham.

Assessment for admission to the RSU

In contrast to the situation in general psychiatry, the assessment of patients for admission is not solely a medical decision. Nursing staff who will have to manage the patient on the ward, and who have security responsibilities, have an important role in assessments. RSU nursing staff in particular bring to the assessment their skills in the management of difficult and violent patients, and their knowledge of the existing patient mix on the RSU. When a referral is made for admission to the RSU, a team of medical and nursing staff, accompanied where relevant by a psychologist, social worker or occupational therapist, visits the patient to make an assessment. Depending on the nature and urgency of the case, a decision can be made immediately, or the case is presented to a clinical team meeting before admission. Most patients are admitted from the courts and from prison (up to 60%). Other large groups come from local psychiatric hospitals (20–25%) and special hospitals (10–15%). A small number of patients are admitted from the community or other RSUs.

Admission criteria

Strict admission criteria are necessary to prevent the RSU silting up and thus becoming an ineffective service. Box 7.2 shows the general criteria for admission. Any patient assessed by the multidisciplinary RSU team and considered too dangerous for the RSU is referred to a special hospital. If a patient is likely to require treatment for longer than two years in the RSU, advice is given to the referral agency and other facilities (if available) are considered. However, within the current services chronicity is often a problem without any simple solution. It is recognised that facilities should

---

Box 7.2   General criteria for admission to a regional secure unit

The patient requires treatment at the level of security provided by the RSU

Where admission is for assessment (e.g. remanded prisoner), it is inappropriate to utilise a lower level of security

The patient must have, or be thought to have, a mental disorder, and is detainable under a relevant section of the Mental Health Act 1983

Occasionally informal patients may be appropriate for admission, such as those on bail with a condition of residence in the secure unit, or readmission of former patients, with their agreement

It is considered likely that the patient will be ready to move on from the RSU within two years

be developed for those who need medium security for over two years. These include patients who are currently considered to be inappropriately placed in special hospitals (Shaw *et al*, 1994).

Source of referral and patient characteristics

Data on the practice of interim secure units have been reviewed by Treasaden (1985). More recently, Bullard & Bond (1988) reported a pattern of use which is likely to be consistent in the permanent units (RSUs) that replaced the interim secure units. They found that, of 105 patients, approximately 42% had committed either homicide or an assault, 12% theft or robbery, 7% arson, 6% sex offences, and 17% were non-offenders. The largest admission group were prisoners who had been on remand (47%); transfers from general psychiatry units, of convicted prisoners, and from special hospitals made up the remainder of the in-patient cohort, apart from a small number of patients who came from police stations or the community. In 63% of the patients the diagnosis was one of schizo-phrenia. Personality disorder and affective psychoses each contributed 15% of the total.

The majority of patients in RSUs are male. The proportion of female patients varies from 15% to 40% (Treasaden, 1985). Smith *et al* (1991) have described the characteristics of female admissions to a RSU. Typically, they were young, had a diagnosis of personality disorder, with a history of childhood sexual abuse, deliberate self-harm and alcohol abuse. Compared with male admissions, they were less violent but more likely to set fires. Such patients frequently stretch the resources of RSUs and present long-term management problems.

A striking feature of admissions to RSUs that provide services to inner-city areas is the high proportion of ethnic minority patients, predominantly Afro-Caribbeans. These patients are typically admitted from prison, are diagnosed as suffering from schizophrenia, have a previous criminal history and a history of previous compulsory admissions (Cope & Ndegwa, 1990). Ethnic issues are discussed in Chapter 3.

Assessment and treatment of non-offenders

Psychotic in-patients in district in-patient units may be transferred to a RSU because of aggression, and are usually acutely psychotic. They may have received high doses of neuroleptic medication in a setting of poor physical security, poor nursing surveillance, and a general lack of confidence and skill in the management of this group. In the RSU it is usually possible to reduce neuroleptic medication significantly, so enabling better assessment of the mental state and its relationship to the aggressive behaviour. Some-times it may be apparent that the patient has been reacting to inappropriate interventions from staff, or to the effects of other patients' behaviour (such

Table 7.5a Remand of accused persons in hospital under the Mental Health Act 1983

Section	Situation	Medical signatories	Authority required	Psychiatric disorder and conditions specified in the Act	Effects of order
35	Remand to hospital for report	Written/oral evidence from one doctor (S.12 approved)	Magistrates' or Crown Court[1]	Reason to suspect mental illness, psychopathic disorder, severe mental impairment or mental impairment. Bed must be available within 7 days	Detention for up to 28 days, renewable for further periods of 28 days, up to 12 weeks
36	Remand to hospital for treatment	Written/oral evidence from two doctors (one S.12 approved)	Crown Court only	Mental illness or severe mental impairment. Bed must be available within 7 days	Detention for up to 28 days, renewable for further periods of 28 days, up to 12 weeks

1. In Crown Court, applies to persons awaiting trial for any offence (including murder) and persons convicted of any offence (excluding murder). In Magistrates' Court, applies to persons charged with, or convicted of, an imprisonable offence, if the Court is satisfied that they did the act, or the person consents.

Table 7.5b Transfer of prisoners to hospital under the Mental Health Act 1983

Section	Situation	Medical signatories	Authority required	Psychiatric disorder and conditions specified in the Act	Effects of order
47[1]	Transfer to hospital of sentenced prisoner	Written evidence of two doctors	Secretary of State (Home Office)	(a) Mental illness or severe mental impairment (b) Psychopathic disorder or mental impairment if treatment will alleviate or prevent deterioration. Bed must be available within 14 days	Detention in hospital as under S. 37. May be returned to prison when treatment no longer necessary. S. 47 expires at earliest date of release from prison, but if still in hospital, the patient is subject to a nominal S. 37
48[1]	Transfer to hospital of remanded prisoner[2]	Written evidence of two doctors	Secretary of State (Home Office)	Mental illness or severe mental impairment	Order may be terminated: (a) by trial (b) by report from RMO that treatment is no longer required or that no effective treatment can be given

1. Restriction order under S. 49 usually applies.
2. Applies to (a) those remanded in custody and charged with any offence; (b) civil prisoners; (c) those detained under the Immigration Act 1971.

as stealing cigarettes). When the patient has settled, transfer is arranged back to the referring district unit. These patients do not require lengthy treatment in the RSU, and the majority can return within weeks.

Assessment and treatment of remand cases

Under Section 35 of the Mental Health Act 1983 (see Table 7.5a), an offender is admitted to hospital, usually an RSU, or occasionally a special hospital for assessment. Section 35 patients are not included in the consent to treatment provisions of Part IV of the Mental Health Act (see Chapter 10); they cannot be given medication unless they consent to treatment. Therefore, it is important to anticipate problems that may occur at the decision-making stage, as an alternative, such as transfer under Section 48, may be more appropriate.

In some cases a forensic psychiatrist advises the court that a bail order with a condition of residence in hospital may be the most appropriate way of assessing a patient. This is a useful method of dealing with certain patients as there is no fixed time limit for the assessment. Again, such patients are informal, but providing that the decision is carefully considered, this may be a useful strategy. If the patient refuses to cooperate and asks to leave, the police must be informed that the patient intends to break the bail conditions.

Section 48 allows transfer of a remand prisoner in need of urgent treatment (see Table 7.5b). There has been a dramatic and welcome increase in the use of this section in recent years, the numbers quadrupling between 1989 and 1992. The courts are not involved but they should be made aware of such transfers. The clinician makes the assessment of urgency, and it is unlikely that the Home Office will prevent the transfer of a mentally ill prisoner to hospital. This section may be appropriate for mentally ill prisoners refusing food or fluids, the floridly ill, those unfit to plead, or following a serious attempt at suicide. The Home Office (C3 Division) can make rapid decisions if necessary, and a warrant can be issued within 24 hours to direct a prisoner to hospital, if Fax machines are available.

Section 36 is another method of admitting a remand prisoner to hospital for treatment, but the patient can only be treated on this section for a maximum of three months and the case must be heard at a Crown Court (see Table 7.5a).

Treatment of convicted offenders

Sections 38, 37, 41 and 47 are dealt with in detail elsewhere (Chapter 5). The patients who receive interim (Section 38) or hospital orders (Section 37) have often spent periods in a RSU under various remand sections. With hospital orders, clinical teams do not work to any tariff equivalent to the length of prison sentence the offender might have received. A discharge to the community from a Section 37 within days of the order being made is theoretically possible, but unlikely in practice. Probation orders with a condition of in-patient treatment are sometimes useful if in-patient stay is unlikely to be prolonged, and where medical and probation supervision in the community is important. Patients in this group are informal with regard to the Mental Health Act 1983, and can only receive treatment with their consent.

Discharge

The average length of stay in a RSU is from 6–9 months. The majority of RSU patients are discharged either to another psychiatric unit or to the community (home or hostel). A small number deemed dangerous may be transferred to special hospital, and some who are no longer mentally disordered may be transferred back to prison. Discharge plans need to be considered at an early stage of admission. If it is likely that the patient will be integrated within a local psychiatry service, the latter should be involved as early as possible. Patients should be enabled to use a degree of freedom, using hospital leave (see below), before being discharged to out-patient follow-up or transferred to an open psychiatric unit.

A careful discharge plan is necessary if the patient is to be followed up by the community forensic psychiatry service. A high standard of aftercare is essential in forensic psychiatric practice. It may be crucial in preventing, or reducing the seriousness of, relapse, and in averting further offending. Aftercare must have regard for the full range of the patient's needs (see Box 7.3). Most forensic psychiatry services make use of ordinary community facilities, but a few have developed drop-in centres and flats supported by the community forensic psychiatry service exclusively for the use of "forensic" patients.

The Department of Health has announced various initiatives in relation to the aftercare of discharged psychiatric patients. These are summarised in Table 7.6 and are discussed further in Chapter 8. To some extent they all flow from the care programme approach, which was designed to ensure that severely mentally ill people do not fall through what has been termed the "safety-net of care" (Kingdon, 1994).

Box 7.3 Factors to be considered in an aftercare programme

Accommodation with an appropriate level of support
Welfare benefits
Occupational activity
Social and recreational needs
Primary care for general health
Psychiatric care for mental health

Table 7.6 Department of Health initiatives for aftercare of the mentally ill

Aftercare	Requirements
Care programme approach	Requires assessment, review and coordination of care for all patients referred to psychiatric services
Section 117, Mental Health Act 1983	Requires health and local authorities to provide aftercare for all patients who have been detained in hospital
Care management	Requires social services departments to assess, review and coordinate care for the elderly, learning disabled, physically disabled, and mentally ill with social care needs
Supervised discharge	Proposed legislation to ensure that certain discharged patients comply with a treatment plan: failure will lead to a review and possibly recall to hospital
Supervision register	Requires all mental health providers to draw up and maintain a register of people with a severe mental illness (including personality disorder) at significant risk of serious violence, suicide or self-neglect

Community forensic psychiatry services

Community forensic psychiatry services are a more recent development than secure units. Forensic staff initially concentrated on the needs of in-patients and their follow-up after discharge. The term "community" is used in this section to include police cells, prisons and courts.

Staffing

Not all members of a multidisciplinary team are involved in the community forensic psychiatry service, which usually consists of medical staff, community forensic nurses, psychologists and forensic social workers. Patients are usually assessed first by a psychiatrist because of the latter's contacts with the various agencies of the criminal justice system. Other team members are involved as necessary in out-patient treatment.

Links with prisons

Community forensic psychiatry services rarely provide a regular service for all the prisons within each RHA, but appropriate staff will visit when required. Most consultant forensic psychiatrists hold regular clinics in the busier local prisons (containing remand prisoners), and work closely with the Health Care Service for Prisoners (see Chapter 9) to assess prisoners and prepare psychiatric court reports after referral by the courts or lawyers. In some cases a remand prisoner requires transfer to hospital for assessment and report (Section 35) or for treatment (Sections 36 or 48, see Tables 7.5a,b). Alternatively, if the prisoner requires treatment and it is reasonable to undertake this in prison, his or her progress may be monitored by a forensic psychiatrist during a regular (often weekly) session in a local prison. Convicted prisoners who may have been mentally ill during a prison sentence can be managed by "out-patient" prison clinic contact or by transfer to hospital (Section 47).

> **Case example 2**
> A male prisoner serving a long prison sentence for robbery, and who was not considered to be mentally ill at the time of sentencing, became disturbed and bizarre in manner. He described hearing the voice of a spirit and believed he had special powers of healing. He had an inappropriate affect and was thought-disordered. He lacked insight and refused to accept medication. He was assessed by a forensic psychiatry team who agreed to accept the prisoner in a RSU. Section 47 medical recommendations were completed by the prison medical officer and the visiting forensic psychiatrist, who offered a RSU bed. Schizophrenia was diagnosed in the RSU and the response to medication was good. The patient, who had a substantial term of his sentence to serve, wished to return to prison after some months in the RSU, and he agreed to continue with neuroleptic medication. The clinical team agreed and reported back to C3 division, which authorised the return to prison. In prison he was followed-up by a visiting forensic psychiatrist.

If one visits a prison on a regular basis it is usually possible to obtain a Home Office identity card which allows for easier passage in and out of the prison. Routine assessment of prisoners has to be done at a time that fits with the prison routine, usually mid-morning or mid-afternoon when prisoner movement can take place. Doctors may see prisoners in special areas or prison hospital interview rooms. Mealtimes and "lock up" times are usually periods when routine clinical work cannot be done. It is usual to contact a health care officer in the prison hospital centre to arrange a convenient time for assessment (see Chapter 9).

Links with courts and lawyers

Many magistrates' and Crown courts look to regional forensic psychiatry services for psychiatric reports. Sometimes cases are referred directly by solicitors for a report on criminal or civil matters. Defendants on bail are seen either at a hospital out-patient clinic or at clinics held in probation offices (see below). General psychiatrists are also involved in the preparation of reports, and may be in the best position to do so for patients already under their care. Mendelson (1992*a,b*) and Hosty *et al* (1994) describe the work of forensic psychiatrists in relation to court and solicitors referrals.

Court liaison and diversion schemes

There have been recent developments to improve liaison, particularly with the busy metropolitan magistrates courts (Blumenthal & Wessely, 1992). Some psychiatrists (Joseph & Potter, 1993*a,b*; Holloway & Shaw, 1993) have established regular clinics in a magistrates court. Offenders on minor charges are seen and assessed within the court building. If appropriate, immediate transfer to a local psychiatric service can be organised. The court either sentences leniently (e.g. by ordering the defendant to be bound over to keep the peace) or the Crown Prosecution Service discontinues charges. Of the 201 cases in Joseph & Potter's (1993*a*) study, 60% were diagnosed as suffering from a psychotic illness, 31 % were recommended for hospital admission and 38% for out-patient treatment. Ten per cent were admitted informally, 12% on a civil section and 9% on either Section 35 or Section 37. Holloway & Shaw (1993) followed up 22 patients diverted to the health care system. After 18 months, all but one of the ten patients admitted to hospital were still being followed up. Over half of those referred to local psychiatry out-patient clinics or other local services still had intermittent or regular contact.

Other services have used community forensic psychiatry nurses as the first-line assessors of cases arrested by the police and remanded overnight (Kennedy & Ward, 1992). Court liaison schemes may be organised and manned by personnel from the forensic or general psychiatric services depending on local geography, the needs of the local population and the range of facilities available. Box 7.4 summarises the common characteristics of patients diverted from custody.

Box 7.4   Characteristics of patients diverted from custody at the magistrates' courts

Predominantly single, homeless men

Recidivist offenders, charged with relatively minor offences such as theft and public order offences

Serious, chronic mental illness

Previous history of in-patient treatment, frequently as detained patients

All but a tiny minority requiring in-patient treatment are admitted to general psychiatry units, forensic services rarely being required.

Links with probation services

Community forensic psychiatry services work closely with the probation service by, for example, holding out-patient clinics in probation offices (Bowden, 1978; Collins *et al*, 1993). They also work with probation officers attached to the courts, prisons and probation hostels. Bail hostels may accommodate people who have mental health problems. Currently there is only one bail hostel facility (in Birmingham) within the criminal justice system specifically for mentally disordered offenders, but it is possible that more will eventually be established in order to prevent such offenders being remanded in prison solely for the purpose of obtaining a psychiatric report.

The usual point of contact between the community forensic psychiatry service and the probation service occurs when a psychiatrist is preparing a report for court on a defendant on whom a pre-sentence report (formerly called a social enquiry report) is being prepared. Liaison between both services and exchange of reports (with the agreement of the solicitor, if relevant) may lead to sentencing recommendations involving both agencies. A probation order can be made in the knowledge that voluntary psychiatric follow-up has been arranged. An offender may be seen by a psychiatrist (not necessarily a forensic psychiatrist) for out-patient treatment, for example, for an alcohol problem, drug abuse, or psycho-therapy. A forensic psychiatrist may choose to see these cases in a probation office to encourage close cooperation between the two agencies.

Alternatively, a court may include in a probation order a specific condition that an offender should submit to treatment by a psychiatrist. In 1991, 44 067 probation orders were made, of which only 903 had a treatment condition; 88% of these psychiatric probation orders were for out-patient treatment and the remainder for treatment in hospital. A written report by the psychiatrist recommending this disposal is necessary under Section 9 (and Schedule 1A) of the Criminal Justice Act 1991. These probation orders can be useful, but treatment cannot be forced upon an unwilling person in the community; attending appointments may be sufficient to show cooperation. Treatment conditions can be varied on application by the probation officer to the supervising court. Psychiatric probation orders appear to be used less often now, falling from 3.5% of the total disposals in 1981 to 0.02% in 1991. If appropriate, the probation officer may seek to establish a breach of the order; the offender is returned to court for sentencing to be reviewed.

Case example 3
A man with a history of recurrent bouts of mania set a number of fires during a relapse of his mental illness. During his remand in prison he accepted medication and improved rapidly, and it would have been inappropriate to keep him in hospital for a lengthy period. Similarly, a prison sentence would not have been reasonable. The

assessing psychiatrist thought that a brief admission followed by close supervision and control in the community was indicated. This was agreed by the probation officer and the court made a three-year probation order with a condition of treatment. After a short admission to a RSU he was discharged and followed up by the community service, and he remains well on lithium.

When a prisoner is released from a sentence on parole, a probation officer supervises the case. Here again a psychiatric treatment condition may be made, usually after the case has been considered by the parole board with the benefit of psychiatric reports. These cases are monitored in the same way as a probation order. Occasionally, people on parole or on probation whose mental state becomes a cause for concern may be referred to a forensic psychiatrist.

Links with the police

The police are the first point of contact between the criminal justice system and a mentally disordered offender. There are a range of relevant powers available to the police. For example, Section 136 of the Mental Health Act 1983 (which is described in Chapter 4) gives a constable authority to remove a person who is considered to be suffering from mental disorder from a public place to a place of safety, usually a hospital. Section 135 empowers a magistrate to authorise a constable to enter specified premises to remove to a place of safety a person believed to be mentally disordered. These cases usually involve general psychiatry rather than forensic psychiatry services. This also applies to those cases where it appears to the police (often in agreement with the Crown Prosecution Service) that a formal caution is more appropriate than bringing charges.

General psychiatry services are involved if a person in police custody requires voluntary treatment, or detention under civil powers in an ordinary hospital. A forensic service may be contacted if security is considered to be necessary, or if specialist advice is needed. Finally, if a mentally disordered person who has been charged remains in police custody for a lengthy period, there needs to be close cooperation between police and forensic psychiatry services. Police cells are not designed for long-term confinement, and are particularly unsuitable for the acutely mentally disturbed. The latter require rapid transfer to hospital.

Links with local psychiatric services

Forensic psychiatry provides a tertiary service, and receives referrals from general psychiatrists when patients cause concern because of violence, or because of behaviour which could lead to offending. Occasionally these patients are admitted to a RSU (see below), but changes in the patient's management and treatment may be recommended (Bond, 1989). Sometimes it may be appropriate for the community forensic psychiatry service to care for these patients and follow them up in the community. Before taking on the care of such a patient, it is wise to anticipate the problems that might occur in the future, being mindful that if the patient will require in-patient care, regional forensic services usually have access only to secure beds and rarely have day hospital facilities.

Follow-up of discharged in-patients

Some patients after discharge from a RSU are followed up in a 'parallel' way by the community forensic psychiatry service (Gunn, 1977) rather than 'integrated' back to local psychiatric services. The decision on whether a patient should be followed up by a forensic service is based on a number of factors (Box 7.5)

In some cases the decision on follow-up is made by the appropriate clinical teams. For restricted patients who are conditionally discharged, a named doctor and social supervisor must be agreed by the C3 Division (see Appendix). The doctor is usually a forensic psychiatrist who has been treating the patient in the RSU. The social supervisor may be a probation officer, or more usually a forensic social worker. Although it is never good practice for too many members of the community forensic team to become involved with a single patient, it may be necessary (for example, with a restricted conditionally discharged patient with schizophrenia) to involve the forensic community nurses who are able to monitor mental state at home and give depot neuroleptic medication. It is common practice for an emergency bed to be kept available in a RSU so that, if necessary, any community staff member can re-admit a deteriorating patient into the secure unit to prevent further violence or other offending. Follow-up in these cases needs to be long-term. Relapse, however long after the index offence, may result in repetition of harm to others, particularly if there is poor follow-up, or if the patient's care has been passed to a general psychiatry service which is only able to offer infrequent supervision by staff who may not appreciate the serious issues at stake.

Box 7.5 Factors favouring follow-up by forensic psychiatry services

More serious offence
Complex psychiatric disorder
History of poor compliance in the community
The need for close and intensive supervision
Legal status of the patient (subject to restriction order)

General adult psychiatry services

There is a group of patients with forensic histories who, for a variety of reasons, fail to maintain regular contact with local general psychiatry services. They drift between hospitals, prison and a precarious existence in the community. When they fall foul of the law they often report themselves to the police (Robertson, 1988) after committing minor offences of theft, non-payment for meals, or criminal damage. All general psychiatry services are asked from time to time to see such patients, who are often held on remand. As yet, only a small number of general psychiatrists have a special interest in, or responsibility for, mentally disordered offenders and for liaison with local criminal justice system agencies. Bowden (1975) showed that general psychiatry services without a locked ward or an intensive care facility were unlikely to admit offender patients. Such patients should generally be referred to local psychiatry services whenever possible.

If a mentally disordered offender is in prison on remand, then arrangements should be made for the psychiatrist providing the service from the offender's home area to visit the prison to assess the case. For homeless offenders there are guidelines to help identify the responsible local service (see Chapter 5).

It may be appropriate to inform the court that hospital out-patient follow-up has been arranged with the local psychiatrist. Occasionally, a probation order with a condition of psychiatric treatment may be a relevant disposal if arrangements have been made for local provision of the treatment. In cases where hospital treatment is necessary but there is no need for security, then admission should be arranged to an ordinary unit under a hospital order (Section 37). There are still some local services who object to admitting hospital order patients, even though there is no legal, administrative or clinical reason why this should be so. To support local services, it may be appropriate to admit initially to an RSU to demonstrate that there is no management problem, and then arrange transfer after a short time to the local unit. This model of cooperation is not found everywhere, and Coid (1988*a*,*b*) has described the problems in moving remanded mentally disordered offenders from a remand prison to appropriate local services.

The independent sector

There are now a number of independent or private hospitals offering an in-patient service for offender patients, but no aftercare. There are currently approximately 600 beds in the independent sector. The hospitals provide a particular treatment approach (e.g. St Andrews Hospital, Northampton, operates a token economy regime on a secure ward) or a service for parts of the country that have inadequate resources for offender patients. Some units cater for chronically ill and disturbed offenders (and non-offenders) who require long-term hospital care in conditions of low security and who do not meet RSU or special hospital admission criteria.

Services for other groups of mentally disordered offenders

Offenders with learning disabilities

The development of special services for offenders with learning disabilities has been uneven. In part this is because the majority of such offenders can be managed in the community under the supervision of ordinary learning disability services and local authority social services, or the probation service when relevant. In some places there are hostels run by the voluntary sector which offer services for this patient group. There is a further group who require in-patient treatment because of clinical need and other issues such as the nature of the offence, dangerousness, and likelihood of attracting a custodial sentence. In some cases, admission to an ordinary, open, learning disability in-patient unit may be adequate. However, in a number of regions, special units for offender patients have been opened by learning disability psychiatry services. Day (1988) described a unit with a moderate degree of security for male offenders, providing close nursing supervision, training in personal and practical skills, and a socialisation (token economy) programme.

Forensic psychiatrists are often involved in the assessment of defendants with a learning disability, particularly when a serious offence has been committed. Patients with a significant disability are not generally admitted to RSUs. Mildly learning disabled patients may occasionally be admitted, such as when a special hospital patient with a learning disability is considered ready for a move to a lower level of security. In some regional forensic psychiatry services, there are special units for patients with a learning disability. Finally, in the most serious cases where maximum security is necessary, a bed can be requested in a special hospital in the usual way.

Juvenile offenders

It is not possible to discuss this large topic in detail here. Those interested should turn to the review by Sheldrick (1990). However, any review, including this one, is likely to soon become out of date, since services for juvenile offenders are currently in a state of flux. Changing childcare philosophies and practices currently emphasised in a number of official inquiries, together with new legislation, bring about change in this area almost on a daily basis. The two most notable current influences are the Children Act 1989 (see also Chapter 10), which is the most important reform in childcare this century, and the Criminal Justice Act 1991 (Chapter 4).

Legislation

The most significant factor in the Children Act 1989 for juvenile offenders is the abolition of the care order on the basis of criminal offending. This has been replaced by a supervision order with specified activities, and may be used only where the young person has failed to respond to previous community-based disposals.

The Criminal Justice Act 1991 was intended to reduce remands in custody for young people by abolishing the old "unruly certificates", whereby a 15-year-old who was male, and charged with an offence which in the case of an adult would attract a custodial sentence of 14 years, could be remanded to prison. It is hoped that an increase in secure beds nationally will support the reduction and eventual abolition of this type of remand.

Young people convicted of grave or serious offences, excluding murder, may be dealt with by imposing a determinate order under Section 53 (ii) of the Children and Young Persons Act 1933. Those under 18 years of age convicted of murder are detained on the indeterminate order Section 53(i). Young people receiving these orders can be held in secure accommodation, youth treatment centres, young offenders institutions, and even prison depending on age, need and availability of resources.

Young people who are persistent absconders and who are at risk of significant harm may be detained in secure accommodation under Section 25 (1) of the Children Act 1989. However, before such an order may be applied for, the young person must either be subject to a full care order, accommodated by the local authority, or remanded into care by the courts.

Services

While current emphasis is on placing juvenile offenders in the community via juvenile justice teams, there are still more applications for secure beds than there are beds available. The availability of places for disordered adolescents in health or social services units is patchy. There is clearly a case for more effective coordination between social services, health, justice and educational agencies, all of whom provide resources.

Social services provide a few community homes with education, although since the implementation of the Children Act there has been a reduction in the number of care places available. There are some establishments which have secure assessment and treatment units. Red Bank School and Aycliffe Centre for children (both in the North of England) are two well known examples; they admit juveniles via secure care legislation and Sections 53(i) and 53(ii). These establishments use the services of visiting adolescent forensic psychiatrists, general psychiatrists, and child and adolescent psychiatrists.

Youth treatment centres are directly managed by the Department of Health. Glenthorne, near Birmingham, is run on a social learning theory model. St Charles, Essex, uses a psychodynamic model. Both establishments are directed by psychologists.

In the NHS, there are two units for older adolescents (males only) at Ashworth Special Hospital. These patients are admitted under mental health legislation. There are some hospitals which admit disordered adolescents, but there is only one Regional Adolescent Forensic Service (in Manchester) which admits patients to a secure unit under mental health legislation, criminal legislation, and secure accommodation orders. The independent sector fills some of the gaps in health service provision. St Andrew's Hospital, Northampton, has two units operating a behavioural treatment programme for young offenders, one for youngsters of normal intelligence, and the other for borderline or mildly learning disabled offenders.

Finally, there are resources in the prison system. Those youths aged from 15–18 years who enter the prison system are now placed in young offender institutions (YOIs) and, if on remand, are kept separate from adults in local prisons, or (in the case of 15 or 16-year-olds) on the hospital wing of a prison. YOIs receive some extremely disturbed offenders. Some YOIs make use of visiting forensic psychiatrists. In one or two institutions, such as Glen Parva YOI in Leicester, some individual and group work is undertaken. Aylesbury YOI has a role in the management of youths serving long sentences. There is further discussion of special facilities in prisons in Chapter 8.

Treatment

In-patient treatment in forensic psychiatry is little different from that in general psychiatry. The full range of treatment approaches are available, but there are some additional strategies which should be considered.

Ward programmes

RSUs have a daily ward programme for each patient, which is usually developed by occupational therapists and nursing staff in consultation with the patient. There is usually more therapeutic activity in an RSU than in a conventional in-patient unit. The programmes make use of all the facilities available on the unit (such as a gymnasium) and all staffing resources, including, for example,` sessional input from an art therapist or remedial teacher. The aim is not simply to occupy the patient, but to use this active multidisciplinary approach to focus on the patient's identified problem areas and to assist the assessment and treatment process. The ward programme complements the individual work undertaken by medical, psychology or nursing staff.

The use of security

Faulk (1985) has written an excellent review of security in psychiatric treatment. Security is provided through physical barriers and staff surveillance. District-based general psychiatry in-patient units can provide a degree of security, even without a locked area, by using psychological techniques, appropriate medication, close nursing care and supervision. However, a violent patient is not easily managed for any length of time on such units, particularly if they are inadequately staffed. There are no simple rules which determine when a patient should move from an open unit to a secure unit. The best philosophy is to try to manage the patient at the lowest level of physical security possible; this should depend on clinical need rather than service inadequacies. There should be consideration of the patient's level of violence and the identification, where possible, of contributory factors. Admission to secure hospitals should not occur because of matters such as low staffing levels or inadequate consideration of medication and other treatment approaches. Changes in management which might prevent transfer to a higher level of security should first be implemented.

> **Case example 4**
> An acutely psychotic patient in a district general hospital unit was violent towards patients and staff, and admission to an RSU was requested because the referring unit was unable to tolerate this behaviour any longer. The RSU assessment team suggested more vigorous treatment with medication. The patient was spitting out oral preparations and it had not been considered appropriate to prescribe regular antipsychotic intramuscular medication such as chlorpromazine. The RSU team suggested a longer acting depot preparation, which allowed the nursing staff to be less confrontational after the initial injection. The change in nursing roles lowered the patient's arousal and the general tension on the ward. The situation became manageable and transfer to the RSU was avoided.

Bond (1989) concluded from his study of patients rejected for admission to an RSU that the majority subsequently received appropriate treatment, and did not present any major management problem. When it is necessary, admission to a secure unit can be a paradoxically liberating experience. It may be possible to reduce the dose of neuroleptic medication. Nursing staff can be used to provide adequate observation, set limits and establish a therapeutic milieu, rather than being involved in giving medication on a regular basis as on the referring unit – a process which in itself can lead to confrontation.

Provision of a therapeutic milieu in a secure setting should be a matter of constant concern and regular review. It is easy for a unit to acquire a "snake-pit" atmosphere with inappropriate reliance on physical security and minimal attention to the individual needs of patients. Conversely, a unit can become excessively lax and permissive in its style. Both failings can have dire consequences for patients and staff. Secure units need to be well organised, yet flexible, with agreed objectives that are well understood by staff. Security can be effective without being pervasive and intrusive. The "atmosphere" of a secure unit is revealed partly by what it looks like, but also by how the staff behave towards the patients, towards each other and towards visitors. There is never room for complacency, and all units have scope for improvement. Staff working in secure units need a genuine sense of involvement and commitment. The most secure of units will become insecure when staff are inadequate, in quality or quantity, or if their principal agenda has little to do with caring for patients. Security should be an integral part of treatment. When security achieves primacy over treatment, institutional problems of the type that led to the Ashworth Inquiry are likely.

Case example 5

The RSU team was asked to assess a patient in a general psychiatric hospital with schizophrenia, who was described as extremely violent, but who was so heavily sedated when seen that he could not be interviewed. It was considered best to admit him to the RSU and to withdraw him from as much medication as possible. The cocktail of major and minor tranquillisers was rationalised. On interview with the patient it was clear that he was responding to the belief that radioactive rays were adversely affecting his body, and the main source of these rays were glasses worn by staff or patients. With this information a nursing strategy was set up which minimised the chance of his experiencing such phenomena. When settled he was transferred back to the referring hospital.

Specialling by nursing staff

Sometimes it is necessary in any in-patient unit to arrange for nursing staff to "special" a patient. This means that one or sometimes two nurses remain with the patient at all times, sometimes even in the bathroom or toilet. It is used to prevent violence or self-injury by very disturbed patients. Specialling is often used in RSUs but the benefits of such an intrusive approach must be balanced against the increase in tension that may result between staff and patient. An alternative strategy is to make use of any day areas, bedroom space, or exercise areas to remove patients into a less stimulating environment. This may be possible in secure units, which tend to have more flexible room space, as well as a secure perimeter, but there is no reason why it cannot also be implemented in an open ward.

Seclusion

Angold (1989) in his recent review said that very little is known about the overall use of seclusion in Britain, in what circumstances it is used, and its effectiveness in different groups of patient. From experience, it is rarely necessary in RSUs to put a patient in seclusion for any reason other than violence. Disturbed or disruptive behaviour, which may lead to seclusion in poorly staffed units, may be dealt with by other means.

All forensic units have specially designed secure rooms in which patients may remain for only a minimum period. Seclusion should be the last resort for the violent patient; sometimes it is necessary if further injury to staff or patients is to be avoided. The decision to place a patient in seclusion is often (in the acute situation) a nursing matter. Medical staff should be contacted at the earliest opportunity and should be involved in the care of such patients. Nursing and medical staff should regularly assess the patient while in seclusion. A joint plan is necessary in order to end seclusion at the earliest opportunity. The *Code of Practice* (Department of Health & Welsh Office, 1993) sets out the type of seclusion policy expected in the National Health Service. Many health care professionals and others who have contact with patients (i.e. the Mental Health Act Commission and MIND) now argue that seclusion has no place in modern psychiatry. Some RSUs, such as the Reaside Clinic in Birmingham, do not use seclusion; an intensive care ward, adequate staffing levels and high calibre staff enable the violent patient to be managed in other ways (Kennedy *et al*, 1994).

Control and restraint

Nursing staff in secure hospitals sometimes use physical restraint to help to control a patient's violent behaviour. The term "control and restraint" refers to a specific procedure in which a team of three nurses use physical intervention skills to restrain the patient (Tarbuck, 1992). RSUs and special hospitals run recognised training courses to teach not only the safe use of these skills, but also how to recognise and defuse potentially violent situations. Staff from other disciplines, including doctors, are encouraged to attend such courses. Alternatively, staff may attend the shorter "breakaway" courses designed to teach people how to disengage from violent situations.

Hospital leave

Hospital leave is the process of increasing a secure unit patient's freedom and responsibility, in order to test the improvement of mental state, behaviour and general level of cooperation in a gradual and careful way. Special hospitals and some RSUs use the term "parole" synonymously with "leave". This should be avoided since it creates confusion with the term as employed in the prison system, and is inappropriate in a hospital context. In RSUs, leave outside the unit starts with escorted (nursing) trips within the grounds of the hospital. If successful, time-limited or unlimited unescorted hospital leave is the next stage, followed by escorted leave outside the hospital, and finally full unescorted leave. The rate of the whole process depends on the patient's progress and the decision-making of the clinical teams in a hospital order case. Restriction order patients progress more slowly because of the required involvement of the Home Office through C3 Division.

While academics may argue about the inaccuracy of predictions of dangerousness, RSU clinical teams must wrestle with such matters in coming to decisions on leave (see also Chapter 8). They need to consider the risk that a patient may become aggressive, re-offend, or abscond on leave. The police and C3 Division (in the case of restricted patients) must be informed if a patient detained under the Mental Health Act absconds.

Psychotherapy

There are few psychotherapy services within the NHS with the special purpose of studying and treating offender patients. An exception is the Portman Clinic in London, which offers a psychoanalytical out-patient treatment service for adults, adolescents and children who have engaged in criminality or sexual deviation. There are a handful of psychotherapists working in forensic psychiatry. In special hospitals Cox (1983, 1990) has written widely, but little has yet been published by regional forensic services, even though some offer psychotherapeutic expertise to individual patients and groups. Because of the scarcity of psychotherapists in forensic work, it is necessary for those working in this field to acquire and develop practical skills (Gallwey, 1990) through experience based on a common-sense approach. Complicated treatments, without supervision or theoretical framework, must be avoided. Misguided psychodynamic or behavioural interpretations in personality disordered or psychotic patients can have dangerous consequences.

The commonest practical approach with in-patients and out-patients is counselling or supportive psychotherapy. Many forensic psychiatrists support a number of out-patients whose offending and general behaviour are positively influenced by regular sessions that give the patient the chance to vent his feelings in a safe environment. Because of the nature of forensic cases, it is often necessary to be more directive than is usual in psychotherapy. In selected cases it may be appropriate to undertake simple explorative or cognitive psychotherapy if supervision is available. Many regional forensic services provide treatment groups for in-patients, for those in the community, and even for prisoners (for example, sex offenders).

A general understanding of defence mechanisms, transference and countertransference issues is helpful in understanding, explaining and exploring interactions between staff and patients, and how this can lead to difficult management situations.

Finally, cognitive–behavioural treatment programmes are well developed in forensic in-patient units, partly because it is often behavioural problems that have led to the involvement of forensic psychiatry services. Consequently, forensic psychologists are skilled in the design and operation of these programmes, often supervising nursing and occupational therapy staff at ward level.

Physical treatments

The use of physical treatments in forensic psychiatry follows the same principles that apply to general psychiatry. Electroconvulsive therapy (ECT) and antipsychotic medication (particularly for psychotic and affective disorders) are used in accordance with accepted clinical and professional standards. In practice, because so many patients in forensic psychiatry suffer from chronic mental illness, it is prudent to observe certain guidelines (see Box 7.6).

Some of the most disturbed and difficult patients in psychiatry are managed in forensic settings. It does not automatically follow that they require heroic doses of antipsychotic medication. They do require careful assessment and management in properly resourced and appropriate facilities. Medication in forensic psychiatry has become a sensitive issue.

Box 7.6 Guidelines for use of medication in forensic psychiatry

Improve the quality of diagnosis and assessment by a period of drug-free observation

Gain familiarity with the use of a small range of preparations

Regularly review medication, and aim to use the minimum dose necessary to control symptoms

Be prepared to explain, repeatedly if necessary, the nature, purpose and effects of treatment and the implications of alternatives

Keep up to date with developments (e.g. the atypical antipsychotic preparations)

Be cautious in use of drugs of dependency (e.g. benzodiazepines and anticholinergics)

Avoid polypharmacy

Comply with legal requirements for consent to treatment

In selecting treatment, be mindful of the need for patient compliance after discharge

Follow the Royal College of Psychiatrists' consensus statement on high-dose antipsychotic medication (Thompson, 1994)

Sudden deaths have been attributed to antipsychotic medication and, with little supporting evidence, to the use of high doses. In addition, there have been a series of deaths of patients in Broadmoor Hospital in which the use of medication has been criticised (Ritchie, 1985; Special Hospitals Service Authority, 1993). In summary, physical treatments should be implemented in accordance with the highest professional standards. The use of antipsychotic medication is not a task to be left to unsupervised junior staff.

Management of violent patients

Nothing tests the skills of the staff of a forensic unit more decisively than the management of an acutely violent in-patient; weaknesses in training, experience, organisation, leadership and morale can be brutally exposed.

Box 7.7 Strategies for the management of violent in-patients

Organisational
- regular staff training in anticipating, avoiding and managing violence
- effective communication with patients
- regular clinical review

Nursing
- adequate staffing with proper skill mix and gender mix
- key (and associate) nurse system
- effective senior support

Medical
- forms part of the overall strategy
- high standards needed in the use of emergency medication

Psychological
- appropriate in individual cases

Physical
- restraint in accordance with professional standards
- control and restraint techniques only by trained staff
- breakaway techniques to disengage from violent situations
- seclusion only in exceptional circumstances, and in accordance with the *Code of Practice*

Monitoring and audit
- regular monitoring and scrutiny of violent incidents, type of intervention and outcome

Staff counselling
- debriefing and support after incidents

Research
- collection and analysis of national data

The task is one of great importance, yet it has attracted surprisingly little discussion. A working party of the Royal College of Psychiatrists is currently examining strategies in the safe management of violent patients. A multi-disciplinary approach is essential, and the aim should be to control the behaviour by the least restrictive means. Action should be taken to identify and minimise possible precipitants to violence. Adequately trained staff and other resources are essential. General measures can have a profound influence on patients' behaviour, such as the nature of the environment, a patient's daily programme, the availability of staff, and the contribution of specific disciplines within the multidisciplinary team.

In the best of units, and even with attention to all these matters, violence will occur. Strategies for dealing with violence have various components (see Box 7.7). It cannot be overemphasised that medication is one part of a variety of measures to be employed. The administration of parenteral medication to a resisting patient, and his immediate care thereafter, calls for the highest standards of skill and vigilance (Pilowsky, 1994). Pharmaco-kinetic changes in a highly aroused patient, who may have elevated cardiac output, can result in unusually high concentrations of drug reaching the brain. Cough reflexes may be impaired, with an increased risk of vomiting and regurgitation. For all these reasons a properly considered approach by trained and experienced staff is vital.

Role of the Department of Health and the Home Office

The relevant functions of the Department of Health and the Home Office are shown in Table 7.7.

Department of Health

In the Department of Health (DoH) the mental health section of the medical division has a responsibility for forensic psychiatry. Here, medical officers work alongside colleagues in the social services inspectorate, in nursing and the priority health service administrative divisions. The DoH no longer has any direct managerial responsibility for clinical services for adult mentally disordered offenders. Before the management reorganisation of the special hospitals in 1989, a unit within the old Department of Health and Social Security (DHSS) was responsible for administering the special hospitals. Now, the role of the DoH is to advise Ministers, monitor services, and develop policy in concert with the relevant sections of the Home Office. It was a joint committee of the Home Office and DHSS – the Butler Committee – whose report in 1975 led to the development of forensic psychiatry as a subspecialty (see Chapter 1).

Table 7.7 Functions of the Department of Health and the Home Office in relation to services and procedures involving mentally disordered offenders (MDO)

	Department of Health	Home Office (C3)
Advise ministers	Yes	Yes
Direct responsibility for patients	Manages youth treatment centres for juvenile offenders	Restricted patients (Sec. 41), Sec. 47, Sec. 48, CP (Insanity and Unfitness to Plead) Act 1991
Monitoring role	All health services involved in assessment and treatment of MDOs	Mental health and criminal legislation, and use made of these in diverting MDOs from the criminal justice system
Policy	Individually and jointly, the review of all services, mental health and criminal legislation leading to policy recommendations which involve both the NHS and the criminal justice system	

Reed Report

In 1990 a DoH and Home Office review of health and social services was established under the chairmanship of Dr John Reed. Much of the work was conducted through a series of advisory groups. Three initial groups were set up to look at services provided by the community, hospitals and prisons. Further advisory groups built on the work of these first working groups to focus on finance, staffing and training, research, and academic developments. The final summary report (DoH & Home Office, 1992) emphasised that mentally disordered offenders should receive care and treatment from health and social services rather than custodial care. The guiding principles of what has now become known as the Reed Report are shown in Box 7.8.

The Reed Report recommendations will be costly, even if implemented gradually. Eighty additional consultant forensic psychiatrist posts were recommended, with an even larger expansion of other consultant posts, all supported by additional training grade posts. An increase in the national target for medium secure unit beds was recommended, from 1000 places (the post-Butler Report target which has not yet been reached) to 1500, and that there should be some provision for those requiring long-term medium security. It was also recommended that in each health region there should be a forensic psychiatrist who takes on the role of regional

---

Box 7.8   Reed Report

The guiding principles state that mentally disordered offenders should be cared for:

- by health and social services
- with regard to the quality of care and proper attention to the needs of the individual
- as far as possible in the community, rather than in institutional settings
- under conditions of security no greater than is justified by the degree of danger they present to themselves or others
- in such a way as to maximise rehabilitation and their chances of sustaining an independent life
- as near as possible to their own homes or families, if they have them

---

forensic advisor, to coordinate hospital, community and other relevant services involved in the management of mentally disordered offenders, including the many agencies involved in the criminal justice system. There are indications of a cautious introduction by the Government of some of the Reed recommendations. It has allocated funding to increase the number of medium secure beds to 1200 by the year 1996. In addition, the review of services for mentally disordered offenders was extended to examine high security care and, separately, psychopathic disorder.

High security and related psychiatric provision

The Reed working group recommended sweeping changes in the way high security care is provided in England and Wales (Department of Health, 1994). It suggested that the services provided by the special hospitals should be delivered by geographically dispersed units, each catering for no more than 200 patients. There should be improved links with other relevant services. The report also called for improved standards and greater sensitivity to the needs of patients generally, and to women and those from ethnic minorities particularly. The Minister is examining the proposals, particularly those relating to new arrangements for funding and managing high security care.

Psychopathic disorder

A joint working group of the Department of Health and Home Office (1994), again under the chairmanship of Dr Reed, drew attention to the lack of knowledge about the nature, aetiology and treatment of psychopathic disorder. It acknowledged the major problems posed to the criminal justice system, to health and social services and to the community by this group of people. The report recommended that diverse service provision is necessary in a variety of settings, and that these should be properly evaluated. A new "hybrid" hospital order should be considered; it was suggested that it would provide courts with greater flexibility between punitive and therapeutic disposals for psychopathically disordered offenders. The Government has put the report out to relevant agencies for consultation.

Home Office

Two Home Office departments are relevant to forensic psychiatry, namely that dealing with the prison service, and the criminal policy department. The prison service is discussed elsewhere (Chapter 9), and only the criminal policy department will be considered here. One of three Ministers of State in the Home Office has responsibility for the criminal policy department. A division known as C3 in the criminal policy department has responsibility for all patients detained under restriction orders in hospital. In 1992 there were 2333 such cases (Home Office, 1994). This division also has responsibilities for a similar number of patients subject to formal supervision by a psychiatrist and a social worker/probation officer following conditional discharge from hospital. The 34 civil servants within C3 are divided into four teams, each responsible for a group of restricted patients determined alphabetically.

The restricted patients detained in hospital can be separated into five groups according to their legal classification (Table 7.8). Until 1990, the largest group was made up of patients admitted on a restriction order (Section 37/41), but more recently the largest group consists of transferred prisoners, especially remanded (Section 48), but also sentenced prisoners (Section 47). See Table 7.5 for an explanation of these sections.

Case files of all restricted patients held in C3 division include information from the court, the police and clinical teams. Permission for increased freedom for these patients is only granted by the Minister on the advice

Table 7.8 Restricted patients admitted to hospital by legal category (Home Office, 1994)

Legal category	1990	1992
Restricted hospital order	154	156
Transferred from prison before sentence	180	393
Transferred from prison after sentence	145	239
Recalled after conditional discharge	43	38
Unfit to plead or not guilty by reason of insanity	20	6

of C3 division which considers detailed written information submitted by the responsible medical officer (RMO). The Home Office issues notes of guidance to psychiatrists who have responsibility for restricted patients (Home Office & Department of Health and Social Security, 1987) (see Appendix). Direct telephone contact can be useful to clear up misunderstandings, or to help clinical teams direct their rehabilitative efforts in a way that will meet with Home Office approval. When restricted patients are conditionally discharged, C3 division requires regular reports from the medical and social work supervisors. If there is evidence of deterioration which could be a risk to others, the patient may be recalled to hospital by officers of C3 division, with or without the support of the supervisors.

Although there are no doctors in C3 division, the experience and expertise of the civil servants dealing with these difficult cases is immense. Their primary concern is the protection of the public, and from time to time their decisions may be influenced by prevailing attitudes to "law and order" issues. When the Home Office disagrees with, or is uncertain about, the recommendation of the RMO for a restricted patient's mental health review tribunal (see Chapter 10), an independent forensic psychiatrist may be instructed to interview the patient and report to C3 division; in this way the Home Office is able to give informed medical advice to the tribunal.

Finally, C3 also advises ministers, monitors the use of mental health and relevant criminal legislation, and develops policy initiatives.

Advisory Board on Restricted Patients

The Minister of State in the Home Office also has available the view of the Advisory Board on Restricted Patients, colloquially but incorrectly known as the Aarvold Board. A working party under the chairmanship of Judge Carl Aarvold was set up in 1972 by the then Home Secretary following the public outcry and reconviction of Graham Young. Some years before he had been convicted of poisoning, but was released from Broadmoor Hospital only to kill by poisoning within a few months. The recommendation of the Aarvold group was that an independent Advisory Board should be set up to give the Minister of State advice on cases where it is difficult to predict the likelihood of serious re-offending. Such cases are usually drawn to the Minister's attention by C3 division, but the formal decision to refer such cases to the Advisory Board rests with the Minister. The Advisory Board currently has two members from the legal profession, two forensic psychiatrists, a social services and probation representative and two additional members chosen for their experience in the criminal justice field. Often a member of the Board (not necessarily a doctor) will interview the patient in hospital. In 1993, a total of 48 cases were considered by the Board. A Mental Health Act category of psychopathic disorder will invariably lead to the case eventually being considered by the Advisory Board. This extra tier of decision-making may contribute to patients spending longer periods in hospital. The Minister will consider all of the information from C3 division and the Advisory Board before making a decision. In 1993, the Board supported the clinical team proposals in 75% of the cases reviewed.

Interrelationship of services

It will be apparent that the relationships between the services described above are highly complex. The interdependence of services are such that a change in the function of one will have a variety of knock-on effects. For example, before the development of RSUs there were few hospital services for offender patients. At that time there was much anecdotal information to suggest that many mentally disordered offenders were in prison because of what the Butler Committee called a "yawning gap" in psychiatric services. The situation was complicated further by the difficulties that the special hospitals were experiencing in trying to transfer patients to other hospital services, who were reluctant to take on this group of patients.

The effect of the Glancy and Butler reports (see Chapter 1) was to introduce regional forensic psychiatry services, with the result that services became more elaborate. Thus far, the evidence suggests that RSUs are filtering some cases that would previously have been admitted to the special hospitals. However, they have also become a bottleneck slowing up the transfer of these patients to lower levels of security. The Home Office and mental health review tribunals expect the transfer of special hospital patients to RSUs to be the first step to the community or other hospital units. Thus, patients from the special hospitals must compete with patients from prison, district general hospitals and the community for a limited number of RSU beds. Special hospital patients are often disadvantaged in this competition for beds because regional forensic psychiatry services must respond to the immediate needs of the courts, prisons and non-offenders who are acutely disturbed and in need of urgent hospital treatment.

Changes in the NHS over the last 10–15 years have led to a further shift in the provision of general services away from work with offenders. Snowden (1987) warned that developments in the field of community care could put RSUs under threat, by isolating them and turning them into locked mini-asylums, as they come under pressure to admit patients from general units who do not really require the security of a RSU, but whose needs are not met by local services. If this happens it will have a profound effect on the way RSUs are able to respond to offender patients who need secure care. However, problems may arise from another source. The policy of diversion from prisons to hospitals, with an increase in the transfer of unsentenced and convicted prisoners, will make it more difficult for patients from general units to be admitted to either RSUs or special hospitals.

There is now clearly a case for the development of continuing-care medium-secure beds for some mentally disordered offenders. Many of these patients are now to be found in the special hospitals, although the independent sector does also provide a service for this group of patients.

Changes in the prison service will also have an effect on hospital services. A review of the prison medical service by the Home Office (1990) suggested a radical solution, namely that prisons should purchase medical services from the NHS (see Chapter 9). An increase in staffing, beds and facilities in RSUs and even special hospitals will be necessary if this is to succeed. Service development in this field must embrace a wide view of the interrelationships described above. Unless this is done, the mistake will again be made of assuming that the system of dealing with mentally disordered offenders can be tinkered with in a piecemeal fashion. Changes in one agency, without regard for the possible effects elsewhere, will only aggravate the problems.

Acknowledgements

Photographs which constitute figures in this chapter are reproduced with the kind permission of the following: Fig. 7.1, General Manager of the State Hospital, Carstairs; Figs 7.2 and 7.3, Clinical Director of the Reaside Clinic, Birmingham.

Appendix

Summary of guidance issued by the Home Office and the Department of Health and Social Security for the multidisciplinary team at the discharging hospital when considering conditional discharge of a restricted patient (Home Office & DHSS, 1987)

(1) Preparation for discharge should begin as soon as such an outcome seems likely.

(2) The multidisciplinary clinical team should instigate an individual programme of treatment and rehabilitation and reach a common view about the patient's expected approximate length of stay.

(3) The hospital social work department should maintain links with outside individuals and agencies who may be able to offer support to the patient after discharge.

(4) The multidisciplinary team should have a clear idea of the arrangements in the community which will best suit the patient.

(5) The potential supervisors should be involved as early as possible in the multidisciplinary team's preparations for the patient's discharge, with an opportunity to attend a case conference and meet the patient.

(6) After the identification of supervision and aftercare arrangements best suited to the patient's needs, nominated members of the multidisciplinary team should be responsible for arranging the various elements to be provided.

(7) Where the choice of supervision between the probation service or the social services department is clear cut, a request for the nomination of an individual social supervisor, accompanied by information about the patient, should be made to the Chief Probation Officer or Director of Social Services, as appropriate.

(8) Where the choice of supervising agency is not clear cut or cannot be resolved quickly, information about the patient should be sent to both the Chief Probation Officer and the Director of Social Services with an invitation to send representatives to a case conference for discussion of the issue.

(9) The responsible medical officer, after consultation with the other members of the multidisciplinary team, is responsible for arranging psychiatric supervision by a local consultant psychiatrist.

(10) Responsibility for arranging suitable accommodation should be allocated by the multidisciplinary team to a named social worker or probation officer.

(11) The views of the multidisciplinary team should be taken into account and the question of accommodation discussed in a pre-discharge case conference, attended by psychiatric and social supervisors.

(12) It is important to identify suitable accommodation and to specify which types of accommodation would not be appropriate for individual patients.

(13) There should be no question of a patient going automatically to unsuitable accommodation simply because a place is available, and equal care is necessary whether the proposal for accommodation is to live with family or friends, or in lodgings or a hostel.

(14) A member of staff of a proposed hostel should meet the patient and discuss the patient's needs with hospital staff.

(15) The patient should visit and possibly spend a period of leave in a hostel before the decision is taken to accept an available place.

(16) The warden of the hostel should be given detailed information about the patient, including information which he may need about medication. He should be encouraged to contact the two supervisors and, if necessary, the social work department of the discharging hospital, for further information or advice.

(17) Certain written information about the patient should be sent by the hospital social work department to supervising and aftercare agencies upon admission, as soon as discharge is in view, and when nomination of a social supervisor is requested.

(18) Supervisors should receive comprehensive, accurate and up-to-date information about a patient before he is discharged to their supervision. A standard package of information should be provided to both social and psychiatric supervisors as soon as they have been nominated.

(19) Copies of supervisors' reports to the Home Office should be sent to the discharging hospital for a period of one year after discharge, generally for information.

(20) After the conditional discharge of a patient, supervisors may some-times seek information, guidance or support from those who know the

patient well. It is hoped that discharging hospitals will be able to respond helpfully to such requests.

References

Angold, A. (1989) Seclusion. *British Journal of Psychiatry*, **154**, 437–444.

Blumenthal, S. & Wessely, S. (1992) National survey of current arrangements for diversion from custody in England and Wales. *British Medical Journal*, **305**, 1322–1325.

Bond, M. (1989) Referrals to a new regional secure unit – what happens to patients refused admission? *Medicine, Science and the Law*, **29**, 329–332.

Bowden, P. (1975) Liberty and psychiatry. *British Medical Journal*, **ii**, 94–96.

—— (1978) A psychiatric clinic in a probation office. *British Journal of Psychiatry*, **133**, 448–451.

Bullard, H. & Bond, M. (1988) Secure units: why they are needed. *Medicine, Science and the Law*, **28**, 312–318.

Close, A. A. & Larkin, E. P. (1994) A survey of referrals to a special hospital (Rampton Hospital). *Psychiatric Bulletin*, **18**, 221–223.

Coid, J. (1988a) Mentally abnormal remands. I: Rejected or accepted by the National Health Service. *British Medical Journal*, **296**, 1779–1782.

—— (1988b) Mentally abnormal prisoners on remand. II: Comparison of services provided by Oxford and Wessex regions. *British Medical Journal*, 1783–1784.

Collins, P., Ball, H. & Costello, A. (1993) The psychiatric probation clinic. *Psychiatric Bulletin*, **17**, 145–146.

Cope, R. & Ndegwa, D. (1990) Ethnic differences in admission to a regional secure unit. *Journal of Forensic Psychiatry*, **1**, 365–378.

Cox, M. (1983) The contribution of dynamic psychotherapy to forensic psychiatry and vice versa. *International Journal of Law and Psychiatry*, **6**, 89–99.

—— (1990) Psychopathology and treatment of psychotic aggression. In *Principles and Practice of Forensic Psychiatry* (eds R. Bluglass & P. Bowden), pp. 1363–1374. Edinburgh: Churchill Livingstone.

Day, K. (1988) A hospital-based treatment programme for male mentally handicapped offenders. *British Journal of Psychiatry*, **153**, 635–644.

Dell, S. (1980) Transfer of special hospital patients to the NHS. *British Journal of Psychiatry*, **136**, 222–234.

Department of Health (1992) *Report of the Committee of Inquiry into Complaints about Ashworth Hospital.* Cm 2028-1-2. London: HMSO.

—— (1994) *Report of the Working Group on High Security and Related Psychiatric Provision.* London: DoH.

—— & Welsh Office (1993) *Code of Practice, Mental Health Act 1983.* London: HMSO.

—— & Home Office (1992) *Review of Health and Social Services for Mentally Disordered Offenders and Others Requiring Similar Services* (Reed Report). Cm 2088. London: HMSO.

—— & —— (1994) *Report of the Working Group on Psychopathic Disorder.* London: DoH & Home Office.

Faulk, M. (1985) Secure facilities in local psychiatric hospitals. In *Secure Provision. A Review of Special Services for the Mentally Ill and Mentally Handicapped in England and Wales* (ed. L. Gostin), pp. 69–83. London: Tavistock.

Gallwey, P. (1990) *Psychotherapy Training for Senior Registrars in Forensic Psychiatry: Notes of Guidance.* London: Forensic Psychiatry Specialist Advisory Committee, Royal College of Psychiatrists.

Gunn, J. (1977) Management of the mentally abnormal offender: integrated or parallel. *Proceedings of the Royal Society of Medicine*, **70**, 877–880.

Hamilton, J. (1990) Special hospitals and the state hospital. In *Principles and Practice of Forensic Psychiatry* (eds R. Bluglass & P. Bowden), pp. 1363–1374. Edinburgh: Churchill Livingstone.

Home Office (1990) *Report on an Efficiency Scrutiny of the Prison Medical Service.* London: HMSO.

—— (1994) *Statistics of Mentally Disordered Offenders in England and Wales 1992.* London: Home Office.

—— & Department of Health and Social Security (1987) *Mental Health Act 1983. Supervision and after-care of conditionally discharged restricted patients.* London: Home Office and DHSS.

Holloway, J. & Shaw, J. (1993) Providing a forensic psychiatry service to a magistrates' court: a follow up study. *Journal of Forensic Psychiatry*, **4**, 575–581.

Hosty, G., Cope, R. & Derham, C. (1994) 1000 forensic out-patients: A descriptive study, *Medicine, Science and the Law*, **34**, 243–246.

Joseph, P. L. A. & Potter, M. (1993a) Diversion from custody. I: Psychiatric assessment at the magistrates' court. *British Journal of Psychiatry*, **162**, 325–330.

—— & —— (1993b) Diversion from custody. II: Effect on hospital and prison resources. *British Journal of Psychiatry*, **162**, 330–334.

Kennedy, N. M. J. & Ward, M. (1992) Training aspects of the Birmingham Diversion Scheme. *Psychiatric Bulletin*, **16**, 630–631.

——, Hillis, J. A., Mawson, D. S., *et al* (1995) A retrospective analysis of violent incidents in a regional secure unit. *Medicine, Science and the Law* (in press).

Kingdon, D. (1994) Care Programme Approach. Recent Government policy and legislation. *Psychiatric Bulletin*, **18**, 68–70.

Mendelson, E. F. (1992a) A survey of practice at a regional forensic service: what do forensic psychiatrists do? I: Characteristics of cases and distribution of work. *British Journal of Psychiatry*, **160**, 769–772.

—— (1992b) A survey of practice at a regional forensic service: what do forensic psychiatrists do? II: Treatment, court reports and outcome. *British Journal of Psychiatry*, **160**, 773–776.

Pilowsky, L. (1994) The pharmacological management of aggressive behaviour. In *Violence and Health Care Professionals* (ed. T. Wykes), pp. 175–188. London: Chapman & Hall.

Ritchie, S. (1985) *Report to the Secretary of State for Social Services Concerning the Death of Mr Michael Martin at Broadmoor Hospital on 6 July 1984* (private circulation).

Robertson, G. (1988) Arrest patterns among mentally disordered offenders. *British Journal of Psychiatry*, **153**, 313–316.

Shaw, J., McKenna, J., Snowden, P., *et al* (1994) The North West Region. 1: Clinical features and placement needs of patients detained in special hospitals. 2: Patient Characteristics in the research panel's recommended placement groups. *Journal of Forensic Psychiatry*, **5**, 93–122.

Sheldrick, C. (1990) Treatment and facilities: child custody. In *Principles and Practice of Forensic Psychiatry* (eds R. Bluglass & P. Bowden), pp. 1041–1049. Edinburgh: Churchill Livingstone.

Smith, J., Parker, J. & Donovan, M. (1991) Female admissions to a regional secure unit. *Journal of Forensic Psychiatry*, **2**, 95–102.

Snowden, P. R. (1985) A survey of the regional secure unit programme. *British Journal of Psychiatry*, **147**, 499–507.

—— (1987) Regional secure units: arriving but under threat. *British Medical Journal*, **294**, 1310–1311.

—— (1990) Regional secure units and forensic services in England and Wales. In *Principles and Practice of Forensic Psychiatry* (eds R. Bluglass & P. Bowden), pp. 1375–1586. Edinburgh: Churchill Livingstone.

Special Hospitals Service Authority (1993) *Report on the Committee of Inquiry into the Death in Broadmoor Hospital of Orville Blackwood and a Review of the Death of Two Other Afro-Caribbean Patients – "Big, Black and Dangerous"*. London: HMSO.

Tarbuck, P. (1992) Use and abuse of control and restraint. *Nursing Standard*, **7**, 27–30.

Thompson, C. (1994) The use of high-dose antipsychotic medication. *British Journal of Psychiatry*, **164**, 448–458.

Treasaden, I. H. (1985) Current practice in regional interim secure units. In *Secure Provision: A Review of Special Services for the Mentally Ill and Mentally Handicapped in England and Wales* (ed. L. Gostin), pp. 176–207. London: Tavistock.

8 Dangerousness
Derek Chiswick

It may seem odd that a condition that cannot be accurately defined, reliably recognised or properly prevented earns a chapter to itself in a forensic psychiatry textbook. Social scientists, criminologists and lawyers agonise over the existence, validity and application of dangerousness. But for psychiatrists, dangerousness is no philosophical exercise; they are required every day to assess dangerousness in their patients, to plan treatment on the basis of their assessment, and to take responsibility for their decisions. Indeed, the topic has undergone something of a rebirth arising from public and political concern about violent behaviour by mentally ill people living in the community. The Government recently reminded psychiatrists of the need to consider the potential for dangerous behaviour when discharging patients from hospital (NHS Executive, 1994). However unfair it may seem, psychiatrists are stuck with dangerousness, and therefore a chapter devoted to it needs no apology.

Dangerousness in theory and in practice has been addressed from many different angles. There have been important reviews of the history (Foucault, 1978), philosophy (Bottoms, 1977), and legal implications (Baker, 1992) of dangerousness. The Butler Report (Home Office & Department of Health and Social Security, 1975) and the Floud Committee (Floud & Young, 1981) provide global reviews of dangerousness from a British perspective. In this chapter we will consider the concept and definitions of dangerousness, its relationship to psychiatric disorder, aspects of its prediction, some issues of law and public policy, and, most importantly, the practical role of psychiatrists in its assessment and management.

Concept and definitions

The word "dangerous" is an ordinary adjective of the English language and, in common with other adjectives like "generous" or "ugly", it cannot be medically defined. It does not depend on medical science for its definition. It is certainly not in the category of medical adjectives like "anaemic" or "hemiplegic", which can be defined in medical terms. It is not even a partly medical term, like "disabled" or "anxious". Hence, to invent a medical definition of dangerousness is a dubious exercise. It implies that dangerousness is a medical condition with a real existence; it reifies the concept into a biological entity which can then be declared either present or absent in a person. It has been elevated (mistakenly) to the status of a condition, and unfortunately there is now no turning back.

To define in scientific terms what is not a scientific entity is bound to be an exercise with limitations, but we can identify some common themes in the various attempts that have been made. Walker (1978) emphasises that the dangerousness of a person is an ascribed rather than an objective quality; what observers think about the person rather than what can be identified or measured in him. Thus a dangerous person is one who:

> "has indicated by word or deed that he is more likely than most people to do serious harm, or act in a way that is likely to result in serious harm." (Walker, 1978)

The Butler Committee defined defined dangerousness as:

> "a propensity to cause serious physical illness or lasting psychological harm." (Home Office & DHSS, 1975)

A problem with the "propensity" definition is that it implies a permanent and constantly exhibited characteristic like left-handedness or blue eyes. People who, for 24 hours a day, and in any situation, are likely to cause harm to others are extremely rare, but the Butler definition implies a concept of dangerousness as a somewhat freakish feature of character. Searching for people with "the propensity" is likely to be a fruitless exercise throwing up many false positives.

Scott (1977) made an important contribution to the dangerousness literature. His definition also suffers from the "propensity problem", although he used the word "tendency" instead:

> "an unpredictable and untreatable tendency to inflict or risk irreversible injury or destruction, or to induce others to do so."

Tidmarsh (1982) has pointed out that the degree of danger may not be reduced, even where the tendency described by Scott is predictable and treatable.

What emerges from these definitions is that dangerousness is about the perception by observers that, on the basis of what the subject has done or said, violent behaviour will result in the future. We make a judgment about what seems likely to happen, rather than what the person is. As Mullen (1984) rightly points out, dangerousness is a quality of an individual's actions rather than of the individual himself. The question psychiatrists need to pose in clinical practice is not "is this patient dangerous?" but rather "might this patient in certain circumstances behave in a dangerous way?" The latter question focuses the psychiatrist's attention on relevant clinical issues, whereas the former leads to a spot-the-propensity approach which is doomed to failure. Unfortunately, there is often pressure on psychiatrists to answer the wrong question. This arises particularly in court-room questioning, or where a "yes/no" statement must be made for statutory purposes (e.g. whether or not a patient meets criteria for a restriction order).

Finally in this section, we should emphasise that dangerousness has a contextual element. We have said that dangerousness is an ascribed quality of someone's acts or behaviour. Such behaviour does not occur in a vacuum; it would be difficult for a person who lived alone on a desert island to be dangerous. Dangerous behaviour, like any other, takes place within a context. In particular it requires a victim (usually) and a set of circumstances. Identification of these contextual factors is of great importance when we discuss the assessment of dangerousness.

Who is assessed and what are the implications?

Only a tiny and highly selected minority of the population is ever likely to be subjected to an assessment of dangerousness. Before leaving the concept and definition of dangerousness, we need to consider precisely who that tiny minority is, why they are selected for this assessment, and the implications of a positive assessment of dangerousness.

The concept of dangerousness is intimately related to the mentally ill and to people who have committed crimes of violence. It is not surprising that society should seek to identify dangerous mentally ill people and dangerous offenders so that it can curtail their freedom; it is a function of government to protect its citizens. This may be done under the guise of providing treatment or supervision, but the essential purpose is protection of the public. This is considered in more detail later in this chapter, but it is introduced here because it is fundamental to an appreciation of dangerousness.

In reality, locking up a few mentally ill people and violent offenders as a means of public protection has no impact on improving the safety of society generally. This is for two reasons. Firstly, violence is so ubiquitous in society that the extra protection afforded by incarcerating a few selected people is insignificant. Secondly, society faces dangers from many sources, often unexpected, that do not depend on the mentally ill or on violent offenders. The most obvious source is from dangerous drivers, but there are others, such as inadequate control of large crowds at major public events, or inadequate supervision of children on adventure holidays. There may be more danger from factory owners, shipping companies and construction firms who ignore safety regulations than there is from the mentally ill. But society has a fear of the mentally ill, and an expectation that violence by the previously violent should be preventable. Whether or not the concept of dangerousness as applied to the mentally ill actually achieves any significant public protection does not seem to matter. It is the perception of the problem that matters, and that is why psychiatrists are inevitably drawn into assessing dangerousness. It is, however, important that they do not exaggerate, either to themselves or to others, their role as protectors of public safety.

Finally, we need to consider the implications of assessing dangerousness for both patient and psychiatrist. A patient who is deemed dangerous will lose his liberty for longer than would otherwise apply. Discharge from hospital will depend on his satisfying others that he is no longer a danger, or at least that the danger can be contained. Proving that he is not a danger is difficult while he is detained in conditions of security. Psychiatrists should not underestimate the implications of a positive assessment of dangerousness. If he errs by detaining 20 patients for ten years longer than was really necessary, the fact is hardly likely to come to light or cause him professional harm, even though he is responsible for 200 years of unnecessary detention. Conversely, if he releases one patient who subsequently commits a violent crime, particularly a random attack on a stranger in the street, he will experience intense public opprobrium and professional scrutiny (Coid & Cordess, 1992). He is likely to face an inquiry, and even disciplinary proceedings or a civil action for professional negligence. Given this situation it is not surprising that psychiatrists err on the side of caution. The assessment of dangerousness inevitably depends not only on the skill and knowledge of the psychiatrist, but also his personal attributes, and in particular his confidence and stamina to cope with making difficult decisions.

Dangerousness and psychiatric disorder

An apparently simple question such as "are the mentally ill more dangerous than the non-mentally ill?" begs another dozen questions, and the answers to those will be hedged with qualifications. The most obvious problems concern the definition of terms (such as "mentally ill", "dangerous" and "violent") and the nature of the cohort under scrutiny. We can consider three questions:

(1) Does psychiatric disorder contribute significantly to dangerousness?
(2) What happens to "dangerous" patients after discharge?
(3) Are there any factors associated with dangerousness?

Does psychiatric disorder contribute significantly to dangerousness?

In an excellent review, Wessely & Taylor (1991) have critically examined what they call the "criminological and the psychiatric" views of crime and the mentally disordered; much of what follows is based on their analysis. The criminological view holds that the well established predictors of offending, such as economic deprivation, criminality in the family, poor parenting, school failure, hyperactivity or attention deficit disorder, and antisocial behaviour in childhood, are such powerful factors that they overshadow any effect due to mental illness. In essence, previous criminality predicts future criminality, whether or not the person is mentally ill.

Even data suggesting increased rates of criminality in discharged psychiatric patients in the US (Rabkin, 1979) may be explained in criminological terms. In particular, an increased rate of offending simply reflects the fact that more psychiatric patients with criminal records are in the community now than 30 years ago (Steadman *et al*, 1978). Thus what Wessely & Taylor (1991) call "artifacts" in the way offenders who may be mentally abnormal are processed by the criminal justice and mental health systems may account for any perceived association between mental illness and criminality, rather than an inherent feature of the illness. Other studies have found little association with mental illness (Sosowsky, 1978; Steadman *et al*, 1978) or only with personality disorder or substance abuse (Guze *et al*, 1974; Guze, 1976). In summary, the criminological view holds that social disadvantage operates as an aetiological factor in criminal behaviour by both the mentally ill and the non-mentally ill.

In contrast, psychiatric research has focused on rates of offending in cohorts of psychiatric patients before, during and after admission to hospital. Pre-admission violence of admitted patients is a common finding, particularly in association with schizophrenia (Johnstone *et al*, 1986; Humphreys *et al*, 1992). Studies, usually retrospective but some prospective, of in-patient populations show high rates of violence, particularly for patients with schizophrenia (Edwards *et al*, 1986; Noble & Rodger, 1989).

Follow-up studies of discharged patients have shown elevated rates of offending in mentally ill patients (Zitrin *et al*, 1976), but this may again be confounded by the factor of an increasing population of patients with criminal records finding their way into the community. Research in cohorts of unselected psychiatric in-patients points to an association between post-discharge violence and schizophrenia.

Perhaps the most interesting results come from large surveys of the general population. A community survey of 10 000 people in three American cities found that the presence of *any* psychiatric disorder was associated with assaultive behaviour, although rates were higher in those with alcohol and drug problems than in those with schizophrenia (Swanson *et al*, 1990).

Perhaps there is little more to be learned from research that compares violence at a particular time in cohorts of mentally ill people with that of controls, because of the rarity of mental illness compared with violent behaviour (Wessely & Taylor, 1991). Longitudinal studies of "criminal careers" over lengthy periods provide more useful data than a cross-sectional approach. Using this method, Lindquist & Allebeck (1990) found the risk of serious violence in schizophrenia to be four times that of normal controls. Similarly, Wessely *et al* (1994), in a longitudinal study of 538 cases of schizophrenia, found that men with this diagnosis were 3.8 times more likely to commit a violent offence than men with other mental disorders.

What happens to "dangerous" patients after discharge?

If there is an association between serious violence and psychiatric disorder, we should expect to find evidence of it in those patients discharged after receiving psychiatric treatment as a consequence of an offence, and particularly those patients subject to restriction orders and/or treated in a special hospital. Reconviction has been the usual outcome criterion to be investigated, but this measure is of limited validity (Robertson, 1989). Conviction requires negotiation of all the stages of the criminal justice system (see Chapter 4) and is likely to be an underestimate of violent behaviour of the cohort under scrutiny.

Walker & McCabe (1973) carried out an important survey of all hospital orders made over 12 months in 1963–1964. In a two year follow-up of 673 patients, they found 23 patients (3.4%) who committed subsequent acts of serious violence. However, a replication study with longer follow-up showed reoffending to have risen to 10% after five years, and 15% after seven years (Soothill *et al*, 1980).

On the basis of the then published research, Bowden (1981) suggested that up to 50% of patients leaving special hospitals are convicted of a subsequent offence, and approximately 10% of a serious offence. These estimates are broadly in accordance with research over the last decade (see Table 8.1). Longer periods of follow-up tend to show higher reconviction rates. Most cohorts have consisted of either all patients discharged, or only those going to the community. The single study (Cope & Ward, 1993) of 51 patients discharged to a regional secure unit (RSU) found the modal figure for serious offending but, surprisingly, no minor offending.

The question of how "dangerous" these former special hospital patients are can only be answered in relative terms. Clearly they are more dangerous than the public at large, but the rate of reoffending among conditionally discharged restriction order patients (most of whom will have come from ordinary hospitals or from RSUs) is almost identical with that found in life-sentenced prisoners released on parole. It is much lower than the average for all those released from prison (Home Office, 1993a). A 5-year follow-up of discharged restriction order patients and of life-sentenced prisoners found that, in both groups, about 25% reoffended and about 5% committed a grave offence (Murray, 1989). In selected groups of prisoners the reoffence rate is much higher. In a 10-year follow-up study of prisoners released from Grendon Underwood (see Chapter 9), Robertson & Gunn (1987) found an

Table 8.1　Patients discharged from special hospitals:
reconviction studies

Author	Cohort	Cohort size	Period of follow-up (years)	Reconviction rate	
				all	serious
Norris (1984)	All discharges	588 M	4–8	20%	9%
Tennent & Way (1984)	All discharges	617 M	12–17	55%	21%
Black (1982)	Patients discharged to community	128 M	5	39%	10%
Home Office (1988)	Restricted patients conditionally discharged	496	5	27%	6%
Bailey & MacCulloch (1992*b*)	Patients discharged to community	112 M	0.5–14	37%	17%
Cope & Ward (1993)	Patients transferred to RSU	38 M 13 F	0.5–10	11%	11%

overall reconviction rate of 92% and a serious offending rate of 20%. Approximately 10% of released life-sentenced prisoners and of conditionally discharged patients are recalled within two years (Home Office, 1993*a*).

Are there any factors associated with dangerousness?

In all research on future violence by the previously-violent, whether or not there is a psychiatric disorder, one factor has primacy as a statistical predictor, namely previous similar behaviour. In a review of studies of discharged special hospital patients, Murray (1989) also identified younger age, shorter length of stay, and absolute (as distinct from conditional) discharge as correlates of subsequent reoffending (see Box 8.1). Murray based his review on studies completed in the 1970s and 1980s. However, in the last decade or so the special hospital admission population has been changing, and so too has the manner of discharge (Home Office,

---

Box 8.1 Correlates of reoffending in patients leaving special hospitals (based on Murray, 1989)

Previous offending: Type and quantity of previous offending are the most powerful predictors of future offending

Age: Younger age is the second strongest correlate for reoffending

Admission offence: Property offenders are most likely to reoffend, violent offenders more likely to reoffend with violence, and homicidal offenders (particularly of "known" victim) are less likely to reoffend than other violent offenders

Length of stay in hospital: Shorter length of stay is associated with greater likelihood of reoffending, but may be confounded by the influence of age

Mode of discharge and aftercare: Less reoffending occurs with conditional discharge than with absolute discharge, and in transfer to another hospital or RSU rather than direct to the community

Psychiatric diagnosis: More offending occurs in psychopathic disorder than in other mental illnesses

Alcohol/drug abuse: Not extensively researched, but probably increases likelihood of reoffending

Ethnic group: In studies this is not clearly separated from socio-economic disadvantage

Employment, family stability, education and intelligence: Unemployed status, an unstable family background and poor education/low intelligence are generally associated with reoffending, but there are few data on discharged special hospital patients

Personality profiles: No unidimensional profile correlates with reoffending but over-controlled psychopaths are more likely to commit acts of extreme aggression

---

1993*b*). The number of patients in the legal category of mental illness has increased, as has the proportion of discharges ordered by mental health review tribunals (MHRTs; not available to restricted patients before 1983).

An important series of recent studies of patients discharged from Park Lane (now Ashworth) Special Hospital has carefully examined the legal categories of the patients and their manner of discharge from maximum security (Bailey & MacCulloch, 1992*a,b*; MacCulloch & Bailey, 1993). These studies indicate that psychopathic disorder patients are reconvicted at twice the rate of other mentally ill patients, and that conditional discharge is associated with halving the reconviction rate in all legal categories. The researchers also found that discharge through a hospital was safer than directly to the community, and that long-term follow-up was important, since patients continued to offend long after discharge.

In summary, the features indicating poor prognosis for patients leaving maximum security include the previous criminal record, the legal category of psychopathic disorder, discharge directly to the community, and short periods of conditional discharge. Early signs of deterioration in mental state enable swift measures to be taken to prevent offending. In psychopathic disorder the first sign of deterioration may be the commission of a serious crime (Cope & Ward, 1993). The importance of the quality of aftercare in preventing relapse (but not always reoffending) cannot be overemphasised, and is taken up later in this chapter.

Finally, it is important to consider the particular clinical aspects of the various psychiatric disorders that are implicated in dangerous behaviour, and these are fully discussed in Chapter 3. Such considerations are particularly important in relation to schizophrenia, the commonest psychiatric illness encountered in forensic psychiatry. It is wrong to imagine that there is a dangerous form of schizophrenia which can be spotted at onset and, conversely, a non-dangerous form. Schizophrenia is a lifelong disorder with its own natural history. Whether or not there is violence depends on what Wessely & Taylor (1991) refer to as a continually changing interaction between the illness, the person and the environment. Mullen (1988) has pointed out that "the majority of violent offences occur in established schizophrenics who have drifted out of any ongoing care and supervision".

Aspects of prediction

Consideration of the prognosis of any disorder is an important part of medical practice. We use our knowledge of the natural history of a disease to give advice and information to patients and their relatives. However, few doctors would predict exactly when a particular disease might occur. While we know that being hypertensive, overweight and a smoker increase the likelihood of suffering a heart attack, it is impossible to say whether an attack will strike because other factors, some unknown and some unpredictable, also operate. In psychiatry the situation is even more difficult. Not only must psychiatrists have knowledge of disease process, but they are drawn into predicting the possibility of a certain behaviour taking place, namely an act of violence, at some unknown time in the future. Many feel that the prediction should never be made nor even the question put, but the questions *are* put, and answering them requires what Pollock (1990) calls "a balance between scientific integrity and social responsibility". This section essentially deals with "scientific integrity".

Predictions of violence: accuracy and methods

Research into the prediction of violence by psychiatrists has been extensively reviewed and summarised by Monahan (1984, 1993*a*). He identifies a shift in the nature of that research over the last 10–15 years, and describes three important conclusions which have been influential for many years. These are that:

(1) for every three patients detained by psychiatrists on the grounds of dangerousness, only one would subsequently commit a violent act
(2) the best predictors of violence for mentally disordered offenders (MDOs) are the same as those for offenders who are not mentally disordered (e.g. previous violence)
(3) diagnosis, severity of disorder and personality traits are the poorest predictors.

Much of the research has been on people released from conditions of maximum security. In the US, changes in law or a decision of the Supreme Court have sometimes led to the automatic release of large numbers of patients who had been detained on the grounds of dangerousness. These circumstances provide the setting for so-called "natural experiments", the most famous of which was that of the Baxstrom patients (Steadman & Cocozza, 1974). Johnnie Baxstrom was sentenced to imprisonment for assault in 1959. In 1966 he was transferred to the Dannemora State Hospital for the criminally insane and detained beyond 1961 when his prison sentence expired. In 1966 the Supreme Court upheld his appeal that his constitutional rights had been violated, and he was transferred to a civil mental hospital along with 966 similarly detained patients. Follow-up of the Baxstrom patients revealed much lower than anticipated rates of offending. Four years after transfer, 3% were detained in a prison or institution for the criminally insane; of the 246 patients who had by then reached the community, only two committed serious crimes of violence. There were similar findings from other institutions (Thornberry & Jacoby, 1979).

Psychiatric predictions have been criticised not only on the grounds of their inaccuracy. Special psychiatric expertise in this task, if it exists, should rely on special methods (i.e. not simply those of any other professional group). Psychiatric predictions should have higher interrater reliability, and be correct more often, than those made by others. Research findings do not support these expectations. Psychiatrists use the same information as other prediction-makers, and agreement between them is no greater than that, for example, between school teachers (Quinsey & Ambtman, 1979; Montandon & Harding, 1984).

Recent research

Monahan (1993a) emphasises that research in the last ten years has challenged the three conclusions described above, but that much of it is inconsistent. He draws attention to serious problems in conducting useful research in this area:

(1) *The nature of the cohort*: It is important to distinguish between diagnostic groups, between hospital and community-based samples, and according to whether or not community-based patients are receiving any support or treatment.

(2) *Inaccuracies in identifying whether violence occurs*: Much violence may be undetected or unreported, and allowance should be made for this.

(3) *Samples from which valid conclusions about diagnostic groups cannot be made*: Hospital-based samples may be subject to institutional suppression of violence (i.e. they are "artificially" less violent) while community samples often consist of patients who have been selected for discharge (i.e. they have reached the community *because* they are non-violent).

(4) *Lack of coordinated research effort*: There is a lack of coordination in the types of predictor variables (i.e. the characteristics that might predict violence and their measurement) and criterion variables (i.e. violence and its measurement). Much research is based on retrospective data collected in a non-standardised manner.

Clinical guidance

With this uncertain theoretical framework, how can psychiatrists maintain clinical integrity in their pronouncements on dangerousness? Pollock (1990) emphasises three principles which should underpin conclusions. Firstly, it is impossible to make any predictions in those who have not previously been violent. In the absence of previous violence the probability of future violence is simply equal to the base rate for violence in that particular society. Secondly, predictions must take into account individual characteristics and environmental or situational variables. This interplay of constitutional/psychiatric features with life circumstances is crucial. Thirdly, the extent to which violence is a constantly exhibited characteristic, or is only present in association with periods of illness, disorganisation, disinhibition or substance abuse should be examined. In other words, the assessment must be based on global considerations because of the multi-factorial nature of violent behaviour. The practical implications of carrying out the task are discussed later in this chapter.

Actuarial guidance

Faced with uncertain theory for predicting dangerousness, decision-makers have turned to actuarial methodology in the hope that it might fill the clinical void. An actuarial model depends on producing contingency tables which give a mathematical probability for the criterion variable (in this case "dangerousness"). The tables are only as good as the data on which they are based; they also require data from large populations. Unfortunately, in relation to dangerousness, the predictor variables and the criterion variables are so poorly defined that it is doubtful if any reliance can be placed on actuarial methods. They may be useful in presenting collective data and in providing information about classes of patients, but they provide no answers in an individual case.

Actuarial methods do, however, have the advantage of uniformity of application. For many years the system in the UK for assessing prisoners for parole (early release) has depended, in part, on a system of scoring the likelihood of reconviction (Nuttall *et al*, 1977). The score is based on 16 weighted variables (e.g. offence, previous offending and sentences, occupational and domestic status), but it does not enable conclusions to be drawn from any individual predictor variable.

Risk management

In recent years the term "risk management" has gained currency (Snowden, 1993), particularly in the context of a business-orientated health service. It is a term borrowed from the insurance industry to describe measures aimed at reducing expenditure on successful claims. It can be applied to any aspect of a hospital (e.g. the safety of its operating theatres or of its heating system) and also to clinical practice. It is, therefore, not a device for prediction but a systematic method of ensuring that risks are recognised in advance and reduced to a minimum. It should result in safe clinical practice, or at least exculpation from blame in the event of disaster. Monahan (1993*b*) has described five elements of risk containment on the basis of the Tarasoff judgment (see Chapter 12), but they have general applicability in forensic psychiatry (see Box 8.2).

One element of risk containment, namely risk assessment, is virtually synonymous with the assessment of dangerousness. However, the term "risk assessment" has a more modern ring to it, implies something systematic that can be monitored, and is very likely to become the favoured term in the future.

The case of Kim Kirkman

Sometimes the task of prediction is impossible and this is exemplified by the case of Kim Kirkman, a man who, after being detained in secure hospitals for 17 years, killed himself in prison while awaiting trial for the murder of a young woman (to which he had confessed). He was 35 years old at the time of his suicide. The murder occurred as Kirkman was being prepared for conditional discharge from a regional secure unit. The legal category for his detention was psychopathic disorder. An independent inquiry found that "Kirkman's dangerous behaviour could not be predicted, in the present state of knowledge" (West Midlands Regional Health Authority, 1991). The killing may have been attributable to aspects of

---

Box 8.2 Principles of risk containment (after Monahan, 1993*b*)

1. Risk assessment:
- become educated in risk assessment, current developments and the law
- review all records of current and previous treatment
- question patients and relevant others about violent acts
  and ideation
- communicate information about violence to relevant staff

2. Risk management:
- review treatment regularly, particularly in cases of concern
- seek opinions of experienced colleagues
- follow up lack of compliance with treatment

3. Documentation:
- record source, content and date of significant information
  on risk
- record content, reason and date of all actions to prevent
  violence

4. Policy:
- develop guidelines for handling risk and submit them to
  clinical and legal review
- educate staff in use of guidelines and audit
- have a method for ensuring compliance with guidelines
- ensure data collection for audit

5. Damage control:
- if disaster occurs, discourage public statements of
  responsibility
- do not tamper with records

Kirkman's personality or to a pre-existing sexual fetish. In either event, observation and assessment failed to reveal outward signs of abnormality at the material time. It is indeed in cases like this (as distinct from patients with a mental illness) where "we simply do not yet have the necessary theoretical and technological sophistication to make reliable clinical predictions based on personality assessment alone" (Pollock, 1990). This fact is probably responsible for much of the general criticism of the psychiatric prediction of dangerousness (Steadman,1983).

We must conclude that clinicians cannot rely upon instruments of proven scientific validity in their assessment of dangerousness. New research may help (Monahan & Steadman, 1994), but at present, psychiatrists must firstly ensure that the questions they are asked are appropriate, and secondly that the answers they give are derived from clinical and theoretical knowledge, drawing upon the results of relevant research .

Issues of law and public policy

There are four general measures which the state can apply to people it perceives as dangerous. It can:

(1) lock them up
(2) lock them up indefinitely
(3) apply special controls to them in the community
(4) execute them.

All four measures currently operate in the Western world, and generally with the assistance of psychiatrists. These measures are applied to the mentally ill and to criminals, and sometimes the distinction between the two groups is blurred. Indeed, Foucault, cited by Bowden (1985), identified the shared squalid conditions for the mad and the bad in 19th century Europe as the reason for society's common approach to both. The extent to which society invokes special measures for the dangerous waxes and wanes. The last quarter-century has seen a rekindling of legislative endeavours to control dangerous people, but it coincides with conflicting contemporary concerns such as consumerism and human rights (Bottoms, 1977; Campbell, 1985). Let us consider how the four measures listed above are applied to the mentally disordered.

"Locking them up"

This phrase is a somewhat emotive substitute for compulsory detention. The dual strands of, firstly, the presence of a mental disorder, and secondly, an undesirable consequence, underpins laws for compulsory hospitalisation in the US, but to a much lesser degree in the UK. Indeed, the Government has recently been at pains to point out that mentally disordered people do *not* need to constitute a danger or a risk (whether to themselves or others) in order to be detained – see Chapter 10 and the *Code of Practice* to the Mental Health Act 1983 (Department of Health & Welsh Office, 1993). Admission "in the interests of [the patient's] own health" will suffice. As for third parties, the 1983 Act simply specifies "the protection of other people" as sufficient grounds. Not so in the US, where most states include stringent criteria of "dangerousness", specifying, for example, that the patient is "likely in the near future to cause physical injury" (Monahan & Shar, 1989).

Locking them up indefinitely

Can an offender deemed dangerous be locked up for longer than another offender who has committed the same crime but is not deemed dangerous? The answer is "yes", if he is also mentally disordered, and "very rarely" if he is not. Indeed, the place of psychiatry in facilitating incarceration of dangerous MDOs in hospitals is of profound importance. Psychiatry may also assist in effecting the rare indefinite imprisonment of dangerous, but non-mentally disordered, offenders.

Indefinite detention of MDOs is achieved by the imposition of a court order restricting discharge under Section 41 of the Mental Health Act 1983 (see Chapter 5). It is applied "to protect the public from serious harm". Discharge of such patients is the responsibility of the government minister responsible for law and order (the Home Secretary), not the minister responsible for health matters. This arrangement survives from the days when Broadmoor Hospital (and the patients within it) were the responsibility of the long-since defunct Prison Commission. The hospital order with restrictions on discharge is the psychiatric life sentence; indeed, the Home Secretary also determines when life-sentenced prisoners are released. Yet the restriction order can be applied for any crime tried in a Crown court, and thus (theoretically) could be imposed for shoplifting. Moreover, it is applied at the discretion of the judge who, although he must hear oral medical evidence on the matter, is not obliged to accept it.

The question of whether psychiatrists should pronounce on the perceived dangerousness of non-mentally disordered offenders is a vexing one. They frequently do, and the result is often the only indefinite or indeterminate sentence available to the court, life imprisonment. This is mandatory for murder but is possible on a discretionary basis for certain other crimes such as manslaughter, attempted murder and rape. This use of psychiatrists to legitimise, on grounds of dangerousness, a punishment imposed for public protection should be deprecated – principally because the prediction of dangerousness is not a matter on which psychiatry can speak with confidence.

Preventive detention (the life sentence apart) has been abolished in the UK, but in various states of the US and in Canada, it flourishes under the general title "dangerous offender legislation". In essence, certain states recognise the "sexual psychopath" as a distinct category of sex offender. As a result they are sent to hospitals or prisons for treatment for an indefinite period. Sometimes treatment does not take place and the offender is simply detained. Sometimes treatment is provided but the sexual deviation remains unchanged. There has been a trend whereby legislation is enacted, repealed and then re-enacted according to public and political whim (Grubin & Prentky, 1993). Psychiatrists have a key role in operating this legislation, as they have in Canada in giving "dangerous offender testimony" (Rogers & Lynett, 1991).

Before leaving this section we should muse on the case of Garry David in Victoria, Australia (Parker, 1991). After committing a string of major violent crimes (none of which, by chance, resulted in death) he was due for release from a 15-year prison sentence in 1990. Public horror at this prospect was such that the Mental Health Act 1986 of Victoria was amended in order that his detention could continue. What cannot be achieved by the criminal law may, with the help of psychiatrists, be possible under mental health law.

Applying special controls in the community

In the same way as the distinction between treatment and incarceration may become blurred, so only a fine line may separate treatment and control in the community. There are five important community measures of relevance for dangerous patients.

(1) *Conditional discharge of restricted patients.* Legal control (or supervision) of dangerous MDOs in the community occurs when patients subject to restriction orders are conditionally discharged. They are required to reside at a place approved by the Home Secretary and to accept psychiatric and social supervision (see Chapter 7). Failure to comply with the conditions may lead to recall to hospital. The supervision is in some respects similar to that of life-sentenced prisoners released on licence, who are also liable to recall to custody.

(2) *Section 117, Mental Health Act 1983.* There is a statutory obligation for health authorities and social services authorities to provide, in cooperation with other agencies, aftercare for all patients who have been detained in hospital for treatment. Section 117 applies to patients in all categories of mental disorder.

(3) *Care programme approach.* Twice in recent years, a killing committed by a mentally ill person has prompted the government to introduce new measures for aftercare. The first of these was the "care programme approach" (CPA) introduced in 1991 in the wake of the killing of a social worker by Sharon Campbell (Department of Health and Social Security, 1988). (The second followed the homicide by Christopher Clunis which is discussed at the end of this chapter). The CPA is broader in its application than Section 117 and applies to all mentally ill patients who are considered for discharge, and also all those accepted for treatment by the specialist mental health services (Kingdon, 1994). In the latter group, only those with severe mental illness require a multidisciplinary assessment and review. The CPA requires:

(a) systematic assessment of health and social care needs
(b) a key worker to coordinate care
(c) a written care plan
(d) regular review
(e) consultation with users and carers.

(4) *Supervised discharge.* The Government intends to amend the Mental Health Act 1983 to include a power of supervised discharge; it is described in Chapter 10. It would apply to detained, but non-restricted, patients who would present a serious risk to their own health or safety, or to the safety of other people.

(5) *Supervision registers.* Since 1 April 1994, the Government has required all health authorities to ensure that provider units establish supervision registers of all people under the care of an NHS unit who are known to pose a significant risk of suicide, severe self-neglect, or serious violence to others (NHS Management Executive, 1994). It may include not only patients with a mental illness, but also those with a personality disorder, including psychopathic disorder. The supervision register is designed to ensure that:

(a) a care plan is provided and regularly reviewed
(b) contact with the patient is maintained
(c) a point of reference exists for relevant staff to make enquiries
(d) planning of resources for this group of patients is facilitated
(e) patients with the highest priority for care and follow-up can be identified.

It is one task to formulate policies to ensure better care for dangerous MDOs in the community, but quite another to allocate sufficient resources to see they are effected. Supervision registers have been criticised by the Royal College of Psychiatrists because of the perceived vagueness of the inclusion criteria, the failure to fund them separately, and their effects on civil liberties (Caldicott, 1994). The medicolegal implications of the registers are profound; psychiatrists may face allegations of professional negligence if a mishap occurs and it can be shown that the guidance on supervision registers was not followed (Harrison & Bartlett, 1994).

Execution

The ultimate sanction for the dangerous offender is execution. The death penalty has been re-introduced by many states in the US. In some states it is reserved for those considered to be dangerous and likely to repeat their offending (Dix, 1984). The involvement of psychiatrists in enabling the state to reach that conclusion is fundamental to the process. The ethical aspects of this practice are discussed in Chapter 12.

Psychiatric assessment of dangerousness

When?

All who work in psychiatry are required in their daily practice to make assessments of dangerousness. Decisions about admission to hospital, leave from the ward, access to sharp objects, supervision of a visit by or to relatives, and countless other day-to-day happenings, may depend on an explicit or implicit assessment of dangerousness. We are essentially making a decision about immediate and short-term management. Decision-making in these cases is the very stuff of in-patient psychiatric practice and, although very important, it is not within the remit of this chapter. Suffice it to say that it requires an effective and well-informed multidisciplinary staff working according to considered policies.

Psychiatrists are required to assess dangerousness, often as part of a wider assessment, in a variety of situations (see Box 8.3). An assessment of dangerousness should address the relevant issue at that particular time, and conclusions should be couched in terms of what is then under consideration. Global statements that a person is (or is not) dangerous should be avoided; they may be misunderstood and precipitate unwarranted action. It is better to identify any particular danger, such as in relationships with women, attitudes towards alcohol, or an inability to accept the need for continuing care.

How?

In the assessment of dangerousness there are no short cuts or trick questions which reveal the answer. The psychiatrist must employ a combination of good clinical skills, thoroughness, attention to detail, common sense, and the ability to step back and take a broad but balanced view. Sometimes

---

Box 8.3 Situations requiring psychiatric assessment of dangerousness

Need for compulsory admission (although "dangerousness" is not specified in the Mental Health Act 1983)
Advice to court concerning disposal of convicted person
Requirement for a restriction order (Section 41, Mental Health Act 1983)
An "incident" arising during the care of a patient
Transfer of an in-patient between different levels of security
Consideration of discharge from hospital
Psychiatric assessment of sentenced prisoner for parole purposes
Advice on management of prisoner

the task may appear impossible, in which case conclusions will necessarily be qualified. This is preferable to dogmatic but unsupported conclusions.

As indicated in Box 8.3, the assessment of dangerousness is usually in respect of a patient who has already behaved in a violent or threatening manner, whether or not this has lead to criminal proceedings. The examiner is looking to the possibility of further violent behaviour in the future. There are three essential steps in the process: (1) collect information; (2) examine the patient; and (3) ask yourself questions.

Collecting information

Information is available from a variety of sources. The most obvious is psychiatric case notes, but police reports and witnesses' statements are also invaluable. Tape recordings of the police interviews may also be helpful. It is unwise to rely on the patient's statement concerning the index behaviour. While he may say that he "just pushed her with the knife" in his hand, the post-mortem report may describe multiple stab wounds. Nursing reports are often more revealing than the medical entries. Interviews with relatives and/or close friends should always be sought. Letters from relatives and any copies of the patient's own correspondence can add a new perspective. Reports from schools, a list of previous convictions, and probation officers' and social workers' reports should be obtained. In short, the examiner must set aside time for a painstaking search of the written records; helpful data may sometimes emerge from unlikely sources. Discussions with staff currently involved with the patient will provide useful information beyond that contained in nursing records, which is sometimes stereotyped in quality.

Examining the patient

Careful clinical examination is essential. It is important to check the validity of the patient's account against other sources. Many factors change with time, and examination may require more than one interview. It is usually best to begin by taking a personal, developmental, social, occupational, medical and family history. In this way a picture of the patient is built up so that a contextual and situational background exists before moving on to discuss previous violent or offending behaviour. The basic material to be obtained is the same as in any psychiatric examination, but detailed enquiry about certain features is crucial (see Box 8.4)

An account of the index event (usually an offence) should give the patient a chance to explain how it came about; not simply what he did, but also what he was thinking, feeling, and perceiving at the time. What he did immediately after the event should also be covered. A full psycho-sexual history is nearly always relevant, as too is a detailed history of alcohol and substance abuse. For all these topics the examiner is paying attention not only to what the patient says, but also to what he reveals

---

Box 8.4   Crucial items in assessment of dangerousness

Index behaviour or event and its antecedents
Use of alcohol and other substances
Psychosexual behaviour and interests
Mental state examination
Attitude to treatment received

   and sometimes . . .
Special clinical tests (e.g. psychological testing, penile plethys-
   mography)

---

about his attitudes. This will be evident not only in the spoken word but by emotional state, posture and other aspects of non-verbal communication. The patient's attitude to treatment so far received is important, particularly when transfer to less secure conditions is under consideration.

Asking yourself questions

The triad of patient, circumstances and victim in the analysis of violent or offending behaviour is of the utmost importance (Scott, 1977). Therefore, after gathering information and examining the patient, a series of questions need to be asked about each of these in turn.

The patient
(1) *What is the nature of the psychiatric disorder and what is its relationship to the violence?*
   It is essential to make a psychiatric diagnosis, but it is also useful to construe the case in a multiaxial fashion. This need not require slavish adherence to DSM–IV criteria (American Psychiatric Association, 1994) but consists rather of itemising the relevant factors. For example:

Psychiatric disorders:	schizophrenia
	substance abuse (alcohol, anticholinergics)
Developmental disorders:	borderline intelligence
Physical conditions:	none
Situational factors:	hostile–dependent relationship with mother;
	defaulted from treatment

This approach encourages a broader view of the case and a more considered appraisal. It is unusual to meet a situation where a psychiatric disorder is the complete explanation for an offence. All violent behaviour occurs within a context, and the task is to tease out the contribution of various factors. Psychiatric disorder, when present, may contribute to an episode of violence on a hypothetical sliding scale of 0–10, rather than by absolute causation. Having said that, assessing the likelihood of future violence is usually more straightforward in patients with mental illness than in those with a psychopathic disorder or learning disability. Mental illness usually runs a predictable course compared with the vagaries of personality disorder. The task of prediction is easier when there is a close causal relationship between illness and behaviour (i.e. 8–10 on the "sliding scale"). The more tenuous the link between illness and behaviour, or the more fragile the diagnosis of an illness, then the more difficult the task.

(2) *Does the patient have any explanation for his index behaviour, and can he accept the psychiatrist's conceptual understanding of it?*

Here, we are essentially concerned with the patient's insight. This is a variable commodity; it is rarely an all-or-none matter and it varies over time. Some patients have a good understanding of the various factors that have contributed to their violence. Many, probably a majority, appear to get on with life after committing a serious offence, and in daily conversation may not seem greatly affected by what they have done. Such self-protective responses are understandable. However, patients who show denial or who remain blameful of others, or who appear completely indifferent to what has gone before, are worrying.

(3) *Has the disorder been modified by treatment, and is clinical change a matter of observation or speculation?*

Many psychotic offenders commit their offences while untreated, or inadequately treated, or even undiagnosed. A good clinical response to appropriate treatment clearly changes the whole picture. Sometimes, particularly with psychotic patients, the improvement is obvious from all aspects of the patient's behaviour. For a patient with personality disorder, improvement is much more difficult to identify in a reliable manner. Self-report as the only indicator of change is of questionable value.

(4) *To what extent does clinical improvement lessen the likelihood of further violence?*

What constitutes clinical improvement, and how it is measured, varies between patients. In patients with personality disorder emphasis is on improved interpersonal relations, stable day-to-day functioning and a willingness to engage in appropriate therapy. But whether, or by how much, improvement in these spheres reduces the likelihood of, say, sexual assault or fire-raising in the future may be difficult to establish.

(5) *Are there complicating factors in the form of premorbid personality, substance abuse or sexual psychopathology?*

Contributory factors to the index behaviour often take a long time to emerge and be appreciated by staff. When patients are treated in secure conditions, the opportunity for adverse personality factors, substance abuse or psychosexual pathology to manifest themselves may be limited. Information relating to these issues should always be further explored.

(6) *Is the patient's inner world accessible to staff, and do his actions match his words?*

It is difficult to be confident that risk can be properly managed in patients whose disorder prevents them from having any meaningful contact with the clinical team. Sometimes this will have to be accepted, but in general it is difficult to work confidently with a patient whose thoughts and emotions are not accessible to staff. Conversely, what the patient says about himself cannot always be taken at face value. It is crucial to be satisfied that the patient's deeds match his words.

(7) *Does he appreciate the need for continuing care, and what is his attitude towards his carers?*

This question is particularly important when considering a move to less secure care or to the community. There should be some indication that the patient accepts the next stage in his treatment as being necessary and appropriate and is willing to work with his carers. Some patients are so embittered, perhaps after years in a special hospital, that it is difficult for them to appear enthusiastic about any change. A good relationship with the prospective carers is essential so that any early signs of deterioration in mental state are likely to be noticed.

(8) *Is your impression of him shared by your colleagues?*

Bringing a fresh perspective on cases can be a valuable service, but it is worrying if the clinician regularly finds that his views are at odds with those of other experienced staff. Psychiatrists should endeavour to discuss difficult cases with colleagues. Peer group scrutiny is a valuable means of assessing one's own clinical judgment.

The circumstances

(1) *Did situational factors contribute to the index behaviour, can they be identified and have they been modified in the new situation?*

Identifying situational factors is important; it may be possible to modify them in any new environment to which the patient might move. Situational factors might include a previous failure to provide (or make use of) appropriate care, social isolation, a stormy relationship with a key person, or a lifestyle dominated by alcohol or drug misuse.

(2) *Will transfer to a new environment provide a style of care such that changes in the patient's mental condition will be noticed?*

Dangerousness may be greatly modified by the provision of good quality aftercare. Skill is required in identifying clinical change, so questions need to be asked about the ability of carers to identify significant signs of change. Sometimes there are serious conceptual differences in the attitudes of different professional groups; these may result in a failure to recognise changes in mental state. It is important that staff understand how deterioration in a patient's condition is likely to manifest itself.

(3) *If changes are observed, what is the likelihood of effective action following?*

If change or deterioration is noted, staff need to know what action to take. Dangerousness can often be ameliorated by early intervention.

Potential victims

(1) *Why was the original victim involved?*

Victims of violent crimes committed by mentally disordered offenders are usually known to the offender; often the nature of the relationship plays an important part in that offence. It is therefore important to know whether the relationship issues have been addressed, whether the type of relationship is likely to be replicated in the future, and what understanding the patient has of these issues.

(2) *Is it possible to identify potential victims in advance, and are they aware of the patient's psychiatric condition?*

This question is of particular importance in patients who have committed a sexual offence or in whom a disorder of passion (e.g. pathological jealousy or over-possessiveness) has been present. The crucial issue is whether staff are likely to know of relationships which the patient may subsequently make. It is always worrying when staff learn only by chance that a patient has formed a significant sexual relationship. For those previously convicted of a sexual offence, all new sexual relationships should be regarded as significant.

(3) *Are potential victims likely to form pathological (or unhelpful) relationships with the patient, and would they seek professional advice if the need arose?*

Some patients form intense relationships and, sometimes by force of personality or by virtue of shared beliefs, conceal their psychiatric history from a partner or minimise its significance. A potential victim who has no effective means of communication with carers is at risk; some patients deliberately engineer such circumstances.

(4) *Are family members or other significant carers likely to support the need for continuing treatment?*

Families of patients vary enormously in their understanding and attitudes, particularly when a family member has been a previous victim. A therapeutic alliance with the patient's family can be a crucial factor in reducing dangerousness. Conversely, families who reinforce a patient's misguided view that he has "done his time", and has no requirement for aftercare, may be increasing the risk of relapse and dangerous behaviour.

Clinical judgment: bringing the strands together

Finally, all these strands (information, results of the examination and investigations, and answers to the questions posed above) must be brought together in what the Kirkman enquiry called "clinical judgment" (West Midlands Regional Health Authority, 1991). It is a fair term: there is no other measuring device available.

Examples

We can now consider some vignettes and make an assessment of dangerousness. They are necessarily abbreviated case histories.

Case example 1
A 34-year-old single man has been detained in a special hospital for eight years following the murder by stabbing of his mother. His family home was stable, and he showed good academic ability at school. However, his performance deteriorated at university; he began mis-using drugs, including amphetamines. There followed eight admissions to psychiatric hospitals with a diagnosis of schizophrenia; he often took his own discharge. He had delusional ideas that members of his family were in league with the National Front. He believed his family reported on him to that organisation.

He was often violent at home. He stabbed his mother during an argument; she was trying to persuade him to visit the family doctor for depot medication. He was initially found unfit to plead, and subsequently of diminished responsibility. In the special hospital his acute symptoms have responded well to depot medication. He accepts he was ill when he stabbed his mother, but does not consider he has schizophrenia. He resents continued medication. He is current-ly studying for an Open University degree. His father and siblings remain in contact but are anxious at the prospect of his discharge.

Task: Consider transfer to a regional secure unit. The diagnosis of schizophrenia is not in doubt. It was not properly treated before the index offence, and all his violence has been in association with the illness. He does not accept the diagnosis, but has a good relationship with staff. Violence is only likely were he to relapse when out of contact with psychia-tric services. Transfer to a regional secure unit poses little risk. The crucial issues are the quality of aftercare and his compliance with it when he is ready to leave the regional secure unit.

Case example 2

A 35-year-old single man has been detained at a special hospital for 18 years following conviction for two serious charges of indecent assault against two teenage girls upon whom he chanced on separate occasions. He came from a broken home; his father was an alcoholic recidivist. He was raised by foster parents. Aged seven, he was referred to a child guidance clinic for temper tantrums. He attended a school for maladjusted children. His full scale IQ is 85. Behavioural problems continued in his youth. He was excluded from attendance at an adult training centre because of his inappropriate sexual behaviour.

His natural parents remain in touch but cannot offer him a home. He has no other community support. In the special hospital he is somewhat disinhibited and engages in opportunistic sexual behaviour with other patients of either sex. His behaviour is otherwise acceptable.

Task: Consider transfer to inpatient unit of a district psychiatric service. He has a developmental disorder with a mild learning disability, significant emotional immaturity and continuing inappropriate sexual behaviour. There is a possibility of behavioural change in a new environment, but this seems unlikely after such a lengthy period in maximum security. There is no foreseeable prospect of his being suitable for a community placement. His opportunistic behaviour requires constant supervision, and it is doubtful if this could be maintained indefinitely within a district psychiatric service.

Case example 3

A 30-year-old single man with previous hospital admissions for a bipolar affective disorder has been admitted to a district general hospital (DGH) psychiatric unit under Section 3 of the Mental Health Act 1983 from a police station. Neighbours had called the police because of the disturbance coming from his flat; he had knocked down two walls in the house and said he was installing central heating using solar energy. His flat contained an assortment of axes and sledge hammers. In the previous month he had presented to his GP and a local casualty department and had been given some chlor-promazine; he had not taken any.

In the ward he was noisy, overbearing and threatening. He shouted at nurses that he had their addresses and if anyone touched him they would die. He said he would be going to the European Court because of staff brutality. Nursing staff said he was dangerous and unmanageable; they asked the doctor to send him to a secure unit.

Task: Consider transfer to a regional secure unit because of dangerousness. This is a newly admitted patient and the first priority is to establish, by usual clinical methods, a working diagnosis. In the absence of any organic features or evidence of substance abuse, a diagnosis of mania was made. He had defaulted from follow-up and earlier opportunities to admit him had not been taken. He is violent only when manic. He is now ill and untreated. The risk of violence is very real but short-term; it is likely to be ameliorated by appropriate treatment. He requires intensive psychiatric care by skilled staff, in a safe and well-organised environment; key issues are the resources available for his immediate management. He does not require security other than that necessary to prevent impulsive absconding. He does need a well-staffed unit where staff are confident of their capacity to administer antipsychotic medication, in spite of the patient's wishes to the contrary. Extra staff were deployed in the DGH unit, medication was initially given parenterally and his mental state had improved after seven days. Transfer to a regional secure unit was not necessary.

Case example 4

A 27-year-old man has served 12 years of a life sentence imposed when he was 15 for the murder of a 14-year-old girl. He had strangled her in a field and then inserted twigs in her vagina and mouth. A psychiatrist has been asked to provide a psychiatric report for a parole review.

The man was the oldest of three children in a stable middle-class family. He had no history of delinquency, contact with psychiatric services or substance abuse. He was of average academic ability, but had few friends at school. At the time of the murder he had never had a girlfriend or any sexual experience. He has progressed through his sentence without disciplinary problems. Early in his sentence he saw a psychiatrist monthly for one year; he had been referred by the prison medical officer in view of the nature of the crime. For two years he has been attending a college of further education two days weekly for a course in electrical engineering. His parents remain supportive and visit him regularly. He corresponds with a female pen-friend.

Task: Consider suitability for release on life licence. Collecting information about the offence and his pre-offence functioning is first necessary. Records of the previous psychiatric intervention in prison, and the observations of prison staff, should be reviewed. Examination of the prisoner should be unhurried. The crime is bizarre and the only explanation the prisoner can offer is that the girl laughed at him and he got angry with her. No evidence of psychiatric disorder nor of significant abnormalities in personality is found. Opinions about his current psychosexual attitudes, clearly a relevant issue, can only be based on his account. Information about his social functioning while at the college should be obtained. His plans for the future should be reviewed.

There emerges nothing to suggest premeditation of the crime, pathological sexual adjustment, or any preoccupations with violent themes. He seems to be more socially competent than he was 12 years ago, and his contrition for the crime seems genuine. He would live with his family and there are sensible proposals for aftercare. The psychiatrist concludes that:

(1) there is no evidence of any psychiatric disorder or psychosexual abnormalities; (2) there are no psychiatric factors which contraindicate a phased release programme leading to release on licence; and (3) there is no indication for psychiatric follow-up on release.

Case example 5

A 30-year-old man has been remanded to a regional secure unit under Section 35 of the Mental Health Act 1983. He had carried a knife into a Department of Social Security office. He shouted at a complete stranger that she was poisoning him, then grabbed her 3-year-old child and held the knife at the child's throat; there was no physical injury. He had three previous admissions to hospital with a diagnosis of schizophrenia; after discharge he had defaulted from follow-up on each occasion. In the regional secure unit he accepted treatment and his symptoms quickly improved.

Task: Consider appropriate recommendation to court. Full assessment confirms the diagnosis of schizophrenia. He carried the knife because of what he calls "system polluters", whom he believes wish him dead. On previous occasions after recovery he has lacked awareness of the nature of his illness, and has never accepted the need for medication in the community. He lives alone and leads an isolated life. He rarely attends an out-patient clinic, and when community psychiatric nurses call, he is either not in or refuses to answer the door.

He fulfils criteria for detention under a hospital order, but the question of an additional restriction order must be considered. His in-patient management presents no difficulties and when under treatment he does not warrant secure conditions. However, he lacks insight and without treatment he is at risk of committing further offences because he carries and has used a knife in a public place. A restriction order would enable him in due course to be conditionally discharged. This would require an appropriate package of care to be formulated, including a requirement of residence (perhaps in supported accommodation). In this way more effective psychiatric follow-up will be possible. The restriction order was recommended and imposed by the judge. Admission was to a regional secure unit during which attention was paid to the patient's social functioning and links were established with the community team.

Case example 6

A 25-year-old woman was discharged from a DGH psychiatric unit to hostel accommodation after an informal admission for six weeks. The diagnosis was schizophrenia. In hospital she had frequently returned to the unit drunk, and had been abusive to staff. The hostel was run on the principle of giving patients responsibility for themselves. She had declined oral or depot medication. Four weeks after her admission to the hostel she set fire to her bed. The DGH unit was reluctant to admit her on the grounds that she was non-cooperative.

A forensic psychiatrist was asked to see her at the local police station. She had not yet been charged with an offence.

Task: Appropriate advice to the police. The first task is to establish a diagnosis and the immediate clinical needs of the patient. On examination she was unkempt, hostile and abusive. She described the hostel staff as evil and made rambling disconnected statements about a "poisoned water system". Discussion with DGH staff confirmed that her conversation was difficult to follow throughout her prevous admission. A working diagnosis of schizophrenia was made, and the clinical view was that she required immediate admission to hospital. She was admitted under Section 3 of the Mental Health Act 1983 to the DGH unit, with one-to-one nursing care. Three days later she punched a nurse in the face and was urgently transferred to the RSU. Within the structured programme of the RSU, with limit-setting and appropriate depot neuroleptic medication, her condition gradually improved. After three months she was returned to the DGH unit for further management.

While she is acutely ill the emphasis should be on immediate care, and not on medium or long-term requirements. She had been inadequately treated in the DGH unit and her aftercare had been inappropriate for her needs. She had not received sustained treatment until her admission to the RSU. Hasty decisions about dangerousness should be avoided until her illness and its response to treatment can be assessed.

Conclusions

There is currently intense public and political concern with dangerous psychiatric patients; the task of assessing, treating and managing such patients, particularly in the long term, is not easy. Set against the large numbers of previously violent patients who are treated without mishap, incidents of major violence are rare. In 1992 the Royal College of Psychiatrists, together with the Department of Health, established a confidential inquiry into the:

> "circumstances leading up to and surrounding homicides and suicides by people under the care of, or recently discharged by, the specialist psychiatric services, to identify factors in the patients' management which may be related to the deaths, and to recommend measures designed to reduce such incidents".

There are between 600 and 700 homicides annually in England and Wales. The confidential inquiry identified 34 cases over 18 months in which there had been psychiatric contact with the offender in the 12 months before the killing. Most were out-patients; schizophrenia predominated among the men, and depressive disorders in the women. Clinicians caring for the patients regarded the homicides as unexpected and unpredictable (Steering Committee of the Confidential Inquiry into Homicides and Suicides by Mentally Ill People, 1994).

Need for effective aftercare

Throughout this chapter the place of good standards of aftercare in preventing violent behaviour by former patients has been emphasised. These issues have been tragically thrown into sharp focus by the killing on 17 December 1992 at a London underground station of Mr Jonathan Zito by Christopher Clunis, a man suffering from paranoid schizophrenia. The report of the inquiry into the care and treatment received by Clunis is a sombre but instructive read (North East and South East Thames Regional Health Authorities, 1994). Clunis had suffered from schizophrenia since 1986 and had almost continuous contact with agencies (medical, psychiatric, social services, housing, police, prison, courts) from then up to and including the day of the killing. All who came into contact with him recognised his illness and his dangerousness, yet this did not prevent him from stabbing a random member of the public waiting for a train at four o'clock one afternoon.

The Clunis inquiry reveals a mishmash of uncertainty, inadequate and uncoordinated services, poor communication, lack of knowledge, and misguided ideology, as contributory factors to the tragedy. Reference has been made earlier in this chapter to some of the Government's pronouncements concerning dangerous MDOs; there have been others concerning the generality of psychiatric care in the community (Burns, 1994; Coid, 1994*a*). Some see these pronouncements as a cynical manoeuvre to deflect blame on to those who are asked to take responsibility for dangerous patients in what is an inappropriately resourced and under-funded service. Prolonged institutional care for Christopher Clunis, and patients like him, has all but disappeared in London and other parts of Britain in the drive towards community care (Coid, 1994*b*).

The safe management of previously violent patients in the community requires careful, well-organised and well-resourced clinical services working in harmony with other agencies. These essential elements may need to be in place before psychiatrists can show the confidence, commitment and assertive approach that is necessary for the safe care of dangerous patients in the community.

References

American Psychiatric Association (1994) *Diagnostic and Statistical Manual of Mental Disorders* (4th edn)(DSM–IV). Washington, DC: APA.

Bailey, J. & MacCulloch, M. (1992*a*) Characteristics of 112 cases discharged directly to the community from a new special hospital and some comparisons of performance. *Journal of Forensic Psychiatry*, **3**, 91–112.

—— & —— (1992*b*) Patterns of reconviction in patients discharged directly to the community from a special hospital: implications for aftercare. *Journal of Forensic Psychiatry*, **3**, 445–461.

Baker, E. (1992) Dangerousness. The neglected gaoler: disorder and risk under the Mental Health Act 1983. *Journal of Forensic Psychiatry*, **3**, 31–52.

Black, D. A. (1982) A 5-year follow up of study of male patients discharged from Broadmoor hospital. In *Abnormal Offenders, Delinquency and the Criminal Justice System* (eds J. Gunn & D. P. Farrington), pp. 307–323. Chichester: John Wiley.

Bottoms, A. E. (1977) Reflections on the renaissance of dangerousness. *Howard League Journal of Penology*, **16**, 70–96.

Bowden, P. (1981) What happens to patients released from special hospitals? *British Journal of Psychiatry*, **138**, 340–354.

—— (1985) Psychiatry and dangerousness: a counter renaissance? In *Secure Provision: a Review of Special Services for the Mentally Ill and Mentally Handicapped in England and Wales* (ed. L. Gostin). London: Tavistock.

Burns, T. (1994) Mrs Bottomley's ten point plan. *Psychiatric Bulletin*, **18**, 129–130.

Caldicott, F. (1994) Supervision registers: the College's response. *Psychiatric Bulletin*, **18**, 385–388.

Campbell, R. J. (1985) Lessons for the future drawn from United States legislation and experience. In *Psychiatry, Human Rights and the Law* (eds M. Roth & R. Bluglass), pp. 43–57. Cambridge: Cambridge University Press.

Coid, J. (1994*a*) Failure in community care: psychiatry's dilemma. *British Medical Journal*, **308**, 805–806.

—— (1994*b*) The Christopher Clunis enquiry. *Psychiatric Bulletin*, **18**, 449–452.

—— & Cordess, C. (1992) Compulsory admission of dangerous psychopaths. *British Medical Journal*, **304**, 1581–1582.

Cope, R. & Ward, M. (1993) What happens to special hospital patients admitted to medium security? *Journal of Forensic Psychiatry*, **4**, 13–24.

Department of Health and Social Security (1988) *Report of the Committee of Inquiry into the Care and Aftercare of Miss Sharon Campbell.* Cm 440. London: HMSO.

Department of Health & Welsh Office (1993) *Code of Practice. Mental Health Act 1983.* London: HMSO.

Dix, G. E. (1984) Psychological abnormality and capital sentencing. *International Journal of Law and Psychiatry*, **7**, 249–267.

Edwards, J. G., Jones, D., Reid, W. H., *et al* (1986) Physical assaults in a psychiatric unit of a general hospital. *American Journal of Psychiatry*, **145**, 1568–1571.

Floud, J. & Young, M. (1981) *Dangerousness and Criminal Justice.* London: Heinemann.

Foucault, M. (1978) About the concept of the "dangerous individual" in 19th-century legal psychiatry. *International Journal of Law and Psychiatry*, **1**, 1–18.

Grubin, D. & Prentky, R. (1993) Sexual psychopathy laws. *Criminal Behaviour and Mental Health*, **3**, 381–392.

Guze, S. B. (1976) *Criminality and Psychiatric Disorders.* Oxford: Oxford University Press.

——, Woodruff, R. A. & Clayton, P. J. (1974) Psychiatric disorders and criminality. *Journal of the American Medical Association*, **227**, 641–642.

Harrison, G. & Bartlett, P. (1994) Supervision registers for mentally ill people. *British Medical Journal*, **309**, 551–552.

Home Office (1988) *Reconvictions and Recalls of Mentally Disordered Offenders, 1986. Home Office Statistical Bulletin 9/88*. London: HMSO.

—— (1993*a*) *Life Licensees and Restricted Offenders Reconvictions: England and Wales 1990*. London: Governmental Statistical Service.

—— (1993*b*) *Statistics of Mentally Disordered Offenders, England and Wales 1991*. London: Government Statistical Service.

—— & Department of Health and Social Security (1975) *Report of the Committee on Mentally Abnormal Offenders* (Butler report). Cmnd 6244. London: HMSO.

Humphreys, M., Johnstone, E., MacMillan, F., *et al* (1992) Dangerous behaviour preceding first admissions for schizophrenia. *British Journal of Psychiatry*, **161**, 501–505.

Johnstone, E. C., Crow, T. J., Johnson, A. L., *et al* (1986) The Northwick Park study of first episodes of schizophrenia. I: presentation of the illness and problems relating to admission. *British Journal of Psychiatry*, **148**, 115–120.

Kingdon, D. (1994) Making care programming work. *Advances in Psychiatric Treatment*, **1**, 41–46.

Lindquist, P. & Allebeck, P. (1990) Schizophrenia and crime. A longitudinal follow-up of 644 schizophrenics in Stockholm. *British Journal of Psychiatry*, **157**, 345–350.

MacCulloch, M. & Bailey, J. (1993) Issues in the management and rehabilitation of patients in maximum secure hospitals. *Journal of Forensic Psychiatry*, **4**, 25–45.

Monahan, J. (1984) The prediction of violent behaviour: toward a second generation of theory and policy. *American Journal of Psychiatry*, **141**, 10–15.

—— (1993*a*) Dangerousness: an American perspective. In *Forensic Psychiatry: Clinical, Legal and Ethical Issues* (eds J. Gunn & P. J. Taylor). Oxford: Butterworth Heinemann.

—— (1993*b*) Limiting therapist exposure to Tarasoff liability: guidelines for risk containment. *American Psychologist*, **48**, 242–250.

—— & Shar, S. A. (1989) Dangerousness and commitment of the mentally disordered in the United States. *Schizophrenia Bulletin*, **15**, 541–553.

—— & Steadman, H. J. (1994) *Violence and Mental Disorder*. Chicago: Chicago University Press.

Montandon, C. & Harding, T. (1984) The reliability of dangerousness assessments: a decision making exercise. *British Journal of Psychiatry*, **144**, 149–155.

Mullen, P. E. (1984) Mental disorder and dangerousness. *Australian and New Zealand Journal of Psychiatry*, **18**, 8–17.

—— (1988) Violence and mental disorder. *British Journal of Hospital Medicine*, **40**, 460–463.

Murray, D. J. (1989) *Review of Research on Re-offending of Mentally Disordered Offenders. Research and Planning Unit Paper 55*. London: Home Office.

NHS Executive (1994) *Guidance on the Discharge of Mentally Disordered People from Hospital and their Continuing Care in the Community*. HSG(94)27. London: DoH.

NHS Management Executive (1994) *Introduction of Supervision Registers for Mentally Ill People from 1 April 1994*. HSG(94)5. London: DoH.

Noble, P. & Rodger, S. (1989) Violence by psychiatric inpatients. *British Journal of Psychiatry*, **155**, 384–390.

Norris, M. (1984) *Integration of Special Hospital Patients into the Community*. Aldershot: Gower.

North East Thames and South East Thames Regional Health Authorities (1994) *The

Report of the Inquiry into the Care and Treatment of Christopher Clunis. London: HMSO.

Nuttall, C. P., Barnard, E. E., Fowles, A. J., *et al* (1977) *Parole in England and Wales.* Home Office Research Study no. 38. London: Home Office.

Parker, N. (1991) The Garry David case. *Australian and New Zealand Journal of Psychiatry*, **25**, 371–374.

Pollock, N. L. (1990) Accounting for predictions of dangerousness. *International Journal of Law and Psychiatry*, **13**, 207–215.

Quinsey, V. L. & Ambtman, R. (1979) Variables affecting psychiatrists' and teachers' assessments of dangerousness of mentally ill offenders. *Journal of Consulting and Clinical Psychology*, **47**, 353–362.

Rabkin, J. G. (1979) Criminal behaviour of discharged mental patients: a critical appraisal of the research. *Psychological Bulletin*, **86**, 1–27.

Robertson, G. (1989) Treatment for offender patients: how should success be measured? *Medicine, Science and the Law*, **29**, 303–307.

—— & Gunn, J. (1987) A ten year follow up of men discharged from Grendon prison. *British Journal of Psychiatry*, **151**, 674–678.

Rogers, R. & Lynett, E. (1991) The role of Canadian psychiatry in dangerous offender testimony. *Canadian Journal of Psychiatry*, **36**, 79–84.

Scott, P. (1977) Assessing dangerousness in criminals. *British Journal of Psychiatry*, **131**, 127–142.

Snowden, P. (1993) Taking risks. *Journal of Forensic Psychiatry*, **4**, 198–200.

Soothill, K. L., Way, C. K. & Gibbens, T. C. N. (1980) Subsequent dangerousness among compulsory hospital patients. *British Journal of Criminology*, **20**, 289–295.

Sosowsky, L. (1978) Crime and violence amongst mental patients reconsidered in view of the new legal relationship between the state and the mentally ill. *American Journal of Psychiatry*, **135**, 33–42.

Steadman, H. J. (1983) Predicting dangerousness among the mentally ill: art, magic and science. *International Journal of Law and Psychiatry*, **6**, 381–390.

—— & Cocozza, J. (1974) *Careers of the Criminally Insane.* Lexington: Lexington Books.

——, —— & Melick, M.E. (1978) Explaining the increased arrest rate among mental patients: the changing clientele of state hospitals. *American Journal of Psychiatry*, **135**, 816–820.

Steering Committee of the Confidential Inquiry into Homicides and Suicides by Mentally Ill People (1994) *A Preliminary Report on Homicide.* London: Confidential Inquiry into Homicides and Suicides by Mentally Ill People.

Swanson, J. W., Holzer, C. E., Ganju, V. K., *et al* (1990) Violence and psychiatric disorder in the community: evidence from the epidemiologic catchment area surveys. *Hospital and Community Psychiatry*, **41**, 761–770.

Tennent, G. & Way, C. (1984) The English special hospital – a 12–17 year follow-up study: a comparison of violent and non-violent re-offenders and non-offenders. *Medicine, Science and the Law*, **24**, 81–91.

Thornberry, T. P. & Jacoby, J. E. (1979) The criminally insane. A community follow-up of mentally ill offenders. Chicago: Chicago University Press.

Tidmarsh, D. (1982) Implications from research studies. In *Dangerousness: Psychiatric Assessment and Management* (eds J. Hamilton & H. Freeman), pp. 12–20. Royal College of Psychiatrists Special Publication No.2. London: Gaskell.

Walker, N. (1978) Dangerous people. *International Journal of Law and Psychiatry*, 11, 37–50.
—— & McCabe, S. (1973) *Crime and Insanity in England, Vol. 2: New Solutions to Old Problems*. Edinburgh: Edinburgh University Press.
Wessely, S. & Taylor, P. J. (1991) Madness and crime: criminology versus psychiatry. *Criminal Behaviour and Mental Health*, 1, 193–228.
——, Castle, D., Douglas, A. J., *et al* (1994) The criminal careers of incident cases of schizophrenia. *Psychological Medicine*, 24, 483–502.
West Midlands Regional Health Authority (1991) *Report of the Panel of Inquiry Appointed by the West Midlands Regional Health Authority, South Birmingham Health Authority and the Special Hospitals Service Authority to Investigate the Case of Kim Kirkman*. Birmingham: West Midlands Regional Health Authority.
Zitrin, A., Hardesty, A. S., Burdock, E. M., *et al* (1976) Crime and violence among mental patients. *American Journal of Psychiatry*, 133, 142–149.

9 Psychiatry in prisons
Derek Chiswick & Enda Dooley

Historical development • Prison riots and the Woolf Inquiry • Types of prison • Health care in prisons • Prevalence of psychiatric disorder in prisons • Practical and ethical issues • Clinical issues • Early release • Special psychiatric facilities in prisons • Addendum on Scotland, Northern Ireland and the Republic of Ireland

---

The UK currently imprisons a greater proportion of its citizens than any European country with the exceptions of Austria and Turkey. Prisons are therefore important as social institutions and especially as a limb of the criminal justice system.

Prisons are relevant institutions for psychiatry for three principal reasons. Firstly, with approximately 130 000 people received per year and an average daily population of nearly 50 000, the likelihood that a significant number of prisoners will have a mental disorder is borne out by both practice and research. Sadly, the high prevalence of psychiatric disorder in prison populations may have much to do with the quality and quantity of psychiatric resources outside prisons.

Secondly, the social punishment of imprisonment brings with it physical and mental punishment. Thus being in prison may contribute to the development of a mental disorder or to aggravation of a pre-existing psychiatric disorder. In either event, prisoners show a high prevalence of reported psychiatric symptoms.

Thirdly, decisions need to be taken about the time of release for certain prisoners, and psychiatrists may have a part to play in those decisions.

This chapter contains a brief historical review of prisons, discussion of what has been described as the current "crisis" in the British prison system, a description of healthcare services for prisoners, and analysis of the prevalence of psychiatric disorders in prison populations. We also consider the role of the prison psychiatrist and some particular clinical issues, such as suicide and self-harm, HIV and AIDS, and sex offenders. The parole system and prison units which provide a treatment setting are also described.

Historical development

The historical development of prisons in Britain helps us to understand their problems today. Many prisons currently in use date from the expansionist period of prison building in the late 19th century. Prison was intended to be punitive; solitary confinement, rules of silence and hard labour were the norm. There were two types of prisons. Firstly, local prisons (the term continues in use) served the locality and took prisoners serving sentences of less than two years. They were the responsibility of local justices of the peace and councillors. Secondly, convict prisons contained those serving in excess of two years and indeterminate sentences of penal servitude. Convict prisons were centrally administered.

Conditions, particularly in the local prisons, were scandalous, and the Prison Act of 1865 laid down rules which, although they were binding on local prison managers, were largely ignored. In 1877 the Prison Act brought about centralised control of prisons under the Home Secretary via a Board of Commissioners. However, public and political concern at prison conditions mounted, and in 1894 a departmental committee (the Gladstone Committee) was established. The pattern of scandal or crisis driving a review, to which there is a variable and often delayed response, is still a recurring feature of the British prison system.

The Gladstone Committee (Home Office, 1895) was of immense importance. It established reform and rehabilitation as the primary objectives of imprisonment. The importance of prisoners' welfare and the need for them to be properly occupied was a central tenet of the Gladstone Report; it contained the famous maxim that prisoners went to prison *as* punishment and not *for* punishment. The resulting Prison Act of 1898 required the introduction of prison rules which, with periodic revision, have persisted. However, the Prison Commission has not survived; it was abolished in 1963 when the Home Secretary, through the Prisons Department, took direct responsibility for prisons in England and Wales. In Scotland and Northern Ireland the respective Secretaries of State have similar responsibilities. The only local involvement in prisons is through local Boards of Visitors who act as "watchdogs" overseeing the treatment of prisoners.

In 1993 the Prison Service was given executive agency status, that is, it executes the policies laid down by the Home Office. Responsibility for running the prisons rests with the Prisons Board headed by a Director-General.

The prison population has undergone relentless expansion in the last 50 years while, over the same period, prison accommodation has remained much as it was in Victorian times. The result has been gross overcrowding, insanitary conditions and a lack of meaningful activity for many prisoners. Indeed, a committee of the Council of Europe (1991), known as the CPT, has said conditions in some British prisons amount to "inhuman and degrading treatment" (*Lancet*, 1991). Notions of reform and rehabilitation have been discarded (if indeed they were ever attainable) and overtaken by the need simply to contain, as humanely as possible, a prison population two to three times greater in size than the available accommodation.

Prison riots and the Woolf Inquiry

Riots in British prisons are nothing new, but on 1 April 1990 at Strangeways Prison, Manchester, there began the longest and most serious riot in the history of prisons in Britain. It lasted for 25 days, caused the death of one prisoner, injuries to another 47 and to 147 prison officers; the cost of the damage caused was in the region of £30 million. "Satellite" riots broke out in five other prisons, while another 30 experienced severe disruption. The riot was unique in receiving extensive "live" media coverage. For a while it seemed as though the Prisons Department at the Home Office had "lost control" of its prisons.

On the fifth day of the riot the Home Secretary announced the setting up of an independent and public inquiry by Lord Justice Woolf, a High Court judge. He was assisted by Judge Stephen Tumim, HM Chief Inspector of Prisons in England and Wales. The report of this inquiry (Home Office, 1991*a*) produced 12 core recommendations. Most importantly it called for:

(1) a "contract" for each prisoner setting out the prisoner's expectations and responsibilities
(2) a national system of accredited prison standards
(3) a public commitment from ministers regarding access to sanitation for inmates
(4) improved links for prisoners with their families and the community
(5) division of prisons into smaller units
(6) improved standards of justice within prisons for prisoners.

In relation to prisoners with psychiatric disorders, including learning disabilities, Woolf recommended that steps should be taken to minimise the number of such people in the prison service by diversion at the court stage to either hospital or hostel. Facilities for MDOs in prison should be improved. The report also recommended treatment facilities for sex offenders – specifically that a further prison similar to Grendon Underwood (see below) should be established – and that assistance should be provided to them to prevent re-offending. It called for improved facilities and services for prisoners with alcohol and drug problems, and for those with HIV infection.

The Government responded with *Custody, Care and Justice* (Home Office, 1991*b*), a glossy report long on generalisations and short on detail. Since then issues of management, privatisation of prisons and the new agency status of the service have drawn government attention away from conditions and standards (Player & Jenkins, 1994). The Woolf report engendered a wave of optimism that, following the crisis in British prisons, they would at last undergo radical change. The Government's response, and a rising prison population resulting from the Criminal Justice Act 1991, have dampened that optimism. Some radical changes are taking place, particularly with regard to prisoners' rights and a new spirit of openness. However, it is too soon to tell whether we will see a new era in British prison conditions (Tumim *et al*, 1993).

Types of prison

Prisons in England and Wales are categorised as local or training (including dispersal) prisons (see Box 9.1). All local prisons (e.g. Brixton and Wandsworth) are closed prisons. They hold people remanded in custody (i.e. awaiting trial or sentence), and in addition they may hold convicted prisoners serving less than two years. Training prisons are either closed (e.g. Long Lartin, Parkhurst and Wormwood Scrubs) or open (e.g. Ford and Kirkham). They should provide training for prisoners serving longer sentences. Security varies with the category of prisoner held. All prisoners are classified on the basis of a system proposed by the *Report of the Inquiry into Prison Escapes and Security* (Home Office, 1966). The system is based solely on security considerations. The highest category is "A" (requiring maximum security and subject to many restrictions) and the lowest is "D" (suitable for open conditions).

There are currently eight maximum security or "dispersal" prisons. These are organised and equipped to accommodate the most dangerous and high risk prisoners. In practice, a number of prisons have dual local and training functions. Prisons providing special psychiatric facilities are discussed later in this chapter.

Female prisoners are accommodated in separate local prisons (e.g. Holloway) and training prisons (e.g. Styal and Cookham Wood). Durham Prison provides a unit for women requiring special security. Some prisons for women (e.g. Holloway and Styal) contain mother and baby units.

Box 9.1 Types of prisons

Local prisons
- closed prisons only
- for people on remand (awaiting trial or sentence)
- may hold convicted prisoners serving less than two years
- service local courts on geographical basis

Training prisons
- may be open or closed
- for prisoners serving more than two years
- some are dispersal prisons for high security risk prisoners

---

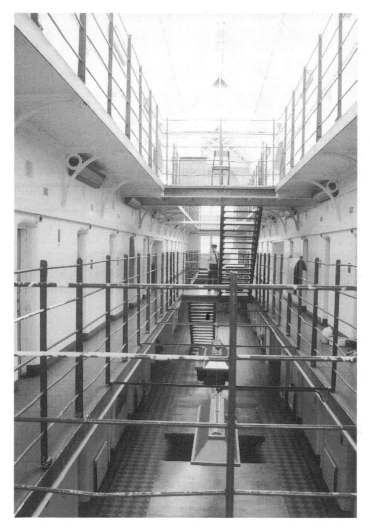

Fig. 9.1 Typical wing on three floors, HM Prison, Edinburgh.

Health care in prisons

For as long as there have been prisons, conditions in them and the health of inmates have given justifiable cause for concern. In 1777 John Howard, the great penal reformer and philanthropist, published his influential work *The State of the Prisons* (Howard, 1777), in which he described the appalling and insanitary conditions of English prisons. In 1779 the Act for Preserving the Health of Prisoners and Preventing the Gaol Distemper required all prisons to appoint a physician who had to report at the Quarter Sessions on the health of prisoners under his care (Ralli, 1994). Implementation of the 1779 Act was patchy because prisons were not then under central control.

1779–1877

The role of the prison doctor was first incorporated in prison rules in 1794 at Shrewsbury Prison (Gray, 1973). His duties required him to examine all prisoners upon admission and every prisoner at least weekly; he was also expected to "enquire into the state of his body and mind" and, after consultation with the chaplain, report adverse findings to the governor. In the 19th century the problem of mentally disturbed prisoners caused much concern. There was some transfer of prisoners to county asylums, but many remained in prisons, such as the one at Millbank, London, which had a medical superintendent. The Criminal Lunatic Asylum Act of 1860 paved the way for the opening of Broadmoor Hospital in 1863 under the management of the Home Office. It was not until the Prison Act of 1877 that central government responsibility for all prisons in England and Wales was established, and the same year marks the birth of the Prison Medical Service (PMS), the oldest civilian medical service.

The Prison Medical Service 1877–1992

The difficulties of delivering decent medical, including psychiatric, care to prisoners should never be underestimated. There is nothing novel about these difficulties. Prisons contain a captive population of people drawn largely, but not exclusively, from the disadvantaged, deprived and dispossessed in the community. Living conditions for prisoners are often appalling and probably beyond the belief of most people. Practising good medicine in an environment that is insanitary, overcrowded and dangerous is not easy.

Prisoners are isolated from society and are therefore vulnerable. The primary aim of the prison is custody of its inmates; institutional practices, rightly or wrongly, dominate the prisoners' day. Doctors therefore find themselves working in an environment whose principal task is not the delivery of medical care. These broad institutional themes are well-recognised as the breeding ground for bad practice, whether in children's homes, boarding schools, the military services, old people's homes or mental hospitals. In these settings the odds may be stacked heavily against doctors making any significant impact; indeed, it is easy for medical work to be substandard and for it to serve the needs of the institution rather than the patient. Thus most of the difficulties of the PMS were not entirely of its own making, and some doctors have made outstanding contributions.

Medical care in prisons is intimately linked with psychiatric care. In this brief review we can only identify important landmarks in the development of psychiatric care in prisons; fuller historical accounts of prison medicine are provided by Gray (1973), Smith (1984) and Ralli (1994). Concern about the mental health of prisoners was reflected in the recommendation of the Gladstone Committee that all prison doctors should have experience in the subject of lunacy.

In 1933 Dr W. H. de B. Hubert was appointed to carry out psycho-therapeutic work with selected prisoners in Wormwood Scrubs prison. In 1939, with Dr Norwood East, he produced an influential report suggesting that psychotherapy as an adjunct to a prison sentence was effective in preventing future antisocial behaviour or offending (East & Hubert, 1939; Bowden, 1991). By 1959 the prison department wanted doctors with psychiatric experience to work with all prisoners. This faith in psychiatry did not find favour with all. Dr Hamblin-Smith (1934), a prison doctor in Birmingham, declared:

> "the strongest objections to combining the ideas of punishment and medical treatment: the subject is certain to look upon the treatment as part of the punishment."

After the Second World War the PMS expanded rapidly. In 1962, nearly a quarter of a century after the East-Hubert report, a psychiatric prison, Grendon Underwood, opened in Buckinghamshire.

The Prison Rules of 1964 place upon the medical officer responsibility for the mental and physical health of the prisoners in his prison. This requires the examination of all inmates on reception and discharge, the examination of prisoners who report sick, and treatment for those who require it. The medical officer is also required to advise management on the maintenance and promotion of the health of prisoners. He must provide reports to the courts as requested, and also volunteer reports if he feels it to be appropriate.

Throughout the last 25 years of its existence, the PMS was the subject of repeated inquiries and reports. The Gwynne Report (Home Office, 1964) urged closer working with the NHS and even toyed with the idea of complete integration. At times the PMS was blamed (unfairly) for its failure to provide proper care for MDOs who should rightfully have been in NHS psychiatric facilities. Problems of accountability, ethics, recruitment and training were recurring issues (Smith, 1984).

Scrutiny of the PMS has gained pace in the last decade with a further series of reports (see Table 9.1). The report of the House of Commons (1986) Social Services Committee and that from the Royal College of Physicians (Home Office & Department of Health, 1990) contained recommendations for improvements in standards and the development of prison medicine as a specialty. Some observers thought it was time to disband the PMS and for its functions to be taken over by the NHS (Bluglass, 1990; Smith, 1992), but radical change has now been recommended and accepted. The driving force has been economic, administrative and managerial;

Table 9.1 The Prison Medical Service: recent reports and
landmarks 1986–1992

Year	Report/landmark	Conclusions/function
1986	House of Commons Social Services Committee	58 recommendations to improve standards
1990	Royal College of Physicians	12 recommendations to develop specialty of prison medicine
1990	Efficiency scrutiny	83 recommendations for greater alignment with NHS; prisons should be purchasers of health care
1990	HM Chief Inspector's inquiry on prison suicides	Radical new approach to managing self-harm and suicide risk
1990	Woolf Report	Improved facilities for MDOs in prison; proposals concerning alcohol/drug misuse and prisoners with HIV
1991	*Custody, Care and Justice*	Equivalent standards to NHS
1991	CPT Report – Council of Europe	Prison "inhuman and degrading treatment"; low standards of medical care
1992	Reed Report	Divert MDOs; contract-in services from NHS
1992	Health Advisory Committee	Provide independent advice on health care in prisons
1992	Health Care Service for Prisoners	Replaced PMS; developing as purchasing agency; promoting health

it is much in line with government policies for the reorganisation of the
NHS.

Efficiency scrutiny, 1990, and the Health Care Service for Prisoners, 1992

Under the title of an "efficiency scrutiny", a small team of civil servants
reviewed all aspects of the PMS with particular regard to its efficiency and

cost-effectiveness (Home Office, 1990*a*). It made 83 recommendations calling for:

(1) closer alignment with the NHS
(2) greater emphasis on promoting health and preventing illness
(3) separation of clinical and managerial tasks
(4) the Prison Service to be a purchaser rather than provider of health care.

Nearly all the recommendations were accepted by the Home Office. In 1992 the PMS was relaunched as the Health Care Service for Prisoners (HCSP) and its first report has been published (Health Care Service for Prisoners, 1993). The efficiency scrutiny did not deal with some crucial issues such as the capacity or willingness of the NHS to provide services to prisons, aspects of industrial relations, and costs. In the last five years, expenditure on health care in prisons has risen by 10.5% compared with an increase of 52% in the NHS budget over the same period. A Health Advisory Committee, chaired by a former Chief Medical Officer at the DoH, has been established to advise on matters affecting the health of prisoners. Change, then, is in the air, but the crucial test is whether the prisoner-patient will notice it. It is now accepted that standards of health care in prisons should be equivalent to those available to other citizens. Setting and monitoring standards, improving facilities, recruiting staff of good calibre, introducing clearer accountability, separating medical care from disciplinary functions, and ensuring confidentiality for patients, all remain huge hurdles to be overcome.

"Reporting sick"

"Reporting sick" is an important, and frequent, activity by prisoners; nearly two million episodes are recorded each year. In most cases prisoners do not have access to over-the-counter remedies and cannot, for example, simply take an aspirin for a headache. In addition, they are likely to have less easy access to a doctor than a free citizen has; requests to go sick are channelled through discipline staff and then a grade of officer known, until recently, as a "hospital officer" (see below). Some prisons have introduced systems for medical consultation much more akin to those of the outside world, with unimpeded access to the doctor through an appointments system. Difficulties in access to a doctor are to the disadvantage of the non-complaining but unwell prisoner; the withdrawn and self-isolating prisoner with a mental illness is likely to escape medical attention.

Hospital officers of the past commonly had no nursing qualifications; they were prison officers who did a special (but non-professional) 24-week training period. They have now been renamed "health care officers". It is planned to enlarge the number of qualified civilian nurses in the service and the aim is to have 75% of all nursing staff with a statutory qualification.

Medical facilities

No prison, or part of a prison, is recognised as a hospital for the purposes of the Mental Health Act 1983. Few prisons have medical facilities comparable to those found in the NHS. In many cases a prison hospital consists of little more than a sick-bay containing a number of cells used for observation. There may be little continuity of staffing. Since the Mental Health Act does not apply in prisons, prisoners cannot be treated without their consent, except in an emergency. This poses serious problems in treating severely psychotic prisoners who lack insight and may refuse treatment. The difficulties are compounded if there is any delay in transferring such a prisoner to hospital in terms of Sections 47 or 48 of the Mental Health Act.

There have, however, been recent examples of improvement. At Brixton Prison, where facilities for MDOs were scandalous, a specially appointed task force has brought about the development of a new psychiatric unit. Here, with better resources, skilled staff, and goodwill, much has been achieved. In accordance with the efficiency scrutiny, prisons in some areas have contracted in a psychiatric service, as opposed to simply buying consultant sessions. The contract is likely to be with the regional forensic psychiatry service. Contracts vary in content, but might include the in-patient care of prisoners in the prison hospital.

Prevalence of psychiatric disorder in prisons

It comes as no surprise that the prison population, drawn as it is from the socially disadvantaged, unemployed, inadequate and rootless sections of society, contains an excess of people who have a psychiatric disorder classifiable in terms of ICD–10. Prisons receive those who are sent to them by the courts. Local and remand facilities in particular receive an unsifted population admitted, especially in urban localities, from the streets. The fact that a large number of prisoners have a mental disorder has been recognised for centuries; some believe passionately that it is currently a direct consequence of government policies, and diminishing resources, for the mentally ill, particularly those who are also homeless (Weller, 1992).

What is less clear is whether the excess is accounted for by people with mental illness, and whether the MDOs in prison should rightfully be in hospital. Recent research based on large cohorts, systematic sampling and improved diagnostic criteria have helped to answer these questions. It is important to consider separately the remanded, or untried population, from the sentenced. The latter will have usually have been through

---

Box 9.2 Psychiatric disorders in prisoners

Psychiatric symptoms are common in the first two months of imprisonment

Between a third and a half may have ICD–10 classifiable psychiatric disorder

Personality disorder and substance abuse are the most common diagnoses

High rates of psychotic disorder exist in prisoners remanded for psychiatric reports

In sentenced prisoners the prevalence of psychotic disorder is similar to that in the general population

---

psychiatric filters at the arrest, pretrial and sentencing stages, and is therefore less likely to contain prisoners with major mental illness. Box 9.2 summarises the nature of psychiatric disorders in prisoners

Studies of remanded populations

Reception into prison is stressful. Loss of freedom, separation from friends and family, uncertainty about the future and the traumas of prison life all play a part. Harding & Zimmermann (1989) measured psychiatric symptoms on the tenth day of remand in 208 male prisoners in Geneva. High levels of symptoms were found, and these correlated with the perceived worries and concerns described by the prisoners. Symptoms had diminished after 60 days. Studies of selected samples of remanded prisoners have, not surprisingly, shown high rates of psychiatric illness. Thus 9% of men charged with violent crimes or located in the hospital at Brixton prison were psychotic (Taylor & Gunn, 1984), and 77% of men remanded in custody in Winchester for medical reports were suffering from acute psychiatric illness (Coid, 1988). These studies demonstrate that remands in custody are made in the hope that immediate medical care will be provided for mentally ill men, many of whom have often been charged with minor offences.

A pilot study of 31 consecutive, adult male remand prisoners showed only one with a psychotic illness, but 15 with problems of substance abuse and four with a personality disorder (Watt *et al*, 1993). A larger study of 698 men and 254 women remanded in custody for medical reports, or who showed evidence of current or previous mental disorder, confirmed that remands in custody were ordered in the hope that psychiatric treatment would thereby be obtained (Dell *et al*, 1991; Robertson *et al*, 1994). In fact, the findings pointed in just the opposite direction; two-thirds of the psychotic men and a third of the psychotic women were rejected for

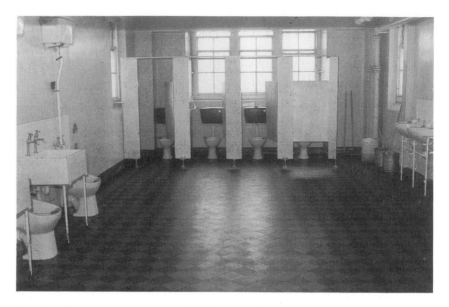

Fig. 9.2 Toilet area on wing of HM Prison, Edinburgh.

hospital admission. In a study using different methodology, Bowden (1978) found that only 10% of a sample of male remands in custody obtained treatment in hospital.

Dell *et al* (1991) conclude that remands in custody are an inefficient, ineffective and inhumane way of securing treatment. They found that prison doctors and catchment area psychiatrists often disagreed about diagnosis, type of treatment, and appropriateness of admission to hospital. Prisoners with chronic psychotic illness, organic brain damage, and learning disabilities are the usual focus of dispute.

Studies of sentenced populations

For many years the annual reports of the PMS drew attention to the number of mentally ill men serving prison sentences. Diagnoses were often disputed and, in any event, assigning a diagnosis says nothing about the need for, and still less the feasibility of, treatment. In a review of 11 important British studies, Coid (1984) concluded that major psychotic illness had a similar prevalence (1–2%) in prisoners as in the population at large. Learning disabilities, epilepsy and neurotic symptoms were probably overrepresented. Better understanding has emerged from an important study by Gunn *et al* (1991*a*). They interviewed a 5% sample of all male prisoners in England (1769 subjects) and found 37% in whom they made a psychiatric diagnosis. Substance abuse, personality disorder, neurosis and sexual deviance together accounted for 90% of the diagnoses. Thirty-four prisoners had a psychotic condition (2% of the total cohort), eight had epilepsy, and only seven had a learning disability. Three per cent were thought to require transfer to hospital, 5% required a therapeutic community and 10% needed further assessment or treatment within prison. Extrapolation from their sample identifies over 1000 prisoners in the UK requiring transfer to hospital, and over 2000 needing a therapeutic community.

Psychiatric disorder in female prisoners

There are approximately 1500 women in prisons in England and Wales, accounting for less than 4% of the prison population. Compared with men they have fewer previous convictions, are less likely to have committed a crime of violence or of burglary, and more likely to have committed a drug offence, theft, fraud or deception (Player, 1994). In recent years there has been a sharp rise in the number of women (40% from overseas) serving long sentences for drug trafficking (d'Orbán, 1993).

Among sentenced women, Gunn et al (1991*b*) found over half to have a psychiatric disorder, most commonly drug abuse or dependency (23%), personality disorder (18%) and neurotic disorder (16%). The prevalence of psychotic disorder was less than 2%. Behavioural disorder has been regarded as more common in women (particularly those on remand or serving short sentences) than in men. Women are put "on report" for offences in prison at twice the rate of men. Self-mutilation by women in prison is common; Wilkins & Coid (1991) found a previous history of self-mutilation in 7.5% of admissions to Holloway Prison. These women, when compared with non-mutilating prisoners, had backgrounds of severe deprivation, greater physical and sexual abuse, and abnormal psychosexual development. They had more extensive records of offending by criminal damage and arson.

Comment

The findings indicate that large numbers of MDOs are received into prison where their requirement for treatment cannot be met. The remand and short-sentence population is most likely to contain mentally ill people. High levels of psychotic disorder seems to be a particular feature in remand prisons serving Greater London, and almost certainly reflects gross inadequacies in the capital in caring for people with serious mental illness who are adrift from their families. Inquiries into the killings committed by Sharon Campbell (Department of Health and Social Security, 1988) and by Christopher Clunis (North East Thames and South East Thames Regional Health Authorities, 1994) provide accounts of the tragic consequences of failures in care.

Substance abuse and personality disorder are the other areas of unmet need, although it may be unrealistic to expect prisons to achieve therapeutic gains that have eluded psychiatry. The emphasis must be on "here-and-now" problems, such as the management of alcohol and drug withdrawal, harm reduction, and other measures relating to general health. These, together with HIV infection and AIDS (see below), are recognised by the HCSP as priority issues.

Reducing the prevalence of psychiatric disorder

There are three approaches to reducing the prevalence of psychiatric disorder in prisons: reducing admission of MDOs; shortening the length of their detention; and providing more effective treatment while in prison. The Reed Report (Department of Health & Home Office, 1992) espoused the central principle that prisoners with psychotic disorders should not be in prison. It identified ways of achieving this, particularly in remand prisons, and called for:

(1) abolition of remands in custody for medical reports
(2) raised awareness of local diversion schemes
(3) links with bail hostels
(4) more use of Section 48 transfer to hospital
(5) a more urgent response from district psychiatric services
(6) closer liaison with regional forensic psychiatry services
(7) better standards of care for mentally ill prisoners awaiting transfer.

These recommendations have major resource implications and, as with the Reed Report generally, come at a time of upheaval in NHS and local authority organisation. The Reed proposals, together with an improved health service within prisons, would clearly do much to alleviate the current problem. However, the mentally ill will always be received into prison notwithstanding improvements in alternative services. The reason is obvious: hospitals control their own gate, while prisons do not. Difficult, disturbed and unpopular MDOs will present to the only facility that cannot say "no" (Coid, 1991), and that is a reflection on psychiatric services rather than prisons.

The important factors in reducing the number of mentally ill people in prison are those very features which constitute a good forensic psychiatry service (see Chapter 7). Effective liaison with the police at the point of arrest and with other agencies, psychiatric bail hostels or other alternatives to custody, and court diversion schemes all play a part. Most importantly, general and forensic psychiatry services need the resources and professional will to admit MDOs to hospital. There is evidence of improvement following the Home Office circular number 66/90 (1990*b*)(see Chapter 7). This stated that MDOs "should never be remanded to prison" simply for a medical assessment. It emphasised the provisions in the Mental Health Act for the transfer of untried and sentenced prisoners under Sections 48 and 47 of the Act respectively. The numbers of such transfers has more than doubled in the five years to 1992, with the steepest increase following publication of the Home Office circular.

Practical and ethical issues

Psychiatrists may provide a sessional service to a prison or be called to see a particular prisoner (e.g. from his catchment area). In 1991–1992 there were nearly 20 000 psychiatric consultations – second in number only to the dentist. What was their purpose? Psychiatrists see prisoners for one of three principal reasons:

(1) to provide a report to the court, which may include an assessment of suitability for hospital admission
(2) to provide assessment and/or treatment at the request of a prison medical officer or, in certain cases, at the request of the prison governor in respect of a prisoner presenting serious, management problems
(3) for certain statutory purposes, such as in relation to parole consideration (see below).

Practical issues

Prisons are not the regular place of work for the psychiatrist; when they attend they are visitors. This can cause problems because the visitor is dependent on the staff to let him in, take him to the patient and then see him out. An internal key is a blessing, but is usually only awarded after years of trouble-free service! Prisons have their routines, and it is usually essential to arrive by appointment. Access to prisoners, who are also visited by lawyers and social workers, is usually confined to 2–3 hours in the morning and afternoon. Good professional relationships with staff make prison work much easier.

It is preferable to see prisoners on their own, but best to be guided by prison staff and common sense. The quality of examination facilities vary. Stories of using the x-ray filing cupboard to interview a patient are not uncommon, but usually there are adequate facilities in the prison hospital. Seeing prisoners on the wings may be a different matter, although it is educational and provides an opportunity to gather information from wing staff. Indeed, if the prisoner is not located in the hospital, it may be very difficult to obtain basic information about his functioning (e.g. is he sleeping, taking meals, seeing visitors, communicating with others?). It may be essential to talk to a relative of the prisoner – remember to ask for the telephone number at the interview as it may not be recorded elsewhere in the prison records. Apart from these practical issues, psychiatric examination follows the normal lines.

Recommendations for hospital admission through the courts are described in Chapters 5 and 7. The transfer of prisoners directly from prison to hospital need not be delayed on grounds of "red tape", although it might for other reasons. The required reports for Section 47 (for sentenced prisoners) and 48 (for untried prisoners) can be faxed to C3 Division at the Home Office (see Chapter 7), and the warrant for transfer faxed to the prison.

Ethical issues

Psychiatric work in a prison is bound to raise ethical dilemmas; issues of confidentiality and consent to treatment are discussed in Chapter 12. There is, however, a broader problem. The psychiatrist is an independent practitioner with principal obligations to the patient. If his work is to be of any benefit to his patients he must relate to the institution in which he and his patients find themselves. Yet the institution is a place of punishment, with staff who do not see themselves as providers of health care (Bernheim, 1993). Psychiatrists who work in prisons are at risk. They may experience a loss of professional esteem by virtue of the work they do, and in turn suffer a loss of self-esteem and autonomy, in much the same way as prisoners lose autonomy (Goldstein, 1983). In these circumstances it is easy to let clinical and ethical standards slip. There is a constant need to ensure that clinical practice is of the best attainable standard within the constraints applied by an environment which may be dehumanising.

Clinical issues

A psychiatrist working in a prison setting will see people with a complete range of psychiatric disorders. There is, however, a miscellaneous collection of phenomena, events, offenders and conditions that are of special relevance in prison psychiatry. In this section there is discussion of suicide and self-harm, HIV and AIDS, sex offenders, and paranoid syndromes commonly seen in prisoners.

Suicide

The annual rate of prison suicides approximately doubled between 1972 and 1987 (Dooley, 1990). Of 71 deaths in prison in 1991–1992, 43 were self-inflicted and coroners recorded 30 of them as suicide; it is easily the commonest mode of death in prison. There have been two investigations by HM Chief Inspector of Prisons in the last ten years (Home Office, 1984, 1990c). The second was precipitated by the increasing suicide rate in the late 1980s in spite of specific preventive steps. The Home Office has been accused of complacency and defensiveness (Smith, 1991).

Box 9.3 Suicide in prisons

The annual rate has doubled in the last seven years
It is the commonest mode of death in prison
The rate is approximately 8–9 times that found in the general
    population
It is nearly always achieved by hanging
Suicide is most common in remanded prisoners
Suicides usually do not differ in antecedants from general prison
    population
The suicide risk in prison is often managed by isolation of the
    prisoner

Prison suicide rates

The crude prison suicide rate in the UK is currently eight times that of the general population. However, the prison population differs significantly from the general population and is composed predominantly of men aged 20 to 30. Compared with the suicide rate in this particular section of the general population, the rate in English prisons is nine times higher (McClure, 1987). In Scotland and the Republic of Ireland prison suicide rates are even higher.

Epidemiology of prison suicide

The prison population contains a significant proportion of people with characteristics associated with suicide in the general population. These include a history of psychiatric disorder, previous self-harm, alcohol and/ or drug misuse, and social isolation. Compounding these underlying risk factors are the cognitive phenomena of uncertainty and powerlessness which accompany imprisonment especially in the remand period (Harding & Zimmermann, 1989). In a study of prison suicides in which there was an attempt to assess motivation, Dooley (1990) considered that there was frequent evidence to suggest that such prisoners had found imprisonment intolerable in some way.

Nearly 50% of suicides take place between 12 midnight and 8 am. The vast majority are by hanging, usually from from the cell window bars (Dooley, 1990). Remanded prisoners are most at risk, but 25% occur in prisoners who have been detained for more than one year. In sentenced prisoners there is an excess among lifers and those convicted of violent crimes. Besides self-inflicted deaths in prison recorded by coroners as suicides, a significant number of other deaths in prison, although not classified as suicide, are similar in method and putative motivation.

Prison suicides commonly have a history of previous psychiatric disorder, alcohol and/or drug abuse, and previous episodes of self-harm, whether in or outside prison. However, most prison suicides are completely unpredictable, and only a minority are suffering from a psychiatric illness. The majority share exactly the same features of vulnerability and situational stress with a large proportion of the prison population. These factors render the task of predicting who will commit suicide in prison "not currently feasible" (Pokorny, 1983). Nonetheless, medical officers and psychiatrists have a major role in the assessment and treatment of psychiatric disorder in prisoners. In some suicides the quality of assessment and treatment has been lamentably poor.

The search for "markers" of potential suicides has diverted attention from what most regard as the crucial factor in self-harm and suicides in prison, namely prison conditions. HM Chief Inspector quotes a prison governor:

> "My own view is that the ethos of an establishment, how inmates are treated, will determine the amount of suicide and self injury . . . Firstly, letting them know that it is part of the culture to demonstrate concern for inmates, and secondly, showing them ways of letting it show." (Home Office, 1990c)

Management of suicide risk

The management of those regarded as at risk is undergoing change. Hitherto, isolation of the prisoner in a strip cell (a cell stripped of all furniture and contents) and passive observation at 15-minute intervals has been the norm. If considered necessary a prisoner could be moved to a prison hospital unit for intensive management, although this was commonly more of the same. The practice of isolating prisoners in a secure strip cell "may still be routinely used" according to Liebling & Hall (1993), in spite of official guidance to the contrary. However, the Director of the HCSP reports a 72% reduction in the use of such facilities over the last year (Wool, 1993).

The report by HM Chief Inspector of Prisons (Home Office, 1990c) made various recommendations aimed at reducing prison suicides. It contrasted the isolation practices in prison with the contact-and-communication approach in psychiatric units. Among the recommendations were improved standards of hygiene (access to sanitation, showers and clean clothing). Regimes should provide at least eight hours per day out of cells, and where this is not possible, in-cell television should be provided. The problem is taken up in *Custody, Care and Justice* (Home Office, 1991b) with commitments to improve training, involve the use of the Samaritans, and establish good standards of practice.

HIV and AIDS

One in ten men and one in four women in prison have been regular users of opiates or stimulants before imprisonment (Maden *et al*, 1990, 1991). At least a third of prisoners in Scotland have injected drugs, and the majority of these have injected in prison (Dye & Isaacs, 1991). It is therefore not surprising that HIV and AIDS is an important issue for prisons. There were 345 reported cases in English prisons between 1985 and 1991. Proportionate figures in some prisons elsewhere (e.g. Edinburgh and Dublin) are higher; there has been an outbreak of HIV infection reported in a Scottish prison (Gore & Bird, 1993). The initial response by prisons to drug misuse, and to the management, control and prevention of HIV and AIDS, was grossly inadequate (Farrell & Strang, 1991). There are signs of recent improvement with drug reduction programmes using substituted methadone, and a more humane approach to the care of prisoners with HIV and AIDS. In particular, the Viral Infectivity Restrictions (VIR), which determined a regime of stark isolation for the infected prisoner, have been reviewed.

Most prisons have now put considerable resources into the prevention and management of HIV and AIDS in prisons. Psychiatrists are unlikely to be involved in general issues of counselling or advice to those who have, or fear they have, the infection. However, the infection runs a well-established course, and there are now a significant number of prisoners with advanced stages of AIDS, who include some serving life or other long sentences. Their day-to-day care is a matter for the prison staff with support from the NHS and other outside agencies. However, psychiatric symptoms, syndromes and disorders (particularly affective) are common in patients with AIDS and may require specialist attention. Neuropsychological impairment heralding HIV-associated dementia may produce behavioural and functional changes, initially subtle in form, which precipitate psychiatric referral. Psychotic disorders require, as for any similar prisoner, transfer to hospital.

Sex offenders

"Programmes will be introduced from this year [1991] to tackle sex offenders' distorted beliefs about their relationships, to make them more aware of the effect of their offences on the victim, and to ensure these prisoners take responsibility for and face up to the consequences of their behaviour." Home Office (1991*b*)

In 1991 the Criminal Justice Act introduced mandatory supervision after release for certain sex offenders. In the words of one observer, "sex offenders have become sexy" (Seven, 1991). The nature of sex offences and offenders is discussed in Chapter 2 where the diversity of people who commit sex offences is emphasised. Once imprisoned there is a public expectation that "something" should be done with the offender which stops him doing it again. What this "treatment" should be is never very clear.

Psychiatrists working in prisons are likely to see a large number of sex offenders. They may be referred for assessment, and perhaps treatment, of sexual deviance, or for other reasons. A few initiate referral themselves, but many attend at the suggestion of another person or agency. Treating sex offenders in prison sounds simple; the patient is captive and there is plenty of time. In practice there are many reasons why treatment is exceedingly difficult. In particular, the prisoner may:

(1) show no clinical evidence of sexual deviance or disorder
(2) deny, wholly or in part, his guilt
(3) be so distressed at imprisonment that he is psychologically not available for therapy
(4) fear breaches of confidentiality to staff or inmates
(5) fear that information disclosed may jeopardise his release.

The institutional factors are real. Many sex offenders spend long periods "on protection" under Rule 43; conditions of deprivation are often appalling. Similarly their anxieties about lack of confidentiality may be justifiable. Even where these factors do not apply, there remains the difficulty of using a talking treatment, which requires inner exploration, in an environment that is completely divorced from real life, its people, relationships and stresses.

However, there are some sex offenders in prison with sufficient insight and understanding to request help. Therapy with such patients must be appropriate for their particular needs and capacities, but common themes are sexuality, childhood sexual experiences, self-perception and interpersonal relationships. It is rarely appropriate to prescribe antilibidinal agents, although if the patient will take them after release then it is wise to begin treatment, with the usual precautions, in prison.

The Home Office has honoured its commitment (see above) and sex offender programmes are being introduced on a large scale (Thornton & Hogue, 1993). There are three types of programmes:

(1) The core programme consists of up to 40 sessions of structured group work to increase motivation and develop relapse prevention strategies.
(2) The extended programme consists of skills-training modules to complement the above.
(3) The booster programme contains both social skills and relapse prevention elements and is instituted before release.

The complexity of the approach shows what can follow when treatment is ordered by government. Whether the prisoner will know, at any given time, what programme he is doing remains to be seen. Under Section 44 of the Criminal Justice Act 1991, sex offenders sentenced to 12 months imprisonment or more may be subject to longer periods of supervision after release than other prisoners.

Paranoid syndromes

The combination of vulnerable personalities, high rates of substance abuse and a threatening environment make it highly likely that paranoid symptoms will be common in prisoners. This is indeed the case, and it is important for the psychiatrist to have a clear understanding of paranoid disorders in prisoners so that treatment is appropriate. Inexperienced practitioners imagine that all prisoners are malingering until proven otherwise. In practice, malingering is unusual in prisoners, and usually easily detected. In a similar vein, the famous Ganser syndrome is more commonly found in the pages of psychiatry textbooks than in prisoners (see below).

Paranoid prisoners are commonly referred to a psychiatrist. Careful assessment on conventional lines is important; particular effort should be directed to obtaining a global view of the prisoner and his premorbid functioning. How does he spend his day? Is there any information about his behaviour with, and if possible from, his visitors?

Paranoid syndromes that are not due to schizophrenia, affective or organic disorder, usually fall into one of three categories, although the boundaries between them are disputed and blurred (World Health Organization, 1992). Men with unstable personalities (perhaps inadequate or antisocial) commonly have paranoid traits which surface on imprisonment. They may complain of feeling under threat from other prisoners or from staff and may be reluctant to leave their cell. Often there is a genuine basis for their fears and it is virtually impossible to know how "paranoid" their reaction is. Such prisoners often request benzodiazepines but these are not appropriate. Most settle with a change in their location or other circumstances.

An acute but transient psychotic disorder may occur with marked delusional and perceptual features that characteristically show variation even from hour to hour. Such patients require observation in the prison hospital, which may of itself be therapeutic. Symptoms do not interfere totally with daily living and features of schizophrenia are absent. These patients usually receive neuroleptic medication for the period of the disorder.

A more clear-cut paranoid psychosis may develop with serious disruption of day-to-day life. Such patients usually require transfer to a psychiatric hospital. Sometimes their symptoms may cease almost upon admission to hospital, only to recur after returning to prison. Many such prisoners oscillate between prison and hospital. Disentangling illness from triggering factors is usually impossible. It is probably helpful for such prisoners to receive maintenance neuroleptic medication but many are unwilling to

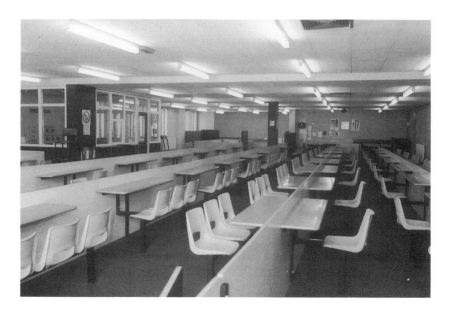

Fig. 9.3 Visiting room in HM Prison, Edinburgh.

do so when well. The management of prisoners with a relapsing paranoid psychosis (some would say schizophrenia) of this type, particularly if they are serving a long sentence, is fraught with difficulties.

The term "Ganser syndrome" is commonly used to describe any behaviour which simulates psychosis or dementia, and is thought to be hysterical in origin. Ganser (1898) described his syndrome in three prisoners awaiting execution; an important element was the giving of approximate answers (i.e. absurd answers which nonetheless indicate understanding of the question). The syndrome has many aetiologies, and whether it is hysterical or malingered is something of a conundrum.

Early release

In 1967 a system of early release from prison, known as parole, was introduced for prisoners in the UK. In essence, prisoners serving fixed sentences (i.e. other than life imprisonment) were eligible for release on parole after serving a third of their sentence. In the community they received supervision by a probation officer, and were subject to recall to prison, until the date when they would have normally been released from their sentence. For prisoners released in the normal way, no supervision was provided. The Home Secretary, who was responsible for the parole system, was advised by the Parole Board, which comprised of approximately 70 members from a wide range of disciplines including psychiatry.

Concern about the parole system, its lack of natural justice, its inconsistency and the fact that it was vulnerable to manipulation on public policy grounds, led to the establishment of the Carlisle Committee (Home Office, 1988) which reviewed parole procedures. Many of the Carlisle Committee recommendations have been embodied in the Criminal Justice Act 1991. Release, either by remission for good behaviour or on parole, has been abolished and in its place there is "early release on licence".

Determinate sentenced prisoners

Early release on licence for prisoners with a specific length of sentence is as follows:

Sentence less than one year:
- release at 50% point
- no supervision
- subject to recall until expiry of full sentence

Sentence 1–4 years:
- release at 50% point
- subject to supervision until 75% point
- subject to recall until expiry of full sentence

Sentence four years or more:
- release between 50% and 66% point: Parole Board if less than seven years
- release between 50% and 66% point: Home Secretary advised by Parole Board if seven years or more
- subject to supervision until 75% point
- subject to recall until expiry of full sentence

If the prisoner does not obtain early release, he is automatically released at the 66% point; thereafter he receives some supervision in the community and is liable to recall until expiry of the full sentence.

Life-sentenced prisoners

Prisoners serving a mandatory life sentence (i.e. imposed for murder) have the tariff (or punitive) element of their sentence determined by the judiciary; the length of time to be served for other reasons is a matter for the Home Secretary advised (but not directed) by the Parole Board. For discretionary life-sentenced prisoners (i.e. imposed for crimes other than murder) the Parole Board sits as a Discretionary Lifer Panel (DLP), when the tariff part of the sentence has been served. In these cases the Board is concerned with risk to the public, and its decision is binding on the

Home Secretary. DLPs have three members: a judge as chairman, a psychiatrist and a third member who is a layman, criminologist, psychologist or probation officer. Prisoners are provided with copies of all the reports (including psychiatric) considered by the DLP; they can have legal representation and may attend the DLP meeting.

Role of psychiatrist in early release

Psychiatrists may provide reports for the Parole Board to give an opinion on any psychiatric factors which are relevant in relation to the protection of the public, the appropriateness of supervision, and the question of any requirement for psychiatric aftercare. Under the new arrangements for discretionary life-sentenced prisoners, psychiatrists may be asked to provide independent reports at the request of the prisoner's solicitor. Finally, the Parole Board continues to have psychiatrist members who are particularly involved when the crime is one of homicide, arson or a sex offence (McGrath, 1987). The new arrangements have been generally welcomed as an improvement on the old parole system (James, 1993).

Special psychiatric facilities in prisons

Grendon Underwood, Buckinghamshire

Grendon Underwood, which opened in 1962, owes its existence to the recommendations of East & Hubert (1939). It was originally intended to be a prison for the investigation and treatment of those with mental disorders, including those with psychopathic disorder. The emphasis has been on group psychotherapy. For 22 years it was run by a doctor who was both governor and medical superintendent. Outcome in Grendon inmates has been carefully evaluated (Gunn *et al*, 1978; Gunn & Robertson, 1982). Inmates show improved self-image, attitudes to staff, and behaviour. Unfortunately the regime does not significantly affect reconviction rates.

Grendon is currently a multipurpose prison for adult males, providing units for assessment and induction, acute psychiatric treatment and sex offenders. Only inmates with at least one year to serve are accepted for admission. There is no equivalent community for women in the prison system. Opinions are polarised between those who see Grendon as an imaginative facility for the psychopath, or a soft option for the discerning prisoner. Genders & Player (1994) provide an account of the establishment. A second unit based on the therapeutic approach of Grendon is planned.

Wormwood Scrubs Hospital Annexe, London

Since 1972 the Hospital annexe at Wormwood Scrubs prison has provided a 40-place therapeutic community for prisoners with problems of personality, substance abuse or sex offending. Admission is usually for about one year before release.

Holloway Prison, London

Holloway is a local prison for women from courts covering much of the south of England. It contains a 90-bedded unit for women with psychiatric problems. It has had a stormy history with frequent reports criticising the environment and the standards of care (d'Orbán, 1993). New staffing and separation from the disciplinary aspects of the prison have had beneficial effects. Standards of care may fluctuate depending on the individual contribution of key personnel.

Parkhurst Prison (Hospital and C wing), Isle of Wight

The prison hospital at Parkhurst has traditionally accommodated up to 50 prisoners, detainable under the Mental Health Act 1983, but awaiting places in special hospitals, regional secure units or district psychiatric services (Cooper, 1990). The management of such patients in these circumstances is difficult. In addition, Parkhurst contains a 25-place unit in C wing for disruptive and disturbed prisoners who have caused management problems in dispersal prisons elsewhere. Many of the inmates are highly dangerous men, some having committed homicide while in prison.

Glen Parva Young Offender Centre, Leicestershire

Glen Parva is a closed young offender institution with hospital facilities including an acute psychiatric admission unit, a small therapeutic community and a unit for youths regarded as inadequate or socially and/or intellectually limited. Such youngsters are highly vulnerable in the ordinary regime of a young offenders institution where they are likely to be targets of abuse, extortion and assault.

Barlinnie Prison Special Unit, Glasgow

The Barlinnie Special Unit acquired fame because some of its former inmates made successful, and publicised, careers in the arts and commerce. It was opened in 1973 in an attempt to defuse serious violence in Scotland's jails. It accommodates ten prisoners who are serving long sentences and are either causing severe disruption, or are approaching the end of their sentence and require pre-release support. There is a complex system for assessing referrals. Individual responsibility, regular (and also ad hoc) group meetings, and close staff–inmate relationships are features. Cooke (1989) reviewed 25 inmates treated in the unit and found lower than expected rates of violence and reoffending. Following a critical government report, the unit will close in 1995.

Comment

All the units described above are special in their own way. They exist because of the diverse nature and needs of the prison population, and the necessity for resources for prisoners with mental disorders. Common themes can be identified in the successful units, namely a well-organised but flexible, sensitive and caring ethos – in fact, the crucial ingredients for any institution charged with the care of others.

Addendum on Scotland, Northern Ireland and the Republic of Ireland

There are no facilities in prisons in Scotland or the Republic of Ireland which are either designated with a psychiatric function or are suitable for the care of prisoners with psychiatric disorders. In Northern Ireland there is a 17-bed psychiatric unit at HM Prison Maghaberry serving prisons throughout the Province. It is not a hospital within the meaning of the Mental Health (Northern Ireland) Order 1986. In Scotland, Northern Ireland and the Republic of Ireland efforts are being made to move mentally disordered prisoners to hospital. There are, however, major difficulties in Northern Ireland in transferring untried prisoners who face serious charges.

In Scotland and the Republic of Ireland, there has been a large increase in the numbers of prisoners with problems of drug misuse and in sex offenders. Special regimes are under development. Prisons in Northern Ireland contain a number of terrorists from paramilitary organisations; they show low rates of consultation with the psychiatric services.

Acknowledgement

The photographs of Figs 9.1, 9.2, and 9.3 are reproduced by kind permission of the Governor of HM Prison, Edinburgh.

References

Bernheim, J. (1993) Medical ethics in prison. *Criminal Behaviour and Mental Health*, **3**, 85–96.
Bluglass, R. (1990) Recruitment and training of prison doctors. *British Medical Journal*, **301**, 249–250.
Bowden, P. (1978) Men remanded into custody for medical reports: the selection for treatment. *British Journal of Psychiatry*, **132**, 320–331.

—— (1991) Pioneers in forensic psychiatry. William Norwood East: the acceptable face of psychiatry. *Journal of Forensic Psychiatry*, **2**, 59–78.

Coid, J. (1984) How many psychiatric patients in prison? *British Journal of Psychiatry*, **145**, 78–86.

—— (1988) Mentally abnormal prisoners on remand: I. Rejected or accepted by the NHS? *British Medical Journal*, **296**, 1779–1782.

—— (1991) "Difficult to place" psychiatric patients. *British Medical Journal*, **302**, 603–604.

Cooke, D. J. (1989) Containing violent prisoners – an analysis of the Barlinnie Special Unit. *British Journal of Criminology*, **29**, 129–143.

Cooper, D. (1990) Parkhurst Prison: C wing. In *Principles and Practice of Forensic Psychiatry* (eds R. Bluglass & P. Bowden), pp. 1329–1331. Edinburgh: Churchill Livingstone.

Council of Europe (1991) *Report of the European Committee for the Prevention of Torture and Inhuman or Degrading Treatment or Punishment (CPT)*. Strasbourg: Council of Europe.

Dell, S., Robertson, G., James, K., *et al* (1991) Remands and psychiatric assessments in Holloway Prison. I: The psychotic population. *British Journal of Psychiatry*, **163**, 634–640.

Department of Health and Social Security (1988) *Report of the Committee of Inquiry into the Care and Aftercare of Miss Sharon Campbell*. Cmnd. 440. London: HMSO.

Department of Health & Home Office (1992) *Review of Health and Social Services for Mentally Disordered Offenders and Others Requiring Similar Services*. Cmnd. 2088. London: HMSO.

Dooley, E. (1990) Prison suicide in England and Wales, 1972–87. *British Journal of Psychiatry*, **156**, 40–45.

D'Orbán, P. T. (1993) Female offenders. In *Forensic Psychiatry: Clinical, Ethical and Legal Issues* (eds J. Gunn & P. Taylor), pp. 599–623. Oxford: Butterworth Heinemann.

Dye, S. & Isaacs, C. (1991) Intravenous drug misuse among prison inmates: implications for spread of HIV. *British Medical Journal*, **302**, 1506.

East, W. N. & Hubert, W. H. De B. (1939) *Report on the Psychological Treatment of Crime*. London: HMSO.

Farrell, M. & Strang, J. (1991) Drugs, HIV, and prisons. *British Medical Journal*, **302**, 1477–1478.

Ganser, S. J. (1898) Ueber einen eigenartigen hysterischen Daemmerzustand. *Archiv fur Psychiatrie und Nervenkrankheiten*, **30**, 633 (trans. C. E. Shorter (1965), *British Journal of Criminology*, **5**, 120).

Genders, E. & Player, E. (1994) *The Therapeutic Prison: A Study of Grendon*. Oxford: Oxford University Press.

Goldstein, N. (1983) Psychiatry in prisons. *Psychiatric Clinics of North America*, **6**, 751–765.

Gore, S. M. & Bird, A. G. (1993) No escape: HIV transmission in jail. *British Medical Journal*, **307**, 147–148.

Gray, W. J. (1973) The English prison medical service: its historical background and more recent developments in medical care of prisoners and detainees. In *16th Ciba Foundation Symposium: Medical Care of Prisoners and Detainees*, pp. 129–136. Amsterdam: Elsevier.

Gunn, J., Robertson, G., Dell, S., *et al* (1978) *Psychiatric Aspects of Imprisonment.* London: Academic Press.

—— & —— (1982) An evaluation of Grendon prison. In *Abnormal Offenders, Delinquency, and the Criminal Justice System* (eds J. Gunn & D. P. Farrington), pp. 285–305. Chichester: John Wiley.

——, Maden, A. & Swinton, M. (1991*a*) Treatment needs of prisoners with psychiatric disorders. *British Medical Journal*, **363**, 338–341.

——, —— & —— (1991*b*) *Mentally Disordered Prisoners.* London: Home Office.

Hamblin-Smith, M. (1934) *Prisons in a Changing Society.* London: John Lane.

Harding, T. & Zimmermann, E. (1989) Psychiatric symptoms, cognitive stress and vulnerability factors: a study in a remand prison. *British Journal of Psychiatry*, **155**, 36–43.

Health Care Service for Prisoners (1993) *First Report of the Director of Health Care for Prisoners.* London: HM Prison Service.

Home Office (1895) *Report from the Departmental Committee on Prisons.* Cmnd. 7702. London: HMSO.

—— (1964) *Report of the Working Party on the Organisation of the Prison Medical Service* (Gwynn Report) London: HMSO.

—— (1966) *Report of a Committee of Inquiry into Prison Escapes and Security.* Cmnd. 3175 (Mountbatten Report). London: HMSO.

—— (1984) *Suicide in Prison. A Report by HM Chief Inspector of Prisons.* London: HMSO.

—— (1988) *The Parole System in England and Wales* (Carlisle Committee). London: HMSO.

—— (1990*a*) *Report of an Efficiency Scrutiny of the Prison Medical Service.* London: HMSO.

—— (1990*b*) *Provision for Mentally Disordered Offenders* (Home Office Circular No. 66/90). London: Home Office.

—— (1990*c*) *Report of a Review by HM Chief Inspector of Prisons for England and Wales of Suicide and Self-Harm in Prison Service Establishments in England and Wales.* London: HMSO.

—— (1991*a*) *Prison Disturbances April 1990. Report of an Inquiry by The Rt Hon. Lord Justice Woolf and His Honour Judge Stephen Tumim.* London: HMSO.

—— (1991*b*) *Custody, Care and Justice: the Way Ahead for the Prison Service in England and Wales.* Cm 1647. London: HMSO.

—— & Department of Health (1990) *The Prison Medical Service in England and Wales – Recruitment and Training of Doctors. (A Report of the Working Party of the Royal College of Physicians to the Chief Medical Officer).* London: Home Office & DoH.

House of Commons (1986) *Third Report from the Social Services Committee Session 1985–86: Prison Medical Service.* London: HMSO.

Howard, J. (1777) *The State of the Prisons in England and Wales*, Warrington (bicentennial edn, 1977). Abingdon: Professional Books.

James, A. (1993) The Criminal Justice Act 1991. Principal provisions and their effect on psychiatric practice. *Journal of Forensic Psychiatry*, **4**, 285–294.

Lancet (1988) Shackled, shameful, and shoddy. Editorial. *Lancet*, **2**, 1402–1403.

—— (1991) A European committee looks at degrading treatment in custody. Editorial. *Lancet*, **338**, 1559–1560.

Liebling, A. & Hall, P. (1993) Seclusion in strip cells. *British Medical Journal*, **307**, 399–400.

Maden, A., Swinton, M. & Gunn, J. (1990) Women in prisons and the use of illicit drugs before arrrest. *British Medical Journal*, **301**, 1133.

——, —— & —— (1991) Drug dependence in prisons. *British Medical Journal*, **302**, 880.

McClure, G. M. G. (1987) Suicide in England and Wales, 1975–1984. *British Journal of Psychiatry*, **150**, 309–314.

McGrath, P. (1987) The psychiatrist on the Parole Board. *Bulletin of the Royal College of Psychiatrists*, **11**, 120–121.

North East Thames & South East Thames Regional Health Authorities (1994) *The Report of the Inquiry into the Care and Treatment of Christopher Clunis*. London: HMSO.

Player, E. (1994) Women's prisons after Woolf. In *Prisons after Woolf: Reform through Riot* (eds E. Player & M. Jenkins), pp. 203–225. London: Routledge.

—— & Jenkins, M. (1994) *Prisons after Woolf: Reform Through Riot*. London: Routledge.

Pokorny, A. (1983) Prediction of suicide in psychiatric patients. *Archives of General Psychiatry*, **40**, 249–257.

Ralli, R. (1994) Health care in prisons. In *Prisons after Woolf: Reform Through Riot* (eds E. Player and M. Jenkins), pp. 125–139. London: Routledge.

Robertson, G., Dell, S., James, K., *et al* (1994) Psychotic men remanded in custody to Brixton Prison. *British Journal of Psychiatry*, **164**, 55–61.

Seven, P. (1991) Treating sex offenders in prison. *Journal of Forensic Psychiatry*, **2**, 8–9.

Smith, R. (1984) *Prison Health Care*. London: British Medical Association.

—— (1991) "Taken from this place and hanged by the neck . . ." *British Medical Journal*, **302**, 54–65.

—— (1992) Prison medicine: beginning again. *British Medical Journal*, **304**, 134–135.

Taylor, P. J. & Gunn, J. (1984) Violence and psychosis I – Risk of violence among psychotic men. *British Medical Journal*, **288**, 1945–1949.

Thornton, D. & Hogue, T. (1993) The large-scale provision of programmes for imprisoned sex offenders: issues, dilemmas and progress. *Criminal Behaviour and Mental Health*, **3**, 371–380.

Tumim, S., Jenkins, D. & Boddis, S (1993) Crying Woolf: has the report impacted on life for prisoners? *Criminal Behaviour and Mental Health*, **3**, 484–490.

Watt, F., Tomison, A. & Torpy, D. (1993) The prevalence of psychiatric disorder in a male remand population: a pilot study. *Journal of Forensic Psychiatry*, **4**, 75–83.

Weller, M. (1992) The objecting or objectional? *Journal of Forensic Psychiatry*, **3**, 400–404.

Wilkins, J. & Coid, J. (1991) Self-mutilation in female remanded prisoners: I. An indication of severe psychopathology. *Criminal Behaviour and Mental Health*, **1**, 247–267.

Wool, R. (1993) Care of suicidal prisoners (letter). *British Medical Journal*, **307**, 805.

World Health Organization (1992) *The ICD–10 Classification of Mental and Behavioural Disorders*. Geneva: WHO.

10 Mental health legislation
Rosemarie Cope

Liberty and constraint • The Mental Health Act 1983 • Consent to treatment • Compulsory treatment in the community • Applications and appeals against detention • The Mental Health Act Commission • Code of Practice • The NHS Health Advisory Service • Addenda for Northern Ireland, Scotland and the Republic of Ireland

---

Psychiatry is the only medical discipline which has special legal powers to detain and treat people against their will. This is because psychiatric disorders may impair decision-making, judgement and behaviour. The laws are necessary to protect the interests of patients, and to protect the public from the possibly serious consequences of mental disorder.

Mental health legislation has existed for over 200 years, and in England and Wales it has been revised about every 25 years. Comparable legislation exists throughout the world, but varies in its complexity, depending, for example, on geographical and economic factors, and the availability of resources. Curran & Harding (1988) have described international comparisons of mental health legislation.

This chapter is concerned with mental health legislation in England and Wales. There are addenda concerning legislation in Northern Ireland, Scotland and the Republic of Ireland.

Liberty and constraint

Before any laws were introduced, "dangerous lunatics" as they were called, were kept in appalling conditions in private madhouses. These came to be controlled by the Act Regulating Madhouses of 1774. Over the next 100 years, successive acts of parliament introduced laws to regulate the activities of the county asylums which replaced the madhouses. Procedures for compulsory admissions were introduced by the Lunacy Act 1890, but it was not until 40 years later that voluntary admission was allowed, under the Mental Treatment Act of 1930. With advances in psychiatric treatment, increasing numbers of patients could be treated on open wards and discharged into the community. The Mental Health Act 1959 encouraged informal admissions, and authority for compulsory detention became a matter for hospitals, doctors and social workers, without involving magistrates as had previously been the case. At the same time, legal control of psychiatric hospitals (formerly vested successively in the Commissioners in Lunacy and the Board of Control) was abolished. Concerns about

272

standards of care were subsequently raised by a number of scandals in psychiatric hospitals (Martin, 1984). Dissatisfaction with the 1959 Act was also expressed by MIND (the National Association of Mental Health) through its legal director, Larry Gostin (Gostin, 1975, 1977). He drew attention to the inadequacies of legal rights for patients, and these concerns eventually led to the amendment of the 1959 Act, now consolidated in the Mental Health Act 1983. Detailed accounts of the 1983 Act are given by Bluglass (1983), Jones (1988) and Hoggett (1990).

Practical aspects of compulsory detention

More than 90% of admissions to psychiatric hospitals are now informal. This means that patients can come to a hospital for psychiatric treatment in the same way as for an operation or investigation for a physical disorder. They can leave hospital when they wish and they have the right to refuse any treatment they do not want.

A patient's first contact with the psychiatrist is normally in the out-patients department following referral by a general practitioner or at home during a domiciliary visit. (Contact via the police or the criminal justice system is dealt with in other chapters). If hospital admission is thought necessary but the patient is reluctant to go into hospital, the psychiatrist should try to allay the patient's fears, and encourage him to accept informal admission. If this is unsuccessful, a clinical decision about the need for compulsory detention in hospital must be made, using the following criteria:

(1) is there a mental disorder as defined within the Act?
(2) is there a risk to the health or safety of the patient (including a risk of deterioration as well as self-harm), or to others?
(3) is admission to hospital necessary to safeguard that risk?

Case example 1
A GP requested a domiciliary visit on a 48-year-old married man with a 2-month history of depression, insomnia and heavy drinking, following the departure of his wife to live with another man. On interview he was tearful and agitated with biological symptoms of depression. He admitted to having thoughts about killing his wife and then himself, using the shotgun which he was known to possess. He could not be persuaded to come into hospital, and compulsory admission was arranged on the grounds that he suffered with a depressive disorder, he presented a risk to himself and his wife, and there was no safe alternative to hospital admission.

Case example 2
A 25-year-old woman who lived with her boyfriend and 2-year-old daughter was referred to the out-patient department with depression and anxiety. On interview she described her unsatisfactory relation-

ship with her cohabitee, financial problems, and difficulties coping with her child. She had presented to casualty departments following overdoses on two occasions in the previous three months, but left before being seen by a psychiatrist. She feared harming her child, whom she admitted hitting too hard on a number of occasions. Hospital admission was offered but she refused. Although she fulfilled the criteria for mental disorder and there was a real risk to the child, she readily agreed to the offer of attendance at a day hospital and involvement of a social worker, which was considered a reasonable alternative to compulsory admission.

The Mental Health Act 1983

Legal categories of mental disorder

The term "mental disorder" is the *sine qua non* of compulsory admission and treatment. The Act makes an important distinction between those sections, notably the short-term detention orders which refer to "mental disorder", and the longer term admission and treatment orders. When applying the latter, it is necessary to state from which of the four specific categories of mental disorder the patient is suffering; these are shown in Box 10.1.

Box 10.1 Mental Health Act 1983

Mental disorder means mental illness, arrested or incomplete development of mind, psychopathic disorder, and any other disorder or disability of mind

Mental illness is not defined

Psychopathic disorder means a persistent disorder or disability of mind (whether or not including significant impairment of intelligence) which results in abnormally aggressive or seriously irresponsible conduct on the part of the person concerned

Mental impairment means a state of arrested or incomplete development of mind (not amounting to severe mental impairment) which includes significant impairment of intelligence and social functioning and is associated with abnormally aggressive or seriously irresponsible conduct on the part of the person concerned

Severe mental impairment means a state of arrested or incomplete development of mind which includes severe impairment of intelligence and social functioning and is associated with abnormally aggressive or seriously irresponsible conduct on the part of the person concerned

Persons suffering from mental disorder by reason only of promiscuity or other immoral conduct, sexual deviancy, or dependence on alcohol or drugs, are excluded

---

The majority of detentions are for mental illness. In 1986 (Department of Health and Social Security, 1986), 91% of all detained patients were under the mental illness category, 5% under mental impairment, and 2% each under psychopathic disorder and severe mental impairment.

Mental illness is not defined in the Act and its application is left entirely to clinical judgement. Attempts to define it include the Butler Committee's (Home Office & DHSS, 1975) definition: "a disorder which has not always existed in the patient but has developed as a condition overlying the sufferer's usual personality". A legal view from the Court of Appeal (in the case of *W v L* ,1974) is that the words "mental illness" have no particular medical or legal significance, but mean what an ordinary sensible person would construe.

The statutory category of psychopathic disorder is a generic description of a disorder rather than any specific clinical condition. The legal definition is based solely on behaviour as distinct from the range of features required for a clinical diagnosis of dissocial personality disorder. Psychiatrists have traditionally expressed dissatisfaction about retaining psychopathic disorder within the Mental Health Act; the legal definition is unsatisfactory and there are doubts about its treatability on an involuntary basis. It is rarely used now for civil commitment, and its use is also declining for the admission of offender patients. The Mental Health (Scotland) Act 1984 and the Mental Health (Northern Ireland) Order 1986 omit the term (see addenda).

The legal definitions of severe mental impairment and mental impairment are hybrid terms, combining elements of the definitions of both mental handicap and psychopathic disorder. In practice, these categories mean that a mentally handicapped patient whose behaviour is not regarded as antisocial cannot be detained on a long-term detention order, nor subjected to guardianship. However, a mentally handicapped patient could be admitted on a short-term order on the grounds of arrested or incomplete development of mind, which is part of the definition of mental disorder.

Compulsory powers under the Act cannot be used to detain a person "by reason only of promiscuity or other immoral conduct, sexual deviancy or dependence on alcohol or drugs". These are regarded as social and behavioural problems, but some alcohol-related conditions (e.g. delirium tremens or a drug-induced psychotic state) would be regarded as mental disorders, namely mental illnesses within the Act.

Compulsory admission under Part II of the Act

This part of the Act is concerned with compulsory admission to hospital under the so-called "civil sections". ("Forensic sections" under Part III of the Act are described in Chapter 5, and the place of safety sections in Chapter 4). Table 10.1 summarises the compulsory admission procedures under Part II of the Act.

Table 10.1 Compulsory admission procedures in England and Wales under Part II of the Mental Health Act 1983

Section	Situation	Medical signatories	Applicant	Psychiatric condition specified in the Act	Duration of detention	Manner of termination[1]	Appeal procedures
2	Admission for assessment	Two doctors, one of whom is approved	Nearest relative or an approved social worker	Mental disorder	28 days	1. Patient discharged or remains informally 2. Application for Section 3 initiated	Mental Health Review Tribunal on application by patient
3	Admission for treatment	Two doctors, one of whom is approved	Nearest relative or an approved social worker	1. Mental illness or severe mental impairment 2. Psychopathic disorder or mental impairment only if "treatable"	6 months, renewable for a further 6 months and then at yearly intervals	1. Patient discharged or remains informally 2. Discharged by the nearest relative unless barred by RMO	Mental Health Review Tribunal on application by patient, nearest relative or automatically by hospital managers
4	Emergency admission	Any doctor	Nearest relative or an approved social worker	Mental disorder	72 hours	1. Patient discharged or remains informally 2. Regraded to Section 2 or application for Section 3 initiated	None

Table10.1 cont.

Section	Situation	Medical signatories	Applicant	Psychiatric condition specified in the Act	Duration of detention	Manner of termination[1]	Appeal procedures
5(2)	Emergency detention of informal patient	The doctor in charge or his nominated deputy	None	None specified	72 hours	1. Patient discharged or remains informally 2. Regraded to Section 2 or application for Section 3 initiated	None
5(4)	Nurse's holding power for informal patients	A first-level trained nurse	None	Mental disorder	6 hours	1. Patient discharged or remains informally 2. Section 5(2) applied by doctor	None

1. The responsible medical officer (RMO) may terminate any of these compulsory admission authorities before the prescribed period of detention. NB Patients absconding from hospital and remaining absent for 28 days are deemed to be "discharged by the process of law" and cannot be recalled to hospital under the same application.

From Chiswick, D. (1993) Forensic psychiatry. In *Companion to Psychiatric Studies* (eds R. E. Kendell & A. K. Zealley)(5th edn), pp. 795. Edinburgh: Churchill Livingstone. Reproduced by kind permission of the author and publisher.

Definitions

An *approved doctor* is a registered medical practitioner approved under Section 12 (2) by the Secretary of State as having special experience in the diagnosis or treatment of mental disorder. In practice, approval is awarded by a regional health authority to doctors with the requisite experience of clinical psychiatry. Psychiatrists who are Members of the Royal College of Psychiatrists would be eligible to apply, although this is not a mandatory requirement. Doctors with three years post-registration clinical experience, including six months in an approved full-time psychiatric training post offering experience in dealing with detained patients would also be considered. Some sections require recommendation from at least one approved doctor.

A *responsible medical officer* (RMO) is a registered medical practitioner in charge of the patient's treatment.

An *approved social worker* (ASW) is an officer of a local social services authority appointed for the purposes of the Act as having appropriate competence in dealing with people suffering from mental disorder. To qualify as an ASW, a social worker must undergo training and assessment at a course arranged by the Central Council for Education and Training in Social Work (CCETSW).

The *nearest relative* is normally determined by the relationship which is first on the statutory *list of relatives* in Section 26(1). This is:

> husband or wife
> son or daughter
> father or mother
> brother or sister
> grandparent
> grandchild
> uncle or aunt
> nephew or niece

There are rules regarding the interpretation of nearest relative; for instance, if a patient has two relatives of the same standing, the elder is considered to be the nearest relative. If a patient lives (or, immediately before his admission, lived) with a relative, that person is the nearest relative. If he has lived with a non-relative as husband or wife for six months, that person is the nearest relative.

Admission

All admissions under civil sections require an application to the hospital managers by either an approved social worker or the nearest relative, supported by one or two medical recommendations. In practice the doctor(s) and ASW complete the necessary statutory forms following an interview with a patient. This allows arrangements to be made for transporting the patient to hospital. The documents should arrive at the same time as the patient, and be handed over to the manager, usually an administrator or senior nurse, who records the time of admission and receipt of documents on a special form. The patient is then regarded as formally detained.

Which section of Part II should be used for admission?

It is now generally regarded as bad practice to use the emergency section for compulsory admission, except in a genuine emergency when it is not possible to find an approved doctor within a reasonable time. It carries the potential disadvantage of a hasty compulsory admission without the benefit of a psychiatric opinion. Whether Section 2 or Section 3 should be used for compulsory admission is a matter of clinical judgement, often hinging on previous knowledge of the patient. The *Code of Practice* (Department of Health & Welsh Office, 1993) makes suggestions about the differing circumstances under which Sections 2 and 3 should be considered (see Box 10.2).

Box 10.2 Which section should be used – 2 or 3?

Section 2 should be considered:
  •   where the diagnosis or prognosis is unclear
  •   where there is a need for in-patient assessment to formulate a treatment plan, or to gauge the effectiveness of compulsory treatment
  •   for re-assessment following a previous admission
  •   where a patient has not previously been admitted to hospital

Section 3 should be considered:
  •   for a known patient with a previous admission and recent assessment who needs compulsory admission for treatment
  •   where further treatment is required after the expiry of Section 2, and the patient is unwilling to remain in hospital informally and to consent to treatment
  •   If an informal patient (who may be willing to remain in hospital) requires electroconvulsive therapy (ECT) or medication but is unable or unwilling to give consent, an application under Section 3 must be made. For ECT, or for medication for more than three months, this must be coupled with a concurring opinion from a second opinion appointed doctor

---

Case example 3
A psychiatrist and social worker were called by a GP to the home of a man known to have schizophrenia who had thrown a brick through a neighbour's window. He had been discharged from hospital a few months previously and it was obvious that he had relapsed after stopping medication. Compulsory admission under Section 3 was appropriate because he was already well known to the psychiatric services, the diagnosis was not in doubt, and admission was necessary to re-start his treatment.

Compulsory detention of patients already in hospital

Section 5 allows the detention of patients already in hospital, and applies to patients in general hospitals as well as those in psychiatric units or hospitals. Out-patients, day patients or those attending accident and emergency (A&E) departments cannot be detained under Section 5. Patients in A&E departments are not eligible for detention under Section 5 as they are not yet admitted to hospital. The two compulsory powers under Section 5 are defined in Table 10.1 and described in the following examples.

Case example 4
An 18-year-old man with a first episode of psychotic illness had been an informal patient for a week. Despite treatment he remained suspicious, admitted to hearing voices and was convinced there was a plot to kill him. Late one night, following a visit from his father whom he tried to assault, he informed the staff nurse on duty that he was going home to "sort out" his father. He could not be persuaded to stay to be seen by the duty doctor, who was busy in another part of the hospital some distance away. The nurse's holding power under Section 5(4) was used to detain the patient until the doctor arrived two hours later. Section 5(2) was then completed and the next morning the consultant and social worker agreed that detention under Section 2 was necessary for further assessment.

Case example 5
A 24-year-old woman was admitted to the A&E department of a district general hospital following an overdose of antidepressant medication. She was unconscious on admission and required treatment in the intensive care unit. When she regained consciousness the next day, she was assessed by a psychiatrist who considered that she remained actively suicidal. She demanded to leave hospital, and was detained under Section (5)2 pending further assessment.

Consent to treatment

The agreement of patients for the treatment they receive is a cornerstone of medical practice. Before a patient can be given any form of treatment, whether for a mental disorder or for a physical condition, valid consent is required. This is sometimes called real or informed consent, and is:

> "the voluntary and continuing permission of the patient to receive a particular treatment, based on an adequate knowledge of the purpose, nature, likely effects and risks of that treatment, including the likelihood of its success and any alternatives to it. Permission given under any unfair or undue pressure is not consent." (Department of Health, 1993*a*)

There are specific problems with consent in psychiatric practice. Some mentally disordered patients may lack the capacity to give consent (e.g. a patient with gross thought disorder or in a stuporose state or with a severe learning disability). Others may refuse treatment because the illness affects their capacity to make an informed decision. The presence of a psychotic disorder does not automatically mean that a patient is unable to give real consent.

Treatment without consent can be given under "common law" but only in special situations (see below) and not where it is specifically overridden by statutory law. "Common law" refers to the law developed by the judiciary, over the centuries, through the doctrine of precedent, as opposed to statutory law which requires legislation by parliament. Part IV of the Mental Health Act 1983 is the statutory law which deals with psychiatric treatment for detained patients. Psychiatric treatment for informal patients is governed by the normal standards for consent to treatment and the common law. Table 10.2 summarises the different categories of treatment and the standards of consent required for mentally disordered patients.

The doctor's duty to disclose information about treatment

The information given to a patient about a proposed treatment will vary according to the capacity of the particular patient and the type of treatment. The explanation should be given in broad terms and the patient must understand the purpose, nature, likely effects and risks of the treatment as well as any alternatives to it. The patient should also be informed of the probable consequences of not having the treatment. It is the responsibility of the doctor giving the information to assess whether the patient can give real consent. The patient should also be informed that he may withdraw his consent to treatment at any time. The amount of information disclosed to the patient, particularly regarding risks, has been legally defined by two important cases. In *Bolam v Friern Hospital Management Committee* (1957), the judge stated that "the test is the standard of the ordinary skilled man professing to have that special skill". This complex phrase is taken to mean that a doctor would not be regarded as negligent if the information disclosed was in accordance with the responsible body of medical opinion. It is often called the "Bolam Test" and has been approved by the House of Lords in *Sidaway v Board of Governors of Bethlem Royal Hospital and the*

Table 10.2 Consent by patients to treatment for mental disorder

Patient	Treatment	Consent
Informal but competent	1. Any psychiatric treatment[1]	Real consent
	2. Urgently necessary psychiatric treatment	Common law
Informal but incompetent	1. Any psychiatric treatment[1]	Common law duty of care or detain under MHA and apply Part IV (see below)
	2. Urgently necessary psychiatric treatment	Common law
Detained	1. Electroconvulsive therapy or 2. Medication for more than three months	Consent *or* second opinion under Section 58 (Part IV)
	3. Psychosurgery or surgical implantation of hormones to reduce male sex drive	Consent *and* second opinion under Section 57 (Part IV)
	4. Urgently necessary psychiatric treatment	Section 62 (Part IV)
	5. Any other psychiatric treatment	No consent required (Section 63)

1. For psychosurgery and implantation of hormones to reduce male sex drive, Section 57 applies.
Based on Chiswick (1993).

Maudsley Hospital (1985). The Law Lords emphasised that although the disclosure of risk is a matter of clinical judgement, no prudent doctor would fail to disclose serious risks. For example, in relation to electroconvulsive therapy (ECT) the doctor should explain that an anaesthetic and muscle relaxant will be given, that the treatment involves the passage of an electrical current through the brain, and that there may be some memory impairment after the treatment.

Common law consent and incompetent patients

Under what circumstances is it possible (and necessary) to dispense with the normal rules of consent? There are three situations where it is permissable to give treatment without consent under common law:

(1) to an unconscious patient to save life, or prevent serious harm unless there is clear evidence that the patient did not want that treatment
(2) to a non-consenting mentally disordered patient to prevent behaviour causing serious danger to himself or others (e.g. an assaultative psychotic patient may be given medication to prevent a serious escalation of violence)
(3) to "incompetent" patients (likely to be informal patients with a learning disability, organic brain disorder or severe depression).

Incompetent patients are so-called because they almost certainly lack the capacity to give real consent. If the proposed treatment is for mental disorder, it is good practice to detain those patients under the Mental Health Act and to apply Part IV. However, the House of Lords in *F v West Berkshire Health Authority* (1982) laid down the common law principles on treatment without consent for incompetent patients. The case in question applied to treatment for a physical condition, and held that treatment could be given to an incompetent patient as long as it was in the patient's best interest, and provided that the doctor acted in accordance with a responsible body of medical opinion. In the case of *F*, the treatment was the sterilisation of a mentally handicapped woman, which the House of Lords declared was a special treatment. Also included in the category of special treatments are abortion and organ transplantation. For these treatments, permission of the High Court is necessary. For less controversial treatments (e.g. an operation to remove a malignant tumour), it is not necessary to involve the courts if it is in the patient's best interest, either to save life, to ensure improvement or to prevent deterioration in physical or mental health. In these cases, it is good practice to discuss the proposed treatment with the patient's relatives.

Case example 6
A 52-year-old man had been an informal patient at a psychiatric hospital for many years with a diagnosis of chronic paranoid schizophrenia. He developed a malignant tumour of the femur. Because of his mental state (he believed doctors had inserted a computer in his affected leg), he was incapable of giving consent to the operation, which was considered necessary to save his life. Not only was the operation lawful, but if it had not been carried out, or had been delayed resulting in the premature death of that patient, the medical staff might have been considered negligent, had the relatives decided to take legal action.

Detained patients

Part IV of the Mental Health Act 1983 gives statutory authority for certain treatments for mental disorder to be given to most detained patients without their consent (see Table 10.2). It also provides specific safeguards for all patients for whom treatments are proposed that give rise to particular concern. Part IV applies only to patients detained in hospital for more than a few days. In particular, it does *not* apply to patients detained under Sections 4, 5, 135 or 136.

Treatments requiring consent or a second opinion: Section 58

Two treatments are currently referred to in this section, namely ECT, and medicines for mental disorder given for more than three months. Other treatments could be included if the Secretary of State so decides.

Giving ECT to detained patients. Before ECT may be given to a detained patient, the RMO must discuss the proposed treatment with the patient. If the patient is able to give real consent, the RMO must complete a certificate of consent (Form 38), which states that the patient is capable of understanding the nature, purpose and likely effects of the treatment. The maximum number of treatments, their frequency and the proposed length of the course should be stated on Form 38. If the patient is unwilling or unable to give consent, ECT may only be given with the agreement of an independent doctor appointed by the Mental Health Act Commission (MHAC). This doctor is referred to as the "second opinion appointed doctor", commonly abbreviated to SOAD. It is also good practice to discuss the proposed treatment with the patient's relatives. In reaching his decision, the SOAD is required to consult two other professionals concerned with the patient's treatment, one a nurse and the other neither a nurse nor a doctor. The SOAD must also consider whether the treatment is likely to alleviate or prevent deterioration of the patients condition. If the SOAD agrees with the treatment he issues Form 39.

> **Case example 7**
> An elderly woman suffering from recurrent depression was admitted to hospital under Section 3. Treatment with antidepressant medication had been ineffective in preventing deterioration. She was retarded, almost mute, had lost two stones in weight and could not be persuaded to eat or drink properly. It was impossible to have any meaningful discussion with her about the proposed ECT. A SOAD agreed to the RMO's treatment plan of ECT given not more than twice weekly up to a maximum of ten treatments over a period of not more than six weeks, and Form 39 (the certificate allowing treatment to be given) was signed.

Giving medication to detained patients. Any detained patient may be given medication for mental disorder without consent, for up to three months. Thereafter medication can be given only with the patient's consent, or with the agreement of a SOAD. Form 38 or 39 must be completed.

The administration of some drugs, such as clozapine and lithium, requires regular blood tests. It is now accepted that if an RMO or SOAD authorises treatment with clozapine, authorisation for the administration of the drug should include the authority for the necessary blood monitoring. If the patient actively refuses to cooperate with the venepuncture, it is a matter for the individual judgement of the RMO, in conjunction with the clinical team, to decide whether or not to proceed with the treatment (Mental Health Act Commission, 1993*a*).

Case example 8
A 30-year-old woman with a diagnosis of schizophrenia had been detained under Section 3 for four months during which time she had improved with oral chlorpromazine. This was her second admission in a year, following relapse after defaulting from treatment with oral medication. Her RMO wished to treat her with a depot neuroleptic but she refused consent because of her concerns about developing tardive dyskinesia, the risks of which had been explained to her by her RMO. Notwithstanding her refusal to give consent, the SOAD agreed with the RMO that treatment by a depot neuroleptic should be given, and Form 39 was completed.

Treatments requiring consent and a second opinion: Section 57

Section 57 applies to treatments which are regarded as hazardous or irreversible. Currently these are only psychosurgery for mental disorder, and the surgical implantation of hormones to reduce male sexual drive. Other treatments could be included if authorised by the Secretary of State. Treatments under Section 57 require both the consent of the patient *and* a second opinion. It applies to *all* patients, whether detained, informal in-patients, or out-patients. These treatments can be given only under the circumstances shown in Box 10.3.

Box 10.3 Treatments under Section 57

These can only be given if:

- the patient has given real consent
- a panel of three people appointed by the Mental Health Act Commission (including an independent doctor) have certified that the patient is capable of understanding the nature, purpose and likely effects of the treatment and has consented to it
- the appointed doctor certifies that, having regard to the likelihood of the treatment alleviating or preventing a deterioration, the treatment should be given
- the appointed doctor, in making the decision, has consulted two other professionals involved with the patient, one a nurse and the other neither a nurse nor a doctor

---

All but one referral to the MHAC under Section 57 have related to psychosurgery. Between 1991 and 1993, there were 46 referrals for psychosurgery, for which 42 certificates were given (Mental Health Act Commission, 1993*b*). The single request to the MHAC for a second opinion concerning treatment by hormone implant was the basis of an important legal ruling (*R v Mental Health Act Commission ex parte W*, 1988). The Commission refused to grant a certificate for the administration of goserelin (a hormone analogue used to treat prostatic cancer) to reduce sexual drive in a paedophile. The Court ruled that goserelin was not a hormone, it was not given by surgical implant, and therefore did not fall within the provisions of Section 57 (*The Times*, 1988; Brahams, 1988).

Urgent treatment: Section 62

If treatment is urgently necessary to save a patient's life, to prevent serious deterioration, to alleviate serious suffering or to prevent behaviour which may be dangerous to the patient or others, the RMO can authorise treatment, providing it is not irreversible or hazardous. The treatments that might come under these categories are not specified in the Act. In these urgent situations it is not necessary to obtain the patient's consent or a second opinion. Section 62 is most often used to give ECT to severely depressed patients who are not eating or drinking, while awaiting a second opinion under Section 58. Most hospitals maintain a central record of the use of Section 62.

Treatments not requiring the patient's consent: Section 63

Medical treatments for mental disorder which are not specifically mentioned in Sections 57 and 58 may be given to detained patients without their consent, although it should always be sought. Such treatments are defined under Section 145 of the Act, and include nursing, but also care, habilitation and rehabilitation under medical supervision. This covers a wide variety of therapeutic activities, such as psychological and social treatments; in practice they could not be carried out without the patient's active cooperation. The Court of Appeal (*The Times*, 1994) recently held that tube feeding of a patient was lawful under Section 63.

The second opinion appointed doctor (SOAD)

In addition to the medical members of the MHAC, the Commission appoints consultant psychiatrists with a minimum of five years experience to provide second opinions under Part IV of the Act. When the RMO requires a second opinion, the RMO's secretary or an administration officer contacts the MHAC office in Nottingham, with details of: the patient's legal status; date of detention; proposed treatment (ECT or medicine); and whether the

---

Box 10.4 SOAD procedure

Peruse the case notes
Interview the patient
Personally discuss the treatment plan with the RMO
Interview a registered mental nurse and another professional
   involved in the patient's treatment (usually a social worker,
   occupational therapist or rarely a psychologist)
If the SOAD considers that the treatment should be given, an
   appropriate certificate will be signed:
   • Form 39 (if the patient is incapable of consenting or refuses
     treatment)
   • Form 38 (if the patient can give valid consent and agrees
     to treatment)
The MHAC monitoring form will be completed and sent, with a
   photocopy of Form 38 or 39, to the MHAC secretariat

---

patient is unable or unwilling to consent. The MHAC will then instruct a
SOAD to visit the hospital at a convenient time. In preparation for the visit,
it is good practice for the RMO to have ready a written treatment plan. Box
10.4 shows the SOAD procedure.

Case example 9
A 38-year-old man with paranoid schizophrenia was admitted on
Section 2 of the Mental Health Act three months earlier and is
currently detained under Section 3. The proposed plan of treatment
is to continue medication with:
(a) one oral antipsychotic preparation from Section 4.2.1. of the
British National Formulary (BNF);
(b) one depot antipsychotic preparation from Section 4.2.2. of the
BNF;
to be given within BNF limits.

Between 1991 and 1993 there were 8839 referrals to the MHAC for second
opinions under Section 58, of which 52.3% were for medicines, 46% for
ECT and 1.7% for both (Mental Health Act Commission, 1993*b*). In about
90% of cases the SOAD agreed a treatment plan with the RMO.

Compulsory treatment in the community

The situation of a psychotic patient who is stable on medication when
detained in hospital, but who defaults from treatment after discharge, is
a familiar one. Relapse causes problems for the patient and his family, and

for those responsible for aftercare. In these circumstances treatment is delayed until the patient deteriorates to such a degree that compulsory detention is again warranted. This cycle of events often causes frustration to the patient's relatives and his carers. Some countries have introduced legislation which provides for compulsory psychiatric treatment in the community (Dedman, 1990; Sensky *et al*, 1991). In Britain, there are currently very limited powers under the 1983 Act for giving compulsory treatment to patients in the community. Some treatment may be compulsorily provided for two groups of patients: (1) those subject to guardianship orders; and (2) formerly detained in-patients on leave of absence. The nature of the treatment that may be given is discussed below.

Guardianship orders

Patients who are subject to guardianship orders may be required to attend for medical treatment but are not compelled to accept it. Guardianship was originally envisaged as the community care equivalent of a compulsory treatment order or hospital order. Its principal function was the protection of vulnerable, mentally disordered individuals from exploitation, ill-treatment or neglect, by appointing a responsible person to offer guidance, control and supervision. In practice, guardianship is infrequently used; there is reluctance by local authority social services departments to take on this time-consuming responsibility. Under the 1959 Act the order was used mostly for mentally handicapped individuals. In 1978 there were a total of 138 guardianship orders, of which 111 were for mentally handicapped persons, and only 37 for the mentally ill or for those suffering from psychopathic disorder.

The 1983 Act altered the rules for guardianship orders and effectively excluded most patients with mental handicap from its provisions. In 1986–1987, of 123 new guardianship orders, only 28 were for the mentally impaired or severely mentally impaired, compared with 93 for mental illness and two for psychopathic disorder. Most guardianship orders fall within Section 7 of Part II of the Act (dealing with civil sections), and only a minority follow conviction (under Section 37: nine such cases in 1986–1987). The great majority of appointed guardians were local authority social workers, and in only five cases were other persons nominated. Wattis *et al* (1990) found that over three-quarters of guardianship orders were used for the elderly, to require residence in an old people's home. For younger people they were used to maintain patients at home and to provide access for treatment. Table 10.3 summarises the powers of guardianship orders.

Formerly detained patients

Patients on leave of absence from hospital (under Section 17) after detention on Section 3 or 37 may receive compulsory treatment after

Table 10.3 Guardianship orders in England and Wales under the Mental Health Act 1983

Section	Situation	Medical signatories	Applicant	Psychiatric condition specified in the Act	Duration of guardianship	Manner of termination	Appeal procedures
7	Guardianship (civil)	Two doctors, one of whom is approved	Nearest relative or an approved social worker	Mental illness, mental impairment, severe mental impairment, psychopathic disorder	6 months, renewable for a further 6 months, then at yearly intervals	Discharge by RMO, social services authority or nearest relative	Mental health review tribunal
37	Guardianship (criminal)	Two doctors, one of whom is approved	Defence, prosecution or court (magistrates' or Crown)	1. Mental illness or severe mental impairment 2. Mental impairment or psychopathic disorder ("only if treatable")	6 months, renewable for a further 6 months, then at yearly intervals	Discharge by RMO or social services authority	Mental health review tribunal

discharge, but only until the section expires. Creative interpretation of the 1959 Act, which had less strict grounds for renewal, led to the widespread practice of renewing detention of known defaulting patients on leave of absence, usually by nominal overnight readmission. The patient would then again be given leave and compulsory treatment in the community would continue. This practice was declared unlawful in 1985, following judicial review of two cases (*R v Hallstrom ex parte W*, and *R v Gardiner and another*, 1986).

There has been extensive debate about the desirability and practicality of a community treatment order, although few would advocate the forced administration of medication to a patient in his own home. Early discussion papers from the Mental Health Act Commission (1986) suggesting an extended form of guardianship, and from the Royal College of Psychiatrists (1987) proposing a community treatment order, produced little impact. More recently, a proposal by the Royal College of Psychiatrists (1993) for a community supervision order has re-opened the debate. The College report recommended a new order, applicable only to patients who regularly defaulted from treatment, which would provide compulsory supervision of the patient in the community. The patient would be required to consent to the order, but if voluntary treatment was refused or supervision rejected, resulting in deterioration in mental state, the patient could be recalled to hospital. Safeguards in the form of appeal to a mental health review tribunal (MHRT) were included in the proposal.

The Government considered but rejected the College proposal. Instead, it announced its intention to introduce new legislation to amend the 1983 Act (Department of Health, 1993*a,b*). There will be a new power of supervised discharge for detained (but non-restricted) patients, who would present a serious risk to their own health or safety, or to the safety of other people, unless their care was supervised. Supervised discharge would incorporate the principles of the care programme approach (Kingdon, 1994), including a named key worker for the patient, a written care plan, and regular multidisciplinary reviews. Failure to cooperate would lead to an immediate review of the case, with the possibility of recall to hospital under the existing provisions of the 1983 Act. Patients would have the same rights of appeal to a MHRT as those detained in hospital. The Government also proposes to extend the duration of Section 17 (leave of absence) from six months to one year. Supervision registers have recently been introduced (Department of Health, 1993*b*)(see also Chapter 8).

Applications and appeals against detention

All detained patients, with the exception of those on short-term sections and certain forensic sections, have the right to appeal against their detention both to the managers of the hospital and to a mental health review tribunal

(MHRT). Under Section 132 of the Act, the managers have a duty to ensure that patients and nearest relatives understand which section of the Act has been applied and the relevant rights of appeal. The Department of Health provides information leaflets on most of the sections. A member of staff, usually a nurse or administrator, is delegated to explain to the patient his rights of appeal against detention. The contents of the leaflet should be explained; this might require several attempts in the case of a seriously psychotic patient. This is often described as "giving the patient his rights". A record should be made that not only has the information been given but that it has been understood by the patient.

Appeals to managers

In the case of NHS hospitals, the managers are members of the district health authority or trust and for special hospitals they are members of the Special Hospitals Service Authority (SHSA). Managers are responsible for administration of the hospital and also have legal responsibility for detaining patients under the Act. They have a duty to nominate an officer, usually a member of the administrative staff, to scrutinise the legal documents, since if they are incorrect the patient cannot be lawfully detained.

Under Section 23 of the Act, managers have the power to order the discharge of a detained patient, if the criteria for detention are not met. These criteria are normally reviewed when the order for detention is renewed, but a patient has the right to ask managers for discharge at any time during the detention. This is called "an appeal to the managers". It is a non-statutory procedure and is not described in the Act. It is not a substitute for a MHRT, but is an additional means for a patient to appeal against detention. Three managers are appointed to hear the appeal. A report from the RMO is normally required and the RMO, and perhaps other professionals, as well as the patient, are usually interviewed. An appeal to the managers rarely results in a patient being discharged because there is reluctance to oppose the RMO's recommendation that the patient should remain in hospital.

Mental health review tribunals

There are 15 regional mental health review tribunals in England and Wales. Tribunal members are appointed by the Lord Chancellor and each tribunal panel has three members: a lawyer, as chairman, a medical member, and a lay member. For restricted patients the legal member must be a judge. Table 10.4 summarises the categories under which an application to the MHRT can be made, who can apply and when, and when renewal of application can be made. Useful accounts of tribunal practice are detailed by Hepworth(1985), Wood(1985) and Peay(1990).

Table 10.4 Rights of application to a mental health review tribunal (by patient or nearest relative)

Section	Patient	Nearest relative	Frequency
Part II			
2	Within 14 days	None	–
3* and 7	Within first 6 months	Within 28 days if notified that RMO has barred nearest relative from discharging patient	During second 6 months, then annually
Part III (unrestricted)			
37 Hospital order	** after first 6 months	Within 28 days if notified that RMO has barred nearest relative from discharging patient	During each subsequent period of one year
37 Guardianship	Within first 6 months	Within one year, then annually after 6 months	During second 6 months, then annually
37 Notional and 47	Within first 6 months	None	During second 6 months, then annually
48	Within first 6 months	Within 28 days if notified that RMO has barred nearest relative from discharging patient	–
Part III (restricted)			
37/41	*** after first 6 months	None	During each subsequent period of one year
47/49	*** within first 6 months	None	During each subsequent period of one year
48/49 and CPA[1]	*** within first 6 months	None	During second 6 months, then annually

1. Criminal Procedure (Insanity and Unfitness to Plead) Act 1991.

*The hospital managers *must* refer the case within six months if the patient has not appealed, *and* if three years have elapsed since the last hearing.
**The hospital managers *must* refer the case if three years have elapsed since the case was last considered.
***The Home Secretary *may* refer the case of a restricted patient to a tribunal at any time, but must refer:
    (a) if three years have elapsed since the last hearing
    (b) within one month of recall of a conditionally discharged patient.

Tribunal procedures

The patient or relative (or someone acting on their behalf such as a nurse or social worker) must apply in writing to the tribunal office for the area. The tribunal must then notify the patient, the nearest relative, the hospital managers, and in restricted cases, the Home Office. The managers are responsible for obtaining reports from the RMO and social worker which must be sent to the tribunal office within three weeks. If applicable, the Home Office may also provide a statement about its views on the suitability of the patient for discharge.

Patients are entitled to have legal representation for their appeal, and may be given a list of appropriate solicitors by the hospital or the Law Society. The solicitor may instruct an independent psychiatrist to provide a report on the patient. Patients are entitled to have legal aid, called "assistance by way of representation" (ABWOR), provided their capital is less than £3000. When reports have been received, a date for the tribunal hearing is set. With the exception of Section 2 hearings, which must take place within 14 days, there is often considerable delay, up to 3–6 months in some cases, and often longer for restricted patients.

Preparing medical reports for tribunals

In preparing the report for the tribunal, the RMO must bear in mind that the patient will read the entire report, unless it is stated that disclosure of all or part of the report "would adversely affect the health or welfare of the patient or others". If the tribunal agrees with the RMO, specified information may be withheld. Some RMOs are reluctant to disclose the contents of their reports to the patient, even regarding diagnosis, believing that this could adversely affect the doctor–patient relationship, but others take a more relaxed view. It is generally considered good practice and beneficial to the therapeutic relationship to discuss the contents of the report and recommendations with the patient. It might be seen as reasonable to withhold information given in confidence by relatives. For example, a patient's mother may make it clear to the hospital that she is frightened of allowing her son to live at home after discharge, although she is unwilling to share her anxieties with her son. Disclosure at a tribunal might have an adverse effect on their relationship.

The tribunal hearing

Shortly before the hearing, the medical member will interview the patient and examine the medical records. Tribunals normally take place at the hospital and usually in private, unless the patient requests a public hearing and the tribunal agrees that this would not be contrary to his interests. Usually the hearing is informal, no oaths are taken and everyone interested in the appeal is invited to attend throughout, unless the tribunal has particular reasons for excluding a participant. In practice, the patient and legal representative, RMO and social worker, a nurse and relatives are present. Other witnesses may also be called. Tribunals vary in their procedures, but usually after introductions, evidence is first heard from the patient, then the RMO, social worker and relatives. The patient's legal representative will usually put questions to the RMO and others. When all the evidence has been heard, the patient, again usually through his representative, will have the opportunity of finally putting his case to the tribunal. The tribunal can be adjourned at any time to obtain further information but must give 14 days notice of the resumed hearing.

Some patients, particularly those who are automatically referred, are anxious or indifferent about attending their tribunal and may refuse to participate. Under these circumstances, tribunal members usually attempt to see the patient on the ward and may later hear evidence in the patient's absence. However, many patients enjoy the procedure and view it as an important opportunity to have their case heard. For some patients, it may provide what is, regrettably, an all-too-rare opportunity to speak in depth to their RMO when interviewed for preparation of the report. For others, the patient may learn for the first time how he is viewed by the consultant and clinical team and what plans there are for his future.

Powers of tribunals

The primary function of the tribunal is to decide whether the patient should continue to be detained in hospital. It is not concerned with the question of whether or not the patient requires treatment. The powers of the tribunal differ according to whether the patient is unrestricted, under guardianship, restricted or transferred from prison.

Unrestricted patients. A tribunal *must* discharge a patient detained for assessment or treatment if it finds that:

(1) the patient is not suffering from mental disorder (Section 2) or mental illness, psychopathic disorder, severe mental impairment or mental impairment (Section 3 or 37); or
(2) the disorder is not of a nature or degree to warrant detention in hospital or assessment for medical treatment; or
(3) detention is not justified in the interests of the patient's health or safety or for the protection of others.

In practice it is for the patient to prove that the grounds for detention do *not* exist, and the tribunal need only be satisfied on the balance of probabilities. Some tribunals place the burden of proof on the hospital. Following a recent court case, it is considered lawful to detain immediately on a fresh section a patient who has been discharged by a mental health review tribunal (*The Times*, 1993).

Guardianship patients. A tribunal *must* discharge a patient subject to guardianship if it is satisfied that:

(1) the patient is not suffering from mental illness, psychopathic disorder, mental impairment or severe mental impairment; or
(2) that it is not necessary in the interests of the patient, or for the protection of others, that he/she should remain under guardianship.

Restricted patients. The criteria for discharging a restricted patient are identical to those for the mandatory discharge of unrestricted patients (see above). The patient can be granted an absolute discharge or, more usually, if the tribunal considers that it is appropriate for the patient to be liable to recall, a conditional discharge. This means that:

(1) the patient may be recalled at any time by the Home Secretary
(2) the patient must comply with any conditions imposed by a tribunal at the time of discharge or imposed at any subsequent time by the Home Secretary; the latter may be varied at any time. The conditions normally include statutory psychiatric and social work supervision, and residing where directed by the social worker. Paradoxically, there is no statutory authority to direct the patient to take medication.

A tribunal can also order a deferred conditional discharge until the necessary arrangements have been made, for example, in obtaining a hostel placement. Although a tribunal has no formal power to recommend leave of absence or transfers in the case of restricted patients, the Home Secretary may take such recommendations into account in his deliberations.

Prisoners transferred with restrictions. In these cases (Section 47 or 48 with 49 restriction) the function of the tribunal is to decide whether or not the patient should remain in hospital. The tribunal must notify the Home Office as to whether the patient would be entitled to an absolute or conditional discharge if he were a restriction order patient. If the patient is entitled to a conditional discharge, the tribunal may recommend that he should stay in hospital rather than return to prison if he is not released. For Section 48 cases, the Home Secretary must transfer the patient back to prison (unless he is entitled only to a conditional discharge and the tribunal has recommended that he should be allowed to stay in hospital). In other cases, the Home Office has 90 days in which to inform the tribunal of its views. If nothing is heard within that time, the managers must return the patient to prison, unless the tribunal has recommended a conditional discharge and continued stay in hospital instead.

The Mental Health Act Commission

From the late 18th century until the Mental Health Act of 1959, there was some form of independent body to inspect and supervise standards of psychiatric care. From 1913 onwards a Board of Control existed, which in addition to its inspectorial function had the authority to discharge patients. The Board of Control was abolished by the 1959 Act. Mental health review tribunals took on the role of appeals and discharge of detained patients, but there was no independent inspectorate of psychiatric institutions in England and Wales from 1959 until the Mental Health Act Commission (MHAC) was established in the Mental Health Act 1983. Its establishment was a landmark in monitoring standards of psychiatric care. The MHAC is a special health authority established under the Mental Health Act 1983. Its functions are shown in Box 10.5.

Members of the Commission are appointed by the Secretary of State. There is a chairman and vice-chairman and about 90 part-time members chosen from the fields of medicine, nursing, social work, law and psychology, and also lay and academic members. The Commission has its office and secretariat in Nottingham, with operational groups which relate to two or three regional health authority areas. There is a central policy committee and a number of standing committees which consider different areas of commission interests. A full account of the Commission's activities is published in the statutory biennial reports. (Mental Health Act Commission, 1993*b*). Curran & Bingley (1994) describe the development, structure and function of the Commission.

Box 10.5 Functions of the Mental Health Act Commission

To keep under review the way in which powers and duties under the Act are carried out in respect of detained patients (the MHAC has no responsibility for informal patients)

To visit and interview patients detained under the Act in hospitals and mental nursing homes

To investigate complaints in certain circumstances

To review decisions to withhold the mail of patients detained in special hospitals

To appoint registered medical practitioners to give second opinions where required by the Act; and others to certify consent under Section 57 of the Act

To maintain the *Code of Practice* and advise Ministers on amendments

To publish a biennial report

To offer advice to Ministers on matters falling within the Commission's remit

The Commission makes annual visits to most hospitals and mental nursing homes with detained patients; special hospitals and regional secure units, which almost exclusively treat detained patients, are visited more frequently. Social services departments and health authorities also receive regular visits. During a hospital visit all detained patients are given the opportunity of a private interview with the commissioners. The number of patients who wish to be interviewed varies. Patients most frequently discuss aspects of their care, particularly concerns about medication and their wish to be discharged, sometimes confusing the role of the Commission with that of a MHRT. Patients may make complaints during visits or by letter, and the Commission investigates those complaints that are within its remit (that is, complaints in respect of matters that occurred during detention under the Act, which had not been satisfactorily dealt with by managers). It receives more than 500 complaints a year.

In preparation for a Commission visit, the hospital administration must provide statistics relating to detained patients. Legal documentation is normally scrutinised and particular attention is paid to forms relating to consent to treatment. Any irregularities are pointed out to RMOs either on the day of the visit or by letter. Most hospitals and staff are positive about Commission visits and perceive them as helpful and often supportive, although occasionally there is criticism about excessive preoccupation with documentation. However, in special hospitals the Commission has made less impact and has not been seen as effective by either staff or patients in preventing malpractice (Department of Health, 1992).

Code of Practice

Section 118 of the Mental Health Act 1983 required the Commission to draft a code of practice on behalf of the Secretary of State, for the guidance of mental health professionals in relation to both the admission of patients and medical treatment of those suffering from mental disorder. After the preparation of two unsatisfactory drafts, a working party at the Department of Health produced a final *Code of Practice* (Department of Health & Welsh Office, 1990), which has been updated by a second edition (Department of Health & Welsh Office, 1993).

All mental health professionals should be familiar with the contents of the *Code of Practice*. Its legal status is uncertain and is not defined in the Mental Health Act. However, the introduction warns: "the Act does not impose a legal duty to comply with the Code, but failure to follow the Code could be referred to in evidence in legal proceedings". To date there have been no legal proceedings for alleged breaches of the Code.

In the introduction, the Code gives several broad principles to be considered when people are assessed for possible admission under the Act or to whom the Act applies (see Box 10.6). The text of the Code refers to:

Box 10.6 *Code of Practice* **principles**

People being assessed for possible admission under the Act, or to whom the Act applies, should:
- receive respect for and consideration of their individual qualities and diverse backgrounds – social, cultural, ethnic and religious
- have their needs taken fully into account, although it is recognised that, within available resources, it may not always be practicable to meet them
- receive any necessary treatment or care in the least controlled and segregated facilities practicable
- be treated or cared for in such a way that promotes to the greatest practicable degree their self-determination and personal responsibility consistent with their needs and wishes
- be discharged from any order under the Act to which they are subject immediately it is no longer necessary

---

assessment before possible admission under the Mental Health Act; admission under the Mental Health Act (to hospital and guardianship); treatment and care in hospital (including patients presenting particular management problems); leaving hospital; and particular groups of patients (those with learning disabilities, and young people under the age of 18).

The NHS Health Advisory Service

This was formerly called the Hospital Advisory Service and was established in 1969 to aid the improvement of the management, organisation and standards of patient care in psychiatric hospitals, and to advise the Secretary of State for Social Services about conditions in hospitals. In 1976 it changed its name to the NHS Health Advisory Service (HAS) and its remit was extended to reviewing community services for mentally ill and elderly people and the links between the services. This was carried out in collaboration with the Social Services Inspectorate (SSI). The NHS Drug Advisory Service (DAS) was established as part of the HAS in 1986 to review district and regional services for problem drug-users. Unlike the MHAC, which deals only with detained patients and the functioning of the Mental Health Act, the role of the HAS has been primarily an inspectorial and advisory one. Visiting teams would spend several weeks in a hospital and/or service. They would gain a comprehensive view of the qualities and shortcomings of the service, and make appropriate recommendations.

Until the end of 1991, the HAS carried out about 40 reviews of health and social services annually, with visits to health authorities approximately every five years. Reports of the visits were sent to the Secretary of State for Health. In 1991 the role of the HAS was again reviewed to take into account the NHS reforms. The HAS now has additional responsibilities for monitoring the quality of health care and the performance of providers in fulfilling contracts set by health authorities. The HAS produces annual reports of its activities (Williams, 1993).

Addendum for Northern Ireland

By Fred Browne

The Mental Health (Northern Ireland) Order 1986 has clearly been influenced by the Mental Health Act 1983 for England and Wales, but it is broader in its scope and has a number of significant differences. The Order is the first piece of UK legislation to define mental illness (Box 10.7). The Order also defines the terms "mental disorder", "mental handicap", "severe mental handicap" and "severe mental impairment". Of the last three of these definitions, only severe mental impairment requires "abnormally aggressive or seriously irresponsible conduct" for inclusion

---

Box 10.7 Mental Health (Northern Ireland) Order 1986

Mental disorder means mental illness, mental handicap and any other disorder or disability of mind

Mental illness means a state of mind which affects a person's thinking, perceiving, emotion or judgement to the extent that he requires care or medical treatment in his own interests or the interests of other persons

Mental handicap means a state of arrested or incomplete development of mind which includes significant impairment of intelligence and social functioning

Severe mental handicap means a state of arrested or incomplete development of mind which includes severe impairment of intelligence and social functioning

Severe mental impairment means a state of arrested or incomplete development of mind which includes severe impairment of intelligence and social functioning and is associated with abnormally aggressive or seriously irresponsible conduct on the part of the person concerned

Psychopathic disorder is not included in the Order

Persons suffering from mental disorder by reason only of personality disorder, promiscuity, or other immoral conduct, sexual deviancy or dependence on alcohol or drugs, are excluded from detention on these grounds alone

---

Table 10.5 Compulsory admission procedures in Northern Ireland under Part II of the Mental Health (NI) Order 1986

Article	Situation	Medical signatories	Applicant	Psychiatric condition specified in the Act	Duration of detention	Manner of termination	Appeal procedures
4	Admission for assessment	Two or three doctors including RMO	Nearest relative or approved social worker	Mental disorder	7 days, renewable to 14 days	Discharged from detention by RMO board or nearest relative Article 12 initiated	Mental health review tribunal on application by patient, nearest relative or certain others
12	Detention for treatment	Signatories to admission for assessment and additional report from RMO	Applicants for admission for assessment	Mental illness or severe mental impairment	6 months, renewable for a further 6 months and then at yearly intervals	Discharged from detention by RMO board or nearest relative	Mental health review tribunal on application by patient, nearest relative or certain others
7(2)	Assessment for patients already in hospital	Medical practitioner on the staff of the hospital	None	Mental disorder	48 hours	Patient discharged from detention or admission for assessment completed	None
7(3)	Nurse's holding power	A first-level trained nurse	None	Mental disorder	6 hours	Patient discharged from detention or Article 7(2) applied by doctor	None

in the category. There is no category of psychopathic disorder, and indeed, personality disorder by itself is specifically excluded as a reason for detention.

Part II of the Order details the procedure for compulsory admission of patients for assessment (Table 10.5). Application for admission is made either by the nearest relative or by an approved social worker, and the application is founded on a medical recommendation which is usually made by the patient's general practitioner. The medical recommendation requires evidence to be adduced not only that the patient suffers from mental disorder warranting assessment in hospital, but also that failure to detain him would create a substantial likelihood of serious physical harm to the patient or to others. Admission for assessment lasts for up to 14 days and may be followed by detention for treatment which is renewable after six months.

Part III of the Order is concerned with patients involved in criminal proceedings or under sentence, Part IV with consent to treatment, and Part V with the mental health review tribunal. Provisions are similar to those in the Mental Health Act 1983, with a few differences in detail. The Mental Health Commission for Northern Ireland has a broad investigative, inspectorial and advisory role which extends beyond patients detained in hospital to include voluntary patients, people on guardianship orders, those in nursing homes, residential homes and hostels – indeed, anyone suffering or even appearing to suffer from mental disorder.

Further details are available in the Order and the accompanying DHSS guide. A *Code of Practice for the Mental Health (NI) Order 1986* has been prepared (DHSS, 1992).

Addendum for Scotland

By Derek Chiswick

The laws of compulsory detention in Scotland are contained in the Mental Health (Scotland) Act 1984, the limited role of the common law having been clarified in a House of Lords judgment, *B v Forsey* (1988). Although broadly similar, the 1984 Act differs in important points of principle and detail from its English counterpart. Table 10.6 contains the compulsory admission procedures under Part V of the Mental Health (Scotland) Act 1984. Applications for detention for more than 28 days require the approval of a sheriff, a legally qualified judge. One in five applications in 1992–1993 proceeded to a judicial hearing, at which the doctors give evidence on oath and are questioned. Delays in obtaining judicial approval caused problems which have been remedied by introduction of the Mental Health (Detention)(Scotland) Act 1991.

Table 10.6 Compulsory admission procedures in Scotland under Part V of the Mental Health (Scotland) Act 1984

Section	Situation	Medical signatories	Applicant	Psychiatric condition specified in the Act	Duration of detention	Manner of termination[1]	Appeal procedures
24	Emergency, any patient unless in hospital	Any doctor	None, but consent of a relative or MHO required	Mental disorder	72 hours	Patient discharged or remains informally Detention under Section 26	None
25(1)	Emergency, any patient in hospital	Any doctor	None, but consent of a relative or MHO required	Mental disorder	72 hours	Patient discharged or remains informally Detention under Section 26	None
25(2)	Emergency, any patient in hospital	Nurse of the prescribed class	None	Mental disorder	2 hours or until arrival of doctor	Patient discharged or remains informally Detention under Section 25(1)	None
26	Patient detained under S.24 or 25(1)	Approved doctor	None, but consent of nearest relative or MHO required	Mental disorder	28 days	Patient discharged or remains informally Discharge by sheriff or by Mental Welfare Commission Detention under Sections 26A or 18	Sheriff or Mental Welfare Commission on application by patient

Table 10.6 cont.

Section	Situation	Medical signatories	Applicant	Psychiatric condition specified in the Act	Duration of detention	Manner of termination[1]	Appeal procedures
26A	Patient detained under S.26	Relevant doctor	None, but consent of nearest relative or MHO required	Mental disorder	3 days, excluding weekends and court holidays	Patient discharged or remains informally Discharge by sheriff or by Mental Welfare Commission Detention under Section 18	Sheriff or Mental Welfare Commission on application by patient
18	Any patient	Two doctors, one of whom is approved	Nearest relative or MHO	Mental illness, including a persistent disorder manifested only by antisocial conduct Mental impairment Severe mental impairment	6 months, renewable for 6 months and then at yearly intervals	Patient discharged or remains informally Discharge by nearest relative unless barred by RMO Discharge by sheriff or by Mental Welfare Commission	Sheriff or Mental Welfare Commission on application by patient

1. The responsible medical officer (RMO) may terminate any of these compulsory admission authorities before the prescribed period of detention.
NB Patients absconding from hospital and remaining absent for 28 days are deemed to be "discharged by the process of law" and cannot be recalled to hospital under the same application.

Box 10.8 shows the categories of mental disorder defined in the Mental Health (Scotland) Act 1984. The term "psychopathic disorder" does not appear in the Scottish Act. Instead, a phrase almost identical to the 1983 Act definition of psychopathic disorder appears as one of the two categories of mental illness. Treatability criteria apply for that disorder and for mental impairment. Guardianship depends on the presence of mental illness or mental handicap (not mental impairment or severe mental impairment as in England). There is no time limit on leave of absence under the 1984 Act, provided the patient remains liable to detention; patients are not routinely recalled to hospital to renew liability to detention. Introduction of a community care order is under discussion.

Consent to treatment provisions are similar to those of England and Wales, except that the mandatory procedures for consent to psychosurgery and the implantation of libido-reducing hormones only apply to detained patients.

Appeals against detention are heard by a sheriff. There are no mental health review tribunals in Scotland, but the Mental Welfare Commission has authority to order discharge; it did so only once in 1992–1993. Notes of guidance on the Act, and a *Code of Practice*, have been published by th Scottish Home and Health Department (1984; 1990). Blackie & Patrick (1990) provide a useful explanation of the Mental Health (Scotland) Act 1984.

Box 10.8 Mental Health (Scotland) Act 1984

Mental disorder means mental illness or mental handicap however caused or manifested

Mental illness – not defined, but includes a mental disorder which is a persistent one manifested only by abnormally aggressive or seriously irresponsible conduct

Mental impairment means a state of arrested or incomplete development of mind, not amounting to severe mental impairment, which includes significant impairment of intelligence and social functioning and is associated with abnormally aggressive or seriously irresponsible conduct on the part of the person concerned

Severe mental impairment means a state of arrested or incomplete development of mind which includes severe impairment of intelligence and social functioning and is associated with abnormally aggressive or seriously irresponsible conduct on the part of the person concerned

Psychopathic disorder does not appear by that name in the Act

Persons suffering from mental disorder by reason only of promiscuity or other immoral conduct, sexual deviancy, or dependence on alcohol or drugs, are excluded from detention on these grounds alone

Mental Welfare Commission for Scotland

The Mental Welfare Commission is a statutory body of at least ten members with a minimum of three doctors and at least one senior lawyer; it must contain a minimum of three female members. It currently has a membership of 20, of whom the majority are on a part-time basis. It has a duty to protect the interests of *all* people with a mental disorder, whether in hospital, nursing home or the community, and whether of detained or informal status. It is required to inquire into any case where there may be ill-treatment or neglect. It has the power to set up a formal inquiry under judicial procedure. It must regularly visit detained patients, whether in hospital or on leave of absence, and those under guardianship. It is notified of all detentions under the 1984 Act and the Criminal Procedure (Scotland) Act 1975 (see Chapter 5). It has authority to discharge detained patients except those subject to restriction orders. It must produce an annual report.

Addendum for the Republic of Ireland

By Enda Dooley

The current law in the Republic of Ireland relating to civil mental health matters is the Mental Treatment Act 1945. This law provides the statutory basis for the organisation of psychiatric hospitals, and for the admission of patients. The Act refers to "mental illness", "persons of unsound mind", and "addict". Only the term "addict" is defined, as a person who: (1) by reason of his addiction to drugs or intoxicants is either dangerous to himself or others, or incapable of managing himself or his affairs, or of ordinary proper conduct; or (2) by reason of his addiction to drugs, intoxicants or perverted conduct is in serious danger of mental disorder.

Unfortunately, the Act says little about the treatment of patients in hospital, or about mechanisms for discharge and aftercare. These shortcomings, in the light of developments in psychiatric practice, have been acknowledged. In 1981 an updated piece of legislation (the Health [Mental Services] Act 1981) was enacted by the Dail (parliament), but because of a number of flaws this legislation was never signed into effect. New mental health legislation is currently under consideration by the Department of Health (Brophy, 1994).

The present legislation allows for admission to hospital on a voluntary basis (Sections 190–192) where the application for admission by the patient (or nearest relative) is supported by a medical recommendation (usually a GP), or on a compulsory basis (Temporary Certification under Sections 184–189) where a mentally ill (including addictions) person is adjudged to require hospital treatment and is unfit to be treated as a voluntary patient. Compulsory detention requires application by the nearest relative (or a

Table 10.7 Compulsory admission procedures in the Republic of Ireland under the Mental Treatment Act 1945

Section	Situation	Medical signatories	Applicant	Psychiatric condition specified in the Act	Duration of detention	Manner of termination	Appeal procedures
184	Admission for treatment	Two doctors, one being the receiving consultant	Nearest relative or involved social worker	Mental illness, addiction	6 months, renewable every 6 months up to a maximum of 2 years	Patient discharged	The High Court (habeas corpus) The Minister for Health

social worker if the relative is unavailable or unwilling) and two medical recommendations, one of whom is the receiving consultant. Compulsory detention in hospital for treatment can last up to six months initially and can be renewed. There are no legal provisions for compulsory treatment in the community.

A voluntary patient cannot have treatment imposed on him against his will. In the case of a compulsorily detained patient, treatment can be given against the will of the patient once the agreement of the nearest relative is obtained. Table 10.7 summarises the compulsory admission procedures.

There are no current provisions for appeal against compulsory detention to an independent body. A patient can appeal to the Minister for Health (who is empowered to have the Inspector of Mental Hospitals investigate the circumstances of the case), or can initiate legal proceedings (habeas corpus) seeking release from hospital. In practice these mechanisms are rarely invoked. Statutory review of the organisation and running of mental hospitals is undertaken by the Inspector of Mental Hospitals who reports to the Minister for Health. There is no code of practice nor equivalent of the Mental Health Act Commission.

Law reports

B v Forsey (1988) *Scots Law Times* 572.

Bolam v Friern Hospital Management Committee (1957) 1 WLR 582; (1957) 2 All ER 118.

F v West Berkshire Health Authority (1992) 2 All E R 454.

R v Hallstrom ex parte W: R v Gardiner ex parte L (1986) 2 WLR 883 (1986) 2 All E R 306.

R v Mental Health Act Commission ex parte W (1988)

Sidaway v Board of Governors of Bethlem Royal Hospital and the Maudsley Hospital (1985) AC 871; (1985) 2 WLR 480; (1985) 1 All ER 643 HL.

W v L (1974) QB711: (1973) 3 WLR 859; 117 SJ 775; 72 LGR 36; 4 Fam Law 134; *sub nom W v L* (Mental Health Patient) (1973) 3 All ER 884 CA.

References

Blackie, J. & Patrick, H. (1990) *Mental Health: a Guide to the Law in Scotland.* Edinburgh: Butterworths, Scottish Legal Education Unit.

Bluglass, R. (1983) *A Guide to the Mental Health Act 1983.* Edinburgh: Churchill Livingstone.

Brahams, D. (1988) Voluntary chemical castration of a mental patient. *Lancet,* June 4th, 1291–1292.

Brophy, J. J. (1994) Forthcoming reforms of Irish Mental Health legislation. *Psychiatric Bulletin,* 18, 100–101.

308   *Cope*

Chiswick, D. (1993) Forensic psychiatry. In *Companion to Psychiatric Studies* (eds R. E. Kendell & A. K. Zealley)(5th edn), pp. 793–816. Edinburgh: Churchill Livingstone.

Curran, C. & Bingley, W. (1994) The Mental Health Act Commission. *Psychiatric Bulletin*, **18**, 328–332.

Curran, W. J. & Harding, T. W. (1988) *The Law and Mental Health: Harmonising Objectives*. Geneva: WHO.

Dedman, P. (1990) Community Treatment Orders in Victoria, Australia. *Psychiatric Bulletin of the Royal College of Psychiatrists*, **14**, 462–464.

Department of Health (1992) *Report of the Committee of Inquiry into Complaints about Ashworth Hospital*. Cm 2028-1-2. London: HMSO.

—— (1993*a*) "Legislation planned to provide for supervised discharge of psychiatric patients". Press release H93/908.

—— (1993*b*) *Legal Powers on the Care of Mentally Ill People in the Community. Report of the Internal Review*. London: DoH.

—— & Welsh Office (1990) *Code of Practice*. London: HMSO.

—— & —— (1993) *Code of Practice*. London: HMSO.

Department of Health and Social Security (1986) *Mental Health Statistics for England 1986*. London: Government Statistical Service.

Department of Health and Social Services (1992) *Code of Practice for the Mental Health (NI) Order*. Belfast: HMSO.

Gostin, L. O. (1975) *A Human Condition 1*. London: National Association for Mental Health.

—— (1977) *A Human Condition 2*. London: National Association for Mental Health.

Hepworth, D. (1985) Dangerousness and the Mental Health Review Tribunal. In *Aggression and Dangerousness* (eds D. P. Farrington & J. Gunn). Chichester: John Wiley.

Hoggett, B. (1990) *Mental Health Law*. London: Sweet & Maxwell.

Home Office & Department of Health and Social Security (1975) *Report of the Committee on Mentally Disordered Offenders* (Butler Report). Cmnd. 6244. London: HMSO.

Jones, R. (1988) *Mental Health Act Manual*. London: Sweet & Maxwell.

Kingdon, D. (1994) Care programme approach. Recent government policy and legislation. *Psychiatric Bulletin*, **18**, 68–70.

Martin, J. P. (1984) *Hospitals in Trouble*. Oxford: Blackwell.

Mental Health Act Commission (1986) *Compulsory Treatment in the Community: A Discussion Paper*. London: MHAC.

—— (1993*a*) Practice Note 1. Guidance on the administration of clozapine and other treatments requiring blood tests under the provisions of Part IV of the Mental Health Act. London: MHAC.

—— (1993*b*) *Fifth Biennial Report*. London: HMSO.

Peay, J. (1990) *Tribunals on Trial: Decision Making under the Mental Health Act 1983*. Oxford: Oxford University Press.

Royal College of Psychiatrists (1987) *Community Treatment Orders – A Discussion Document*. London: Royal College of Psychiatrists.

—— (1993) *Community Supervision Orders*. CR18. London: Royal College of Psychiatrists.

Scottish Home and Health Department (1984) *Mental Health (Scotland) Act 1984: Notes on the Act*. Edinburgh: Scottish Home and Health Department.

—— (1990) *Mental Health (Scotland) Act 1984: Code of Practice*. Edinburgh: HMSO.

Sensky, T., Hughes, T. & Hirsch, S. (1991) Compulsory psychiatric treatment in the community. I. A controlled study of compulsory community treatment with extended leave under the Mental Health Act: special characteristics of patients treated and impact of treatment. *British Journal of Psychiatry*, **158**, 792–798.

The Times (1988) Law report. 27 May.

—— (1993) Law report. 27 January.

—— (1994) Law report. 1 December.

Wattis, J. P., Grant, W., Trayner, J., *et al* (1990) Use of guardianship under the 1983 Mental Health Act. *Medicine, Science & the Law*, **30**, 313–316.

Williams, R. (1993) The NHS Health Advisory Service: the annual report of the Director for 1992–93. London: HMSO.

Wood, J. C. (1985) Detention of patients: administrative problems facing mental health review tribunals. In *Psychiatry, Human Rights and the Law* (eds M. Roth & R. Bluglass), pp. 114–122. Cambridge: Cambridge University Press.

11 Civil matters
Rosemarie Cope & Martin Humphreys

Civil rights in public law • Civil rights in personal affairs • Civil rights in financial matters • Addenda for Northern Ireland, Scotland and the Republic of Ireland

---

All people have legal rights: for example, to get married at the age of 16, to drive a car at the age of 17, and to vote at the age of 18. A list of common civil rights is given in Box 11.1.

Unless the contrary is proved, it is assumed that people are mentally capable of entering into these legal transactions. However, mental disorder can affect a person's legal capacity to make such decisions. The simple test of a person's mental capacity is that he must understand in broad terms what he is agreeing to, and its likely consequences. It is immaterial whether the person is in hospital, either informal or detained, or whether he can carry out the transaction sensibly.

Only when there are grounds to support incapacity do certain statutory powers come into play. Psychiatrists may be involved in the assessment of the subject's mental state and his competence for the particular task in question. These issues form the basis of this chapter. The format is based on Hoggett (1990), to which readers are referred for a fuller account.

Box 11.2 summarises the civil courts in England and Wales, which deal with most of the matters described.

Box 11.1 Civil rights

Public
- standing and voting in elections
- serving on juries
- driving

Personal
- getting married and divorced
- looking after children

Financial
- making a will (testamentary capacity)
- owning property and managing affairs
- entering into contracts

Box 11.2 The civil courts in England and Wales

County Court
- deals with most civil cases

High Court
- deals with more serious cases
- most are heard before a single High Court judge, without a jury
  The High Court has three divisions:
  - *Queens Bench Division*: deals with most common law cases on contracts, damages, points of law and procedure
  - *Chancery Division*: deals with wills, trusts, companies and tax
  - *Family Division*: deals with adoption, divorce and wardship matters

Court of Appeal (Civil Division)
- hears appeals from any of these Courts

House of Lords
- may hear further appeals

Civil rights in public law

Voting

"Persons of unsound mind" as well as "lunatics" and "idiots" are prevented from voting or standing in elections by common law. Only a broad understanding of the general procedure is necessary to vote, and in practice this consists of giving a name and address and confirming that one has not already voted. However, in order to vote the citizen must be registered on the Electoral Roll. Detained patients may not register to vote; all others can. Until recently, informal patients whose only place of residence was a psychiatric or mental handicap hospital were effectively disenfranchised, because such hospitals were not recognised for electoral registration purposes. A series of legal test cases and a Speaker's conference on the subject led to reform of the law. Section 7 of the Representation of the People Act 1983 makes provision for long-term informal patients to vote.

Clinical staff of a hospital are expected to identify, by a particular date each year, all informal patients who might be resident in hospital during the course of the next 12 months, although not necessarily for that entire period, who have no alternative residence, and who therefore might be eligible to register to vote. Each patient who then wishes to register must complete a patient's declaration form, without assistance from others, unless prevented by physical disability alone (e.g. blindness). The form must then be attested by a designated member of hospital staff, and sent to the relevant electoral registration officer. The ability to complete the declaration constitutes an implicit test of the patient's capacity to vote and is clearly more rigorous than anything required of the ordinary citizen.

Before the reform of the law, fears were expressed by some members of Parliament that large numbers of patients voting in one constituency might have a distorting effect on the result of the ballot. In fact, there is evidence that few patients who are identified as eligible actually choose to register, and an even smaller proportion of these then go on to vote (Humphreys & Chiswick, 1993).

Mentally ill Members of Parliament

It is unlikely that a legally incapable person would ever be elected to parliament, but a sitting Member of Parliament (MP) might subsequently become incapable. If an MP is compulsorily detained in hospital for more than six months because of mental illness, Section 141 of the Mental Health Act 1983 allows his removal. There is no equivalent provision in the House of Lords. Any doctor recommending the detention of an MP on the grounds of mental illness is required to inform the Speaker of the House of Commons.

Jury service

Every private citizen has both the right and duty to serve on a jury. However, Section 1 of the Juries Act 1974 excludes a large number of the mentally disordered. A person suffering from mental disorder who is either resident in hospital, or other similar institution, or who regularly attends a doctor for treatment of mental disorder, is prevented from taking on jury duties. Also, those subject to guardianship orders or judged incapable of managing their own property and affairs are ineligible to sit on a jury.

Driving

Anyone applying for a driving licence, or who holds a licence, must disclose whether he has ever suffered from, or develops, what is described as either a "relevant" or "prospective" disability (Road Traffic Act 1972). Individuals with either disability will have their licence refused or revoked. Relevant mental disabilities include: epilepsy (unless there have been no seizures for two years or seizures only when asleep for three years); severe learning disability; or any other disorder deemed likely to render the applicant a danger to the public when driving (e.g. dementia). The side-effects of psychotropic medication may also impair driving ability, and the patient should be advised about this, and warned that even small amounts of alcohol may increase the risks.

A prospective disability may be a relapsing and remitting condition, or one that is progressive over time, thus affecting the person's fitness to drive in the future. This may include a recurrent or chronic psychotic illness or severe bipolar affective disorder. Only in exceptional circumstances might a severe degree of neurotic disorder or personality disorder be considered a prospective disability. In some cases a limited licence (for 1, 2 or 3 years) may be issued, although only after a specified period of stability and evidence of compliance with treatment. This may require the written support of the doctor concerned.

More stringent conditions apply to drivers of heavy goods vehicles, taxis and other public service vehicles (Royal College of Psychiatrists, 1993). It is important to advise patients not to drive if they might place themselves or others at risk. If this advice is not accepted, it may be necessary to inform the Driver and Vehicle Licensing Authority (DVLA). This body has recently published a guide to current medical standards of fitness to drive, covering the whole range of physical and psychiatric disorders (Medical Advisory Branch, DVLA, 1993). The General Medical Council (1993) has published guidelines on disclosure without patient consent in the public interest (see Chapter 12), and these are relevant in relation to questions of mental fitness to drive.

Civil rights in personal affairs

Marriage

Marriage is a life-long voluntary contract between two people which carries certain mutual rights and obligations. It is commonly terminated by divorce and rarely annulment.

Annulment

Annulment is rare but the question may arise in relation to a mentally disordered partner for one of two reasons. Firstly, consent to marriage may be rendered invalid because of "unsoundness of mind" (Matrimonial Causes Act 1973) at the time of the wedding itself. The degree of incapacity must have been severe enough to have prevented an appreciation of the nature of the contract of marriage and its basic duties. However, marriage and its obligations are so widely understood that few people would fail to have some understanding of them. Secondly, although consent to the marriage may be valid, annulment is possible where one partner was suffering from a mental disorder within the meaning of the Mental Health

Act 1983, "of such a kind or to such an extent as to be unfitted for marriage" (Matrimonial Causes Act 1973). Either party may apply for annulment and psychiatric evidence may be required. If the grounds exist the marriage may be annulled at the request of the mentally disordered person or the spouse, providing that both are still living, if either feels that their situation has been exploited. The Marriage Act 1983 enables patients subject to long-term powers of compulsory detention to be married at the hospital, even against medical advice.

Divorce

The criteria for an individual to be capable of agreeing to a divorce are the same as those necessary to give valid consent to marriage; that is, understanding the nature, effects and outcome of the agreement. This is independent of any other incapacity, such as the capacity to manage property and affairs. A person may be incapable of handling affairs for himself and yet still retain the ability to marry or divorce.

A marriage may fail as a result of mental disorder in one partner. For patients in long-term care, divorce may be granted after two years separation if both parties agree and are competent to give consent, or after five years whether or not both parties consent. Only if the divorce is likely to cause the respondent particular hardship is there reason for its refusal, and this is unlikely to apply in the case of a patient in hospital.

An immediate divorce may be granted where one partner has behaved in a way such that it is unreasonable for the other to go on living with them. This may be related to mental disorder. If mental illness has supervened, neither partner is deemed responsible, and belongings and effects are dealt with accordingly. If a report is requested by representatives of either party, it should include a description of the person's disorder and any associated disturbance of behaviour. It is also important to describe the person's current needs and plans for future care to enable the court to decide if undue suffering may be caused if the divorce is granted.

Parental responsibility and the care of children

Parents are responsible for looking after their children. If the parents are married to each other, both have responsibility; otherwise the law gives this responsibility to the mother unless the court says otherwise, or the mother makes a formal agreement to this effect with the father. Parents do not lose parental responsibility unless the child is adopted (or freed for adoption). The law relating to the welfare of children is now contained in the Children Act 1989, which came into force in October 1991. The Act promotes the principle that children should be cared for within their own families through the exercise of parental responsibility, and that the state should intervene only if necessary to safeguard the welfare of the child.

Williams (1992) gives a concise guide to the Act and there are useful accounts by Black *et al* (1991) and the Department of Health (1991).

The child's welfare is regarded as paramount when the court makes any decision about its upbringing. In private and public law proceedings, the court must now establish a timetable and give directions for the expeditious handling of the case, on the grounds that any delay might prejudice the welfare of the child. It must always consider a checklist which covers the child's circumstances. The court must have regard to:

(1) the ascertainable wishes and feelings of the child (considered in the light of his age and understanding)
(2) his physical, emotional and educational needs
(3) the likely effect on him of any change in his circumstances
(4) his age, background and any characteristics of his which the court considers relevant
(5) any harm which he has suffered or is at risk of suffering
(6) how capable each of his parents, and any other person in relation to whom the court considers the question to be relevant, is of meeting his needs
(7) the range of powers available to the court in the proceedings in question.

In court proceedings there are four different types of orders available under the Children Act 1989. These replace the concepts of custody, care, control and access. They are shown in Box 11.3.

Local authority services

Part III of the 1989 Act gives local authorities powers and duties to provide services for children and their families, and for children in need and disabled children. Children are 'in need' if they are:

> "unlikely to achieve or maintain, or to have the opportunity of achieving or maintaining, a reasonable standard of health and development without the provision of services by a local authority, or if their health or development is likely to be significantly impaired or further impaired, without the provision of such services, or if they are disabled." (Children Act 1989)

In practice, the local authority must provide family support where appropriate, for example by advice, counselling or home help, and also make day care available where appropriate. For some children in need the local authority has a duty to provide accommodation, preferably in agreement with the parents, but if this cannot be achieved the child is normally placed with foster parents, since residential care is now avoided, particularly for younger children.

Box 11.3 Orders available under the Children Act 1989
(based on Williams, 1992)

Private Law Orders: *Residence* (states with whom child
(Section 8: law affecting   will live)
family arrangements)   *Contact* (allows child to visit or stay
                                 with parent(s) or others)
                                 Specific issue (covers specific
                                 aspects of parental responsibility,
                                 such as medical treatment,
                                 education, religion, etc)
                                 Prohibited steps (restrains a person
                                 with parental responsibility from
                                 taking any steps specified in the
                                 order, such as removing the child
                                 from the country)

Public Law Orders: Care, supervision and education
(law involving the   supervision orders
family and the State)

Orders for the protection   Child assessment, emergency
of children: protection, and police protection
                                 orders

Wardship: May be available in certain
                                 circumstances

The official solicitor

The Supreme Court Act 1981 gives certain powers and duties to the official solicitor. A major role is acting as next friend or guardian *ad litem* to psychiatric patients involved in civil proceedings where there is no one able or willing to act in that capacity. He acts on behalf of minors in wardship and adoption proceedings, and also on behalf of others in such proceedings, for example, a mentally disordered mother.

Psychiatric assessment of parents in childcare proceedings

As would be expected, child psychiatrists are more frequently involved in assessments for childcare proceedings than general or forensic psychiatrists. However, an opinion from a general psychiatrist may be requested if there is evidence or suspicion of serious mental disorder in a parent; a forensic psychiatrist is more likely to be involved if the child has been the victim of serious physical or sexual abuse. The request for assessment may come from a local authority, the guardian *ad litem* (a person appointed by the court to safeguard the interests of the child, usually a social worker), or a solicitor representing the parent/s or other parties involved.

Forensic and general psychiatrists do not usually have the skills to assess parenting abilities, and do not normally interview the child. Their assessment is specifically concerned with the mental state of the parent, the nature of any mental disorder and its possible effect on the parent's capacity to care for the child. As part of the assessment it is important to have access to any previous psychiatric records, reports from the local authority and any other relevant information. The partner should always be interviewed, and other relatives as appropriate.

Case example 1

A 30-year-old single woman had been caring for her nine and six-year-old daughters with occasional support from her parents. At the age of 24 she developed symptoms of an affective disorder. During the next six years she received treatment as an out-patient for two episodes of depressive illness and she also had three compulsory admissions for hypomanic episodes. When euthymic, her care of the children was exemplary. When depressed, she had sufficient insight to request help from her mother. However, when hypomanic she behaved irresponsibly, neglected the children, sometimes leaving them alone at night, and she developed casual relationships with men whom she sometimes brought home.

An independent psychiatric opinion was requested by the local authority with regard to her current mental state, the prognosis and the effect of her mental disorder on her capacity to provide adequate care for her children. At the time assessment was requested she had been discharged from hospital having defaulted from treatment, the children were with foster parents, and the local authority had allowed her increasing access with a view to allowing the children home for a trial period. During interview she was irritable and hostile, her mood was labile, there was pressure of talk, and she spoke with bitterness about her involvement with psychiatrists and social workers. She showed no real appreciation of the effect of her behaviour on her children when ill and stated that the children were able to look after her when she was unwell. She adamantly refused to consider taking lithium or any other prophylactic medication. The prognosis was considered poor with the likelihood of further relapses, during which she would not be able to provide adequate care for her children.

Case example 2

A 25-year-old man was referred for a risk assessment by the local authority. His 16-year-old girlfriend, who was herself under the care of the local authority, was expecting his child. His parents were divorced, his father was described as an alcoholic who used to physically abuse all the boys in the family, and he and his siblings were made the subject of care orders when he was ten years old. He had acquired a lengthy criminal history, with four convictions for assault, including two against previous girlfriends. He was a heavy drinker and was frequently involved in pub brawls. He described losing his temper easily, with or without alcohol, and admitted he had hit his girlfriend on several occasions when he thought she was looking at other men.

The opinion was that he had a disorder of personality, in that he was volatile, explosive, immature and had poor impulse control. He had a history of aggression which was exacerbated by alcohol. Under the circumstances, the local authority placed the couple in a family assessment centre and monitored the quality of the relationship and parenting abilities after the child was born.

Civil rights in financial matters

Testamentary capacity

Testamentary capacity is the ability to make a valid will. This requires the testator (the person who makes the will) to be of "sound disposing mind and memory". This means that the testator must understand the nature and purpose of a will, he must know broadly the extent of the property and possessions to be disposed of, and the people who might justifiably expect to benefit. For the vast majority of the population, testamentary capacity is never questioned. A will may be challenged in cases of extreme old age, apparent eccentricity, mental illness or learning disability, or if the will seems idiosyncratic. Capacity may fluctuate and wills may be made during a "lucid interval". A psychiatric report concerning testamentary capacity may be requested when a will is made or amended, or when its validity is challenged after death. The criteria for assessing testamentary capacity are legal and not clinical, and the question of competency is decided by the Court.

Assessing testamentary capacity

The testator should be interviewed alone to avoid any suggestion of interference or coercion by others. The assessment must include questions relating to the understanding of the principle of making a will, for example: "what property are you leaving" and "what are the names of your children and close relatives". These facts should be obtained from independent sources before the interview and checked with the account given.

Mental state examination should aim to identify and describe any specific symptoms of major mental disorder, in particular those which might have a direct bearing on the capacity to make a will (e.g. delusions concerning family members or imperative hallucinations), as well as any evidence of disorientation or impairment of memory. The contents of the will itself should be reviewed with the testator and any apparently inconsistent or unusual inclusions or omissions discussed during the interview. The report should include a statement about the presence or absence of mental disorder, and any clinical diagnosis and its likely effects.

When the testator is no longer alive a psychiatrist might be asked to conduct what is essentially a "psychiatric post-mortem". This requires a careful review of all available documentary evidence including medical and psychiatric case notes, other records and any personal papers. In addition, as many family members and friends as possible should be interviewed. As is the case when the testator is still living, the substance of any report relating to testamentary capacity should be based only on what can be established from sources of information; these may be somewhat limited.

Case example 3

A 74-year-old spinster who lived alone died from cancer of the breast with widespread secondary metastases. One month before her death she instructed her solicitor to make a will in which she left her estate (her house and some capital) to a friend who had visited her regularly for many years. A nephew, who had had no contact with the deceased for many years, challenged the will on the grounds that his aunt was of unsound mind when she made it and that she had been manipulated by the friend. He relied heavily on her medical records which included letters by a surgeon and an oncologist, who had both treated the old lady before her death, in which they referred to her as "decidedly odd . . . and demented". The surgeon wrote "I was never convinced that I had managed to communicate satisfactorily with her".

A psychiatrist was instructed by the beneficiary's solicitor and was given access to all the medical records and the statements of various witnesses who had known the deceased, some of whom he was able to interview. It became clear that mental symptoms had been manifested, but only in the last few weeks of her life, and that these consisted of episodes of fluctuating confusion with transient misidentification of people. Until a month prior to her death, although physically ill, she had been alert with intact memory, good self-care and nothing to suggest a progressive dementing illness. The psychiatrist suggested that the mental abnormality was probably due to episodes of subacute confusion (perhaps related to metastases in her brain) and not dementia. He pointed out that there was no evidence available to indicate her state of mind on the day she made the will other than the notes of the solicitor, which did not refer to any abnormality in her mental functioning. The nephew eventually withdrew the application.

A person may have the capacity to make a will, even if he is otherwise incapable of managing his affairs. In England and Wales the Court of

Protection may make a will only if the person does not have the required testamentary capacity, but this is not the case in Scotland where no one may act in this way on behalf of another.

Managing property and affairs

There are three legal mechanisms available for the protection, management and administration of the property and affairs of mentally incapable people. These are: the Court of Protection; appointeeship; and enduring power of attorney. Comprehensive accounts are given by Bingley (1990) and Hoggett (1990).

(1) *Court of Protection*

The Court of Protection is an office of the Supreme Court, whose function is to take responsibility for people whose mental disorder affects their capacity to manage their property and affairs. Currently there are about 28 000 people whose affairs are under the Court's control. Seventy per cent are female, of whom the majority are aged over 70, with a diagnosis of dementia. Approximately half live in private nursing homes, a fifth in NHS hospitals, and the remainder live at home or in sheltered accommodation.

The Court of Protection Rules 1984 govern the Court's proceedings, and its functions and powers are defined in Part VII of the Mental Health Act 1983. Anyone may make an application to the Court of Protection but usually it is the nearest relative, or sometimes a solicitor or social worker. Under Section 94 of the 1983 Act, a Judge of the Court must decide if:

> "after considering medical evidence, he is satisfied that a person is incapable, by reason of mental disorder, of managing and administering his property and affairs".

This refers to the broad definition of mental disorder in Part I of the Act: "mental illness, arrested or incomplete development of mind, psychopathic disorder and any other disorder or disability of mind". This definition is wider than that required for long-term compulsory detention (see Chapter 10). A criticism of the Court's powers is that it can make a decision based on a single medical report from any medical practitioner, for example the general practitioner, who need not necessarily have any specialist psychiatric experience.

Once the Court has received the application, the patient has seven days, or until the hearing date (whichever is the later), in which to object to or contest the evidence. However, if the Court considers that a patient is incapable of understanding the procedure or that it might be harmful to his health, the patient would not be notified, and therefore would have no opportunity to comment upon the application. If the Court has any doubts about the patient's capacity, it may ask a medical visitor, appointed by the Lord Chancellor, to examine him and report to the Court. Visitors, who may be lay, legal or medical, according to the needs of the case, visit patients and investigate the ability of the patient to manage his affairs or any other aspect of the Court's function. The Royal College of Psychiatrists (1983) has issued guidelines to assist doctors who may be involved in preparing medical certificates for the Court of Protection. MacFarlane (1985) describes the role of medical evidence in the Court of Protection, and Carr (1988) gives an account of the work of medical visitors.

> **Case example 4**
> A 50-year-old company engineer suffered from a bipolar affective disorder with two previous admissions to hospital in a hypomanic state. He accepted voluntary redundancy at work and received a substantial redundancy payment. An episode of depression on ceasing work was followed by elevation in mood, whereupon he pursued a variety of wild business ventures. He made long-distance telephone calls at all hours of the day and night, bought advertising space in local newspapers, and was in the process of hiring a sports arena for a pop concert. His wife made an application, supported by a medical recommendation from the patient's consultant, to the Court of Protection for appointment of a receiver which was duly made. His illness ran a protracted course over some years. Eventually his condition stabilised. He maintained regular contact with psychiatric services and showed good insight. The Court of Protection was eventually able to terminate the appointment of a receiver.

The powers of the Court of Protection. Once the patient is subject to the Court's jurisdiction, it has total control over all his property and affairs. Unless the patient has limited assets, the Court appoints a receiver under Section 99 of the Act. This is usually a close relative, often the person who applied to the Court, but it could be a solicitor or a local authority. If there is difficulty in finding a receiver, an official solicitor can be appointed. The Court may sell the patient's property, acquire new property for him, make settlements or provide for members of his family, make a will, make arrangements to carry on his business or profession, carry out a contract, dissolve a partnership or conduct legal proceedings on his behalf.

Discharge from the Court of Protection. Because the great majority of people under the jurisdiction of the Court are elderly, very few apply for discharge (there were only 40 successful cases in 1992). There is no automatic review of the need for the Court's intervention. If a patient recovers his mental capacity, it is a matter for the patient or his solicitor to apply to the Court for discharge, with a supporting medical report.

(2) *Appointeeship*

The Court of Protection is expensive; there are Court fees as well as any due to the receiver or a solicitor, all of which must be met from the patient's funds. It is, therefore, of little practical value in dealing with the affairs of the less well off. Appointeeship, described as "the poor man's Court of Protection", is available for dealing with social security and other benefits due to those "unable to act" for themselves (Social Security [Claims and Payments] Regulations 1981). It is the most commonly used legal intervention for people who are incapable of managing their property and affairs.

Approximately 47 000 appointeeships are made by the Department of Social Security (DSS) in an average year (Bingley, 1990). The Secretary of State for Social Security nominates the appointee, who is usually a close relative, to "act on behalf of a claimant who is unable to manage his own affairs", but whose incapacity need not necessarily be permanent. With the growing number of elderly people, particularly the elderly mentally ill in private nursing homes, it is often the manager of the nursing home who takes on the role of appointee. The appointee may exercise the rights due to any social security beneficiary and also has the right of appeal if such matters are in dispute. It is for the local DSS office, on receipt of an application, to make enquiries about the alleged inability of the beneficiary and also the suitability of the potential appointee. They are under no obligation to obtain medical evidence, although they may do so in either case. Appointeeship is entirely independent of the Court of Protection and is potentially open to abuse in the case of particularly vulnerable individuals who may be made even more so by lack of close family or friends.

(3) *Enduring power of attorney*

Under a relatively new law, the Enduring Powers of Attorney Act 1985, people can now make plans for the management of their property and affairs should they become incapable at some time in the future. Before this Act was passed, there existed only a general power of attorney (Powers of Attorney Act 1971). This allows one person (called the donor) to nominate another person (called the donee or attorney) to manage his property and affairs on his behalf. With this general power of attorney, if the donor becomes mentally incapable, the attorney's authority to act is invalidated.

The Enduring Powers of Attorney Act 1985 has made it possible for the donor to appoint an attorney, providing he has the necessary legal capacity at the time and understands the nature and effect of the power. If, later on, the attorney has reason to believe that the donor is becoming mentally incapable, he must notify the donor and apply to the Court of Protection for registration of the enduring power of attorney. About 15 000 Court of

Protection cases are registered under the enduring power of attorney. The relatives should also be notified and they have the opportunity of objecting to registration by the Court of Protection. Although the attorney acts under the supervision of the Court of Protection, the Court does not have direct or unlimited jurisdiction over the patient's assets.

Contracts

A contract is an agreement between two parties, consisting of an offer and its acceptance. A person's capacity to make a contract is governed by similar principles to those required for making a will. It depends on whether the person can understand the nature and effect of the contract. However, even an incapacitated person is bound by the terms of any contract he has made, unless he can show that the other person had reason to be aware of his incapacity. A contract may not be legitimate if the incapacity was so obvious or severe that the man in the street might have recognised it, as, for example, in the case of severe learning disability. With the exception of these cases, a person is under no obligation to establish if someone with whom they make a contract is capable of acting on their own behalf.

The only exception applies to "necessaries"; these include not only goods but also services such as accommodation which are appropriate to the circumstances and situation of the person at that particular time in his life. The Sale of Goods Act 1979 gives protection to mentally incompetent people. It requires that he should pay a reasonable price for any goods or services, which prevents exploitation by overcharging.

Addendum for Northern Ireland

By Fred Browne

Dickson (1989) provides a useful introduction to the structure of the civil courts in Northern Ireland, their procedures and the civil legislation. The system is broadly similar to that in England and Wales, although there are a number of differences in detail. For example, it is not possible to obtain a divorce by post in Northern Ireland, whereas this can be done in England and Wales.

The Abortion Act 1967 does not apply to Northern Ireland. Instead, following the case of Bourne (1939), a doctor may carry out an abortion if he acts in good faith to preserve the life of the mother. In practice this more restrictive regulation means that each year an estimated 1500 women travel to England to have abortions performed under the Abortion Act 1967.

Many of the legal protections offered to children in Northern Ireland are detailed by O'Halloran (1988) in his book on wardship. In wardship issues the 'paramountcy principle' (that the welfare of the child is of paramount importance) applies in Northern Ireland as it does in England and Wales. The Children (NI) Order is due to be laid before Parliament, and is expected to receive parliamentary approval in 1994. Its provisions are similar to the Children Act 1989.

The mentally disordered who are unable to manage their property and affairs are catered for by the Office of Care and Protection under the direction of the Master of Care and Protection. The scheme under Part VIII of the Mental Health (NI) Order 1986 is similar to that under Part VII of the Mental Health Act 1983. The same criteria for testamentary capacity apply in Northern Ireland as in England and Wales.

Compensation for the victims of crimes has proven to be of particular importance in Northern Ireland because of the civil strife. There is a scheme for compensating the victims of criminal damage under the Criminal Damage (Compensation)(NI) Order 1977, and another for the victims of criminal injuries under the Criminal Injuries (Compensation)(NI) Order 1988. Compensation can also be claimed by people whose property is damaged under the emergency powers legislation. The subject is covered comprehensively by Greer (1990).

Addendum for Scotland

By Derek Chiswick

Most of the issues discussed in this chapter are governed by laws applicable to Great Britain. In particular, the law and procedures concerning competence in relation to voting, jury service, marriage and divorce are essentially the same in Scotland as in England and Wales. There are, however, differences concerning the welfare of children, and in some aspects of managing property and affairs.

Box 11.4 summarises the civil courts in Scotland. Most civil litigation (e.g. contracts, damages, divorce and custody of children) in Scotland is dealt with in the sheriff court; sheriffs in Scotland are legally qualified judges. The country is divided for this purpose into six sheriffdoms (each presided over by a sheriff principal) and further divided into sheriff court districts. Appeals from a sheriff court are to the sheriff principal and then to the Court of Session in Edinburgh. For civil matters only, there is ultimate appeal to the House of Lords.

Children and parental responsibility

Only minor parts of the Children Act 1989 apply in Scotland (e.g. concerning child minding and day care), and the principal legislation concerning the care and welfare of children remains the Social Work (Scotland) Act 1968.

Box 11.4 Civil courts in Scotland

Sheriff courts: Scotland is divided into six sheriffdoms, each headed by a sheriff principal
- deal with bulk of civil litigation (debt, contract, property and custody of children)
- consider applications for civil detention under Section 18, Mental Health (Scotland) Act 1984
- shared jurisdiction with Court of Session for divorce action
- sheriff principal can hear cases on appeal from other sheriffs

Court of Session
- supreme civil court in Scotland
- sits in Edinburgh
- court of first instance *and* hears appeals from sheriff courts
- cases heard by single judge except for appeals

House of Lords
- can hear civil cases on appeal from Court of Session

Children's hearings
- established under Social Work (Scotland) Act 1968
- lay tribunals composed of three members (male and female) drawn from the children's panel
- deal with children under 16 who commit offences or are in need of care and protection
- referrals made to the reporter who conducts initial investigation
- have the authority to impose compulsory measures of care
- decisions can be appealed to a sheriff

A pivotal part of this Act is the children's hearing, which has power to order compulsory measures of care (supervision with or without conditions of residence). In the first instance the child who may be in need of care is referred to the reporter to the children's panel. The reporter is a legally qualified, full-time appointee of the local authority. He may refer the case to a hearing, a tribunal of three ordinary citizens drawn from a list (the children's panel) which each local authority is required to establish. Panel members receive special training. The hearing is intended to be a discussion between the child, his parents and the panel members.

Psychiatrists are commonly asked to provide reports to the panel, usually concerning the child and sometimes the parents. Decisions of the hearing, and indeed the grounds for referral of the case to it, may be appealed to a sheriff. The Children (Scotland) Bill currently before Parliament contains important proposals for dealing with children who are victims of abuse. The system of children's hearings is generally regarded as satisfactory (HMSO, 1993).

Managing property and affairs

The equivalent functions of a receiver appointed by the Court of Protection are, in Scotland, carried out by a *curator bonis* appointed by the Court of Session or a sheriff court; there are approximately 400 appointed each year. Any person may petition the court for appointment of a *curator* but the local authority must, and the Mental Welfare Commission for Scotland may, if a *curator* seems necessary. The petition to the court is accompanied by two supporting medical recommendations.

Hospital managers may look after money (currently up to £5000) belonging to an in-patient and spend it for his benefit if the doctor certifies that the patient is incapable or *incapax* (Section 94, Mental Health (Scotland) Act 1984). For sums over £5000, the managers must obtain approval from the Mental Welfare Commission. If the assets of an *incapax* in-patient are more than £20 000, the appointment of a *curator bonis* should be considered (Mental Welfare Commission for Scotland, 1993).

Arrangements for powers of attorney and appointees are similar in Scotland to those in England. The criteria for testamentary capacity in Scotland are also the same.

Addendum for the Republic of Ireland

By Enda Dooley

The structure of the civil courts in the Republic of Ireland is shown in Box 11.5.

Family matters

The Republic of Ireland recognises the importance of the family unit, and the State is committed to defending the institution of marriage. The criteria for a mentally disordered person to make a valid marriage are essentially the same as for the UK. However, legal divorce does not exist in the Republic of Ireland. In certain circumstances, a judicial decree of nullity can be granted. A marriage contract may be considered void (that is, it never had legal effect) or voidable (that is, valid until it is annulled by a decree of nullity). A marriage may be voidable on the grounds that either party did not have the mental capacity to marry.

Box 11.5 The civil courts in the Republic of Ireland

District Court
- can award damages up to £2500 in contract and civil wrong cases

Circuit Court
- original jurisdiction limited to £15 000
- can hear appeals from the District Court

High Court
- can award unlimited damages
- has wide original jurisdiction covering such matters as succession, trusts, and wards of court
- has considerable supervisory jurisdiction
- can hear appeals from the Circuit Court and exercises consultative jurisdiction over the District Court by means of Case Stated

Supreme Court
- has no original jurisdiction over civil cases
- hears appeals from the High Court and has consultative jurisdiction over the Circuit and High Courts by way of Case Stated

---

The Constitution of Ireland safeguards the rights of parents to raise their children. The Child Care Act 1991 now provides the legislation in relation to children and the family, and its principles are similar to the UK laws. Although divorce does not exist, there is provision for legal separation, which raises issues with regard to access, custody and care arrangements.

Financial affairs

A mentally incapacitated person may be made a ward of court by the High Court. There must be sufficient evidence that the person is of unsound mind, and is incapable of managing his personal property and affairs. The Court then has responsibility for the welfare of the individual. In Irish Law, the ability to make a valid will, as in the UK, requires that the testator be of sound disposing mind. Regarding legally binding contracts, a mentally incapable person must have, at the time, the capacity to understand the contract and that the contract would have had the possibility of performance.

References

Bingley, W. (1990) The Court of Protection. In *Principles and Practice of Forensic Psychiatry* (eds R. Bluglass & P. Bowden). Edinburgh: Churchill Livingstone.

Black, D., Wolkind, S. & Harris Hendriks, J. (eds)(1991) *Child Psychiatry and the Law* (2nd edn). London: Gaskell.

Carr, E. F. (1988) The work of the Lord Chancellor's medical visitors. *Medicine, Science and the Law*, 28, 6–8.

Department of Health (1991) *The Children Act 1989 – An Introductory Guide for the NHS*. London: HMSO.

Dickson, B. (1989) *The Legal System of Northern Ireland*. Belfast: SLS Legal Publications.

General Medical Council (1993) *Professional Conduct and Discipline: Fitness to Practice*. London: GMC.

Greer, D. S. (1990) *Compensation for Criminal Injury*. Belfast: SLS Legal Publications.

Hoggett, B. (1990) *Mental Health Law*. London: Sweet & Maxwell.

HMSO (1993) *Scotland's Children: Proposals for Child Care Policy and Law*. Social Work Services Group. Edinburgh: HMSO.

Humphreys, M. & Chiswick, D. (1993) Getting psychiatric patients to the polls in the 1992 general election. *Psychiatric Bulletin*, **17**, 18–19.

MacFarlane (1985) Medical evidence in the Court of Protection. *Bulletin of the Royal College of Psychiatrists*, **9**, 26–28.

Medical Advisory Branch, DVLA (1993) *At a Glance Guide to the Current Medical Standards of Fitness to Drive*. Swansea: Driver and Vehicle Licensing Authority.

Mental Welfare Commission for Scotland (1993) *Annual Report 1992–93*. Edinburgh: Mental Welfare Commission for Scotland.

O'Halloran, K. (1988) *Wardship in Northern Ireland*. Belfast: SLS Legal Publications.

Royal College of Psychiatrists (1983) Medical visitors and the Court of Protection. *Bulletin of the Royal College of Psychiatrists*, **7**, 34–35.

—— (1993) *Psychiatric Standards of Fitness to Drive Large Goods Vehicles (LGV's) and Passenger Carrying Vehicles (PCV's)*. **17**, 631–632.

Scottish Law Commission (1991) *Mentally Disabled Adults: Legal Arrangements for Managing their Welfare and Finances*. Discussion Paper No 94. Edinburgh: Scottish Law Commission.

Williams, R. (ed.) (1992) *A Concise Guide to the Children Act 1989*. London: Gaskell.

12 Ethical issues in forensic psychiatry

Rosemarie Cope & Derek Chiswick

Confidentiality • Patients' access to their psychiatric records •
Psychiatric practice with dual obligations • Capital punishment •
Working in secure environments

Ethics is a branch of philosophy concerned with the rules of behaviour that are acceptable within a given society. The term 'medical ethics' means the accepted code of conduct within the medical profession. "Ethical" has a different meaning from "lawful" (the latter relating to statute) in that it is possible to act within the law while behaving unethically. For example, it may be lawful to discharge a detained mentally ill patient who no longer fulfils the criteria for detention, but unethical to turn him out on the streets without any accommodation or aftercare arrangements.

Ethical standards in medicine are regulated by the General Medical Council (GMC). This is an independent statutory body founded under the Medical Act 1858. It has a membership of medical practitioners with some lay members to represent the general public. It is responsible to the Privy Council, a body made up of politicians, judges and prominent lay people. The GMC provides guidance to doctors on ethical matters through the so-called "Blue Book" on professional conduct and discipline and upon fitness to practise (GMC, 1993). The Central Ethical Committee of the British Medical Association (BMA) also offers ethical advice to the medical profession (BMA, 1993). Within the Royal College of Psychiatrists there is an Ethics Working Group which produces guidelines from time to time on subjects of ethical importance in psychiatry.

This chapter is about ethical issues that are common to all fields of psychiatry, and indeed to medicine in general, such as confidentiality and consent to treatment. It also deals with matters that present special problems in forensic psychiatry, which, more than any other psychiatric discipline, is practised in coercive settings such as secure psychiatric hospitals and prisons. Doctor–patient contact is frequently initiated by the interests of society rather than by and for the individual patient. This places the doctor in a position of dual obligation.

329

Box 12.1 Exceptions to the duty of confidentiality

The patient or his legal advisor gives valid consent
If it is undesirable on medical grounds to seek the patient's
    consent, information may be given to a relative or other
    person
The information is required by law
In exceptional situations, disclosure in the public interest, for
    example, where the patient or someone else would be at risk
    of death or serious harm
For medical research, where this has been approved by a
    recognised ethics committee

Confidentiality

Patients have a right to expect that whatever they tell their doctor will be
held in confidence. However, modern medical practice, in which a number
of health professionals may be involved in treatment, can threaten
confidentiality. This is a particular problem in psychiatric practice where
multidisciplinary care is the norm. For those working in forensic psychiatry
settings, ethical dilemmas in relation to confidentiality arise with regularity.
The GMC's "Blue Book" gives guidelines for doctors on professional confidence (GMC, 1993). This states that doctors must not disclose information
about a patient obtained in a professional capacity to any third party,
even after the death of the patient. There are some exceptions; see Box
12.1.

A doctor should always be prepared to justify the decision to disclose
confidential information. When in doubt, it is sensible to discuss the matter
with an experienced colleague or to seek advice from a medical defence
organisation or the GMC. It is good practice to obtain a patient's written
consent to disclosure, and if consent is not forthcoming, an attempt should
be made to persuade the patient. If this is unsuccessful, the patient should
be told what information will be divulged, to whom, and the reasons for
the disclosure. A clear account should be written in the case notes. The
Royal College of Psychiatrists' position statement on confidentiality (1990)
gives a comprehensive account of the problems encountered in psychiatry.

Consent to disclosure

It is permissible to disclose information if the patient gives valid consent;
that is, the patient understands the nature and consequences of disclosure.
The patient must be told exactly what will be disclosed and under what
circumstances. It is good practice to record in the case notes that informed
consent has been given. If the patient is unable to consent because of, for

example, psychosis or learning disability, then disclosure can be made if it is in the best interests of the patient. Patient consent may be implied in the sharing of information with other professionals involved in the patient's clinical care. However, the doctor has a positive duty to ensure that colleagues keep all information confidential. This rule also applies to information given in clinical case conferences and for other teaching purposes.

Confidentiality and child abuse

The GMC (1993) has issued revised guidance on confidentiality and child abuse. The "Blue Book" states:

> "Deciding whether or not to disclose information is particularly difficult in cases where a patient cannot be judged capable of giving or withholding consent to disclosure. One such situation may arise where a doctor believes that a patient may be the victim of abuse or neglect. In such circumstances the patient's interests are paramount and will usually require the doctor to disclose information to an appropriate, responsible person or an officer of a statutory agency."

Depending on the situation, the appropriate person will be a social worker or a police officer. As in other circumstances, when a doctor has doubts about the disclosure of information, it is good practice to obtain advice from peers or a defence organisation.

Information required by law

(1) Information about a patient may be required by statute, for example, the notification of drug addicts or the provision of statutory reports to the Home Office about patients detained on a restriction order under Section 37/41 of the Mental Health Act 1983. Patient consent is not required in these situations. In the case of restricted patients, disclosure of information about them could have severe consequences.

Case example 1
A conditionally discharged restricted patient with a diagnosis of psychopathic disorder revealed to her RMO that she was having thoughts of self-harm and setting fires. The index offence had been one of arson. The RMO offered informal admission, which was accepted. However, when the Home Office was informed, a decision was made to recall the patient, against the advice of the RMO. Fortunately the warrant for recall had not been signed, and it was possible to dissuade the Home Office from taking such draconian measures. This was on the grounds that formal recall was unnecessary as the patient was accepting help and recall could have disastrous consequences for the therapeutic relationship.

(2) A judge, coroner or procurator fiscal may order (subpoena) a doctor to disclose information about a patient, either orally in court and/or by releasing medical notes. The GMC (1993) advises that the doctor should establish what information is required and should not hesitate to object to the proposed disclosure, particularly regarding the release of third party information. However, failure to comply may result in the doctor being held in contempt of court.

(3) Medical reports are required for mental health review tribunals and for managers' appeals. Patients' permission for disclosure of information or access to their records is not required.

(4) The Mental Health Act Commission has access to case notes of all detained patients and, again, patient consent is not required.

Medical research and audit

Guidelines are available about the ethics of research, including confidentiality (e.g. Medical Research Council, 1985). All research involving patients should be referred to an established ethics committee (Department of Health, 1991). Doctors are now required to undertake medical audit, and regular reports must be submitted to managers and health authorities. In order to preserve patient confidentiality, no record of an audit meeting should contain any information that could lead to identification of a patient, clinician or other hospital staff (Conference of Medical Royal Colleges, 1992).

Disclosure in the public interest

The leading case on this issue is *W v Egdell* (1990). W was convicted of the manslaughter of five of his neighbours. He was diagnosed as suffering from paranoid schizophrenia and the court ordered his detention in a special hospital under a restriction order. Some ten years later, his solicitors instructed an independent psychiatrist to prepare a report in support of his application to a mental health review tribunal. The report was unfavourable and W's solicitors withdrew the tribunal application. When the psychiatrist discovered that his report had been suppressed, he sent a copy to the hospital and a copy of this eventually reached the Home Office. W brought an action for breach of confidentiality. In dismissing the action, the Court of Appeal held that disclosure of the report was justified because there was a real risk of danger to the public. The psychiatrist had become aware of new information and it was his opinion that without disclosure, the tribunal might make a decision to discharge the patient based on inadequate information.

The duty to warn

Does a psychiatrist have a duty to warn or protect individuals whom his patient has threatened to harm? In the UK there is no statute that covers this situation, but in the US, failure to warn a potential victim resulted in litigation followed by legislation. This was the case of *Tarasoff v Regents of the University of California* (1976). In 1969 a Mr Poddar, a student at the University of California, told his psychotherapist that he intended killing Miss Titiana Tarasoff, a young woman who had rejected him. The therapist informed the police, but no action was taken and two months later Poddar committed the murder. Her parents sued the University, the therapist and the police, claiming that they had been negligent in not warning their daughter of the threat against her.

When the case was first heard in 1974, the California Supreme Court held that a doctor had a legal duty to warn a potential victim that a patient had threatened to harm. This caused consternation among psychiatrists, and the case was reheard in 1976. This time the duty of the psychiatrist was defined more broadly, and the court held that a therapist had a duty to use reasonable care to protect third parties against danger posed by the patient. This could include notifying the intended victim or others, contacting the police or hospitalising the patient, or taking whatever other steps might be necessary under the circumstances. This ruling has been adopted in several states in the US, but recent statutes have attempted to reduce liability to cases where a patient has made a serious threat of physical violence to a named victim. Although the ruling does not apply in the UK, it is easy to forsee the problems that such a ruling might produce. For example, it might affect the patient's willingness to confide in the therapist.

> **Case example 2**
> A man became depressed after his wife left him. He was admitted informally to hospital and soon revealed detailed plans to kill his wife, towards whom there was a long history of violence. He was uncooperative with any therapeutic input and there were no grounds to detain him under the Mental Health Act. Because of the real risk to his wife, the consultant told him that he would have to inform his wife and the police about the threats. Although initially angry, it was possible to persuade him that this was a necessary course of action, and his consent to disclosure was reluctantly given. However, even if consent had not been forthcoming, disclosure would have been justified in the public interest.
>
> **Case example 3**
> A man with a history of indecent exposure was receiving out-patient treatment with some benefit. During therapy he revealed his habit of following women, coupled with violent and sadistic sexual fantasies about them. Although he was considered to present a risk to women,

his therapist, having discussed the case with a colleague, decided that disclosure was not justified. This opinion was based on the fact that the patient was responding to treatment, there was no history of aggression, and there was no definite victim. Keeping the patient in therapy, in an atmosphere of trust, was considered to be the safest option.

Patients' access to their psychiatric records

Traditionally doctors in the UK have adopted a paternalistic attitude in deciding what information should be divulged to their patients about their illnesses. This has resulted in restricted access to medical records, especially in psychiatry. Psychiatric records are regarded as particularly sensitive because of the recording of opinions as well as facts, the nature of the diagnosis, the possible adverse response of the patient to disclosure, and the frequent inclusion of third party information. However, psychiatric patients have always had access to reports about them in certain circumstances, for example, psychiatric reports for mental health review tribunals, solicitors or employers. Legislation over the past decade has formalised the rights of patients to have access to their own medical and social services records (see Box 12.2). Cowley (1994) gives a detailed account of the relevant issues.

The Access to Health Records Act 1990 came into force on 1 November 1991and the legislation applies only to notes written after this date. Access to records gives the patient an opportunity to correct or refute any incorrect information about them.

Information can be withheld if:

(1) disclosure is "likely to cause serious harm to the physical or mental health of the patient or any other individual"; or
(2) the information is "relating to, or provided by, an individual other than the patient, who could be identified by that information", unless the third party has consented.

Box 12.2 Patients' access to records

Data Protection Act 1984 – gave patients access to computerised medical records
Access to Personal Files Act 1987 – gave patients access to social services records
Access to Medical Reports Act 1988 – gave people the right to see medical reports prepared on them for insurance purposes
Access to Health Records Act 1990 – gave patients access to their written medical records

---

In a recent test case in the Court of Appeal (*The Times*, 1994) the view of a consultant psychiatrist and a health authority was upheld, that the patient could be denied access to his medical records on the grounds that disclosure would be detrimental to him.

The Royal College of Psychiatrists (1992*a*) has issued guidelines on the Act. In particular, inaccurate and offensive derogatory comments have no place in psychiatric case notes. All health professionals should be aware that the Act applies to them, and it is recommended that information from different sources should be recorded in separate sections of the notes. Careful judgement is needed when deciding whether to disclose information to a patient suffering from a paranoid illness. Patients with a learning disability may also present problems, unless the information is presented at an appropriate level. Generally it is regarded as good practice to allow patients to know what is written about them. When giving patients access to their notes, the psychiatrist or other relevant professional should be present to go through the records with the patient in order to explain and interpret them and to answer any questions the patient might have.

Forensic in-patients with severe mental illnesses who were allowed daily access to their records were very positive about this (Parrott *et al*, 1988). They appreciated knowing what staff thought about them, and access facilitated discussion and therapeutic intervention. There was no evidence of harmful consequences such as paranoia or antagonism towards staff. However, giving patients access to notes when staff are not available for discussion is less successful. Bernadt *et al* (1991) sent general adult patients a copy of their admission summary or out-patient letter. Only about half the patients found the information helpful and over a quarter were upset by what they had read. All psychiatric units should have a policy for access to health records. Box 12.3 gives an example of such a policy.

Psychiatric practice with dual obligations

Medico-legal work

Much of the day-to-day work of a forensic psychiatrist involves the assessment of individuals to assist the court. Unlike usual doctor–patient interactions, the individual does not see the doctor at his own request about any problems he may have for which he wants treatment or advice. He attends because he has been ordered to do so, whether it is at the behest of the court or his solicitor. He is then expected to cooperate with a lengthy psychiatric interview, in which he is asked to reveal information, not only about himself, but also about his family and others. Finally, no assurance will be given about the confidentiality of that information. The patient does have the right to refuse to cooperate with the interview, although the consequences may be severe. For example, the court might order a remand in custody for failure to attend as an out-patient while on

---

Box 12.3 Policy for access to health records

1. The patient should be advised to make the request directly to the professionals responsible for the particular notes he wishes to see
2. No healthcare professional may give access to records written by another member of staff without prior consultation and agreement
3. The patient should be allowed to read the entry made by a particular member of staff in the presence of that member of staff. A photocopy of any entry or part-entry should be made available free of charge to the patient*
4. Where multiple entries have been made on one page, entries made by other professionals should be covered before the patient is allowed sight of the page
5. Reports written by third parties from other services or agencies should not be disclosed to the patient without the authors' consent
6. In the event of a member of staff having doubts about disclosure causing harm to a patient they should first consult with the RMO
7. Should any patient feel that their legal rights are not being satisfied, they should complain formally to the administration department and action should be taken to ensure that the patient's rights are met

* People applying under the Access to Health Records Act 1990 may be charged a fee

---

bail. In practice, most defendants are surprisingly cooperative, but if not it is important to consider whether lack of cooperation may be related to any psychiatric disorder.

At the beginning of any interview for a court report, it is important to tell the patient who you are, who requested you to see him, and the exact purpose of the interview and subsequent report, stressing that the latter will not be confidential. It is not uncommon for patients to express surprise at seeing a psychiatrist and they may wrongly assume that the purpose of the interview is solely to establish their sanity. Once any report has been sent to court there is no control over its distribution and reports may find their way into various places including prison records, probation and social services records, special hospitals and the Home Office. It is also important to remember that, if reports are used in evidence, they are not the property of one side or the other. Crown Court rules make provision for disclosure of expert evidence that may be used in court proceedings. Sensitive material may be included with the written qualification "not to be revealed in open court", but no guarantee can be given that this request will be respected. Whether a report has been requested by the prosecution or defence, the author should remember that the patient may be given a copy. He should, where possible, allow the patient to know the content of the report and advise him about protecting its confidentiality. Reference to identifiable relatives or victims should be avoided.

Psychiatric testimony

One of the most important tasks of a forensic psychiatrist is to provide psychiatric testimony to the courts: writing reports and giving evidence in courts. The latter may sometimes be as an "expert witness" (i.e. the witness is chosen because of his particular knowledge or because of some special feature of the case). Drife (1989) has argued that such experts may "have no reputation outside the lawyers' offices", yet what they say may be highly influential. This criticism strikes at the heart of legal work: it has a different function from clinical work and operates according to different rules and procedures. The difference between clinical and legal tasks raises ethical problems for the psychiatric witness, particularly in criminal cases (Stone, 1984; Chiswick, 1985). Three aspects of psychiatric testimony are mentioned here: what is said, how it is presented, and how it is obtained.

What is said

Psychiatric witnesses are asked to give evidence on matters outside their expertise and knowledge. The diagnosis of psychiatric disorders is the only task for which psychiatrists have unique skills, yet in court they answer questions about a person's responsibility for his actions (Chapter 5) and his dangerousness (Chapter 8). Some have argued that psychiatrists should restrict their opinions to clinical matters, and not give what the American literature calls "ultimate issue" testimony. This position is extremely difficult to maintain and may be unfair on the defendant. The psychiatrist whose ethical principles prevent him from answering questions about, say, diminished responsibility, should probably not be in the witness box.

On the other hand, so-called expert testimony on dangerousness may have far-reaching consequences for the defendant and his freedom. This need not be ethically unprincipled if the evidence concerns a psychiatric matter, such as the requirement for a restriction order under the Mental Health Act 1983, and if it is based on sound clinical assessment and knowledge. However, if the issue concerns the punishment (and in some countries this may be by the death penalty – see below) of a convicted person, the psychiatrist would do well to ask himself why he is there. The use by the courts of a psychiatrist to legitimise a decision they wish to take for punitive reasons should be resisted.

How it is presented

In clinical work, thorny questions (e.g. about a diagnosis) are commonly discussed in the setting of a case conference. There is a wide canvassing of all views. By contrast, courts operate in an adversarial climate. Each of two sides seeks to persuade judge and jury that his version of the truth is absolutely correct and the other side's is absolutely incorrect. Psychiatric witnesses are therefore required to adopt extreme positions or to give unwarranted importance to what may be a minor element of the clinical picture. In short, the witness is not employed to present a broad consideration of the case; he will not be thanked for pointing out the weaknesses of his own evidence – although the good witness will be all too aware of them. It may not sound impressive if he suggests that other experts might take a completely different view of things. Thus the adversarial nature of the proceedings encourages a degree of selectivity by the witness which conflicts with normal clinical practice.

How it is obtained

The most important ethical dilemma arises because the psychiatric examination of a defendant for the court takes place outside the normal doctor–patient relationship. The psychiatrist is hired by a third party (prosecution, defence or sentencer) to investigate and report. The defendant has been sent to him: he is not a patient who presents with symptoms seeking medical advice. Yet to carry out his task the psychiatrist relies on clinical skills to obtain information from the defendant. He tries to create rapport, as this will encourage self-revelation by the defendant and ultimately produce a better report. The psychiatrist then conveys that report to the agent who hired him and is paying him. In this situation, ethical obligations of the doctor to the patient can be forgotten.

It is necessary in court to be aware of all these ethical dilemmas. Defendants need to be informed why they are being examined, what will happen to the report, and should be given the opportunity to decline to be interviewed. Clinical opinions need to be based on accepted psychiatric knowledge; the tendency for idiosyncratic views and personal bias to creep into a report should be acknowledged. Stone (1984) described the risks of "prostituting" the profession by presenting psychiatric testimony that serves other purposes. He emphasised the need for ethical standards, scientific understanding, honesty, and adversarial debate.

Working with the police

Under certain circumstances the police may request information about a psychiatric patient during a criminal investigation. It would be ethical to disclose information to a senior investigating officer in the case of an investigation into a grave or very serious crime (homicide, grievous bodily harm, rape and similar crimes) where enquiries would be hampered if information were withheld. Any enquiry by a police officer about a patient should be referred to the patient's RMO or another consultant. Information should never be given over the telephone. The case notes or information contained within them should be disclosed only by a doctor and not by managers. Case notes should never be handed over unless there is a subpoena from the court, in which case they would go directly to the court and not to the police.

Working in prisons

Doctors working in prisons include full- and part-time medical officers and visiting psychiatrists. Bowden (1976) has described the ethical problems that arise from the dual role of the prison doctor towards the needs of the institution and the patient. Punishment and maintenance of discipline are the primary consideration of the governor, but these may be incompatible with promoting healthcare. For example, prison doctors are sometimes asked to collude with the system in certifying that a prisoner is fit for punishment.

Imprisonment means that individuals lose autonomy and certain rights. However, prisoners have the right to medical care of a standard available to the general population, that is, the standard provided by the NHS (Royal College of Psychiatrists, 1992*b*). This ideal is often compromised by appalling conditions in prisons, pointed out with regularity in reports by the Chief Inspector of Prisons (Her Majesty's Chief Inspector of Prisons for England and Wales, 1990), and also by the European Committee for the Prevention of Torture and Inhuman or Degrading Treatment (Harding, 1989). Remanded, but not convicted, prisoners have the right to consult a doctor (or dentist) of their choice. This is normally arranged through the individual's solicitor and with the assistance of the prison medical officer.

Consent to medication in prisons

It is important to remember that treatment cannot be given to prisoners without their consent. This is especially important with regard to acutely psychotic prisoners to whom the consent to treatment provisions of the Mental Health Act 1983 do not apply. Treatment can be given under common law in an emergency to prevent serious harm to the patient or others. If psychiatric treatment is required, a hospital rather than a prison is the proper setting, and psychiatric assessment with a view to transfer to hospital should be expedited.

Confidentiality in prisons

Doctors working in prisons have an ethical duty to keep independent, confidential medical records. In some prisons this is difficult because of organisational and storage problems, which are outside the control of the doctor. Visiting psychiatrists who work in prisons on a sessional basis experience similar problems. However, prison medical officers face additional ethical dilemmas; as appointees of the Directorate of Health Care Services for Prisoners, they have an obligation to disclose information about inmates in order to maintain their security and safety. Even so, personal health information should not be disclosed without consent, except in the interests of the prisoner on on a strict "need to know" basis. Prisoners have the same rights of access to their medical records as other citizens under the Access to Health Records Act 1990. The same standard of care with regard to protection of third party information applies.

Hunger strikes

The Declaration of Tokyo (World Psychiatric Association 1989) stated:

> "When a prisoner refuses nourishment and is considered by the doctor as capable of forming an unimpaired and rational judgement concerning the consequences of such a voluntary refusal of nourishment, he or she shall not be fed artificially. The decision as to the capacity of the prisoner to form such a judgement should be confirmed by at least one other independent doctor. The consequences of the refusal of nourishment shall be explained by the doctor to the prisoner."

It is important that the doctor explains the policy regarding resuscitation during hunger strikes to the prisoner at the beginning of the strike, and to respect the prisoner's wishes if these are known. In the case of an unconscious prisoner, or if the prisoner's intention is unknown, the doctor would be expected to use resuscitation. Prisoners who are on alleged hunger strike should be seen by a psychiatrist. They may refuse to eat and/or drink because they are mentally ill. In these cases, the appropriate action is to arrange speedy transfer to a psychiatric hospital under the provisions of Section 47 or 48 of the Mental Health Act 1983.

> **Case example 4**
> Within two weeks of a remand in custody following arrest for assault, a prisoner became mute and refused to eat or drink. He was referred for an urgent psychiatric opinion and was observed to be filthy, markedly dehydrated and inaccessible during an attempt to interview him. Enquiries revealed a previous psychiatric history with an admission for an acute psychotic illness. He was transferred to hospital under Section 48 the following day. Without any specific treatment, he began eating and drinking and started to express delusions of poisoning and persecution.

"Whistle-blowing"

All medical practitioners have not only a right but an ethical duty to disclose situations which they believe to be detrimental to the standards of care for their patients. This principle applies to psychiatrists working in NHS settings, in special hospitals and in prisons. Appropriate channels exist for making complaints, but recent guidelines from the Department of Health (NHS Management Executive, 1993) make it clear that there is a "gagging clause". Neither this nor the Official Secrets Act 1911 (which psychiatrists working in prisons are sometimes required to observe) should deter doctors from making disclosures. Both the BMA and the Royal College of Psychiatrists (1992*b*) record their policy to support and not discriminate against doctors who speak out about unacceptable standards of care. NHS hospitals and trusts may demand a duty of loyalty from all employees and attempt to enforce this by contract. This can cause real dilemmas for doctors and other health professionals in dealing with the conflict between contractual responsibilities and disclosure of information in the public interest (Greene & Cooper, 1992). The consequence of public disclosure was shown by the case of a nurse who was charged with a breach of confidentiality in 1990. He informed the media about his concern for the welfare of geriatric patients in a dangerously understaffed ward, and was subsequently dismissed.

Capital punishment

Psychiatrists as citizens may have personal views about the death penalty. However, for psychiatrists practising in countries which retain the death penalty there are also acute professional and ethical considerations. The issues have been extensively articulated in the US where 39 states currently retain the death penalty, mostly for first degree murder; nearly 3000 prisoners are on "death row". The UK (with the exceptions of the Isle of Man, and as a penalty for treason) has been without the death penalty since 1965.

The British Medical Association (1993) has said that medical ethics not only forbids the act of injecting a lethal substance but also any participation in the execution process; it also recommends that the medical certification of such deaths should take place away from the site of execution. In the US doctors have been involved in the gruesome task of monitoring executions to determine whether or not more electricity or gas was needed to complete the process.

The situation in the US is further complicated by certain constitutional requirements (Sadoff, 1990). Thus the death penalty can only be carried out if the condemned person is competent to be executed. He must understand the nature, purpose and extent of the punishment, and be able to instruct his lawyer on possible aspects of his case which would render the punishment unjust. Finally, many states have lists of mitigating or aggravating factors which respectively determine whether life imprisonment or execution should apply. In Texas, for example, the criterion of dangerousness is an automatic aggravating factor which, if present, is bound to lead to execution (see Chapter 8). In spite of opposition from the American Psychiatric Association, the Supreme Court has ruled that dangerousness testimony for this purpose is in order (Showalter, 1990).

The role of psychiatrists in the death penalty is therefore more extensive than might at first be appreciated. Although participation of psychiatrists in the death penalty has been condemned by the World Psychiatric Association (1989), much depends on what is meant by "participation". The Royal College of Psychiatrists (1992c) has resolved to support psychiatrists in conflict with the authorities concerning their involvement in the death penalty. It has produced guidelines which identify the stages at which psychiatrists might be involved (Box 12.4).

The ethical dilemmas are profound. Some psychiatrists would wish to have no involvement whatsoever with any case in which the death penalty was a possible outcome, although this might leave an insane defendant without a defence. In relation to the treatment of a condemned person, it would be reasonable to provide treatment which the person was able to accept on a voluntary basis. Compulsory treatment is more difficult. Should the psychotic condemned man be left untreated, or treated in the knowledge that it would hasten execution? It would seem unethical to provide treatment on the specific understanding that it is necessary in order to expedite the execution process. Psychiatrists should play no part in the execution process nor in certifying fitness for execution.

This brief discussion leads inevitably to the conclusion that, leaving aside personal views as citizens, most psychiatrists would find that the death penalty and professional ethics are incompatible. Many feel that psychiatric professional bodies should declare public opposition on clinical

---

Box 12.4 The death penalty: stages at which there might be psychiatric involvement

Legal proceedings before and during trial
- investigatory tasks
- assessment of fitness for trial
- assessments for the court to enable the appropriate verdict to be made

Post-sentencing stage
- treatment of the condemned person
- during the execution process
- confirmation of death

and ethical grounds (*Lancet,* 1993) on the basis that there is a limit to what the state can reasonably expect of its doctors. Studies of those awaiting execution make grim reading. Neuropsychiatric assessment of 14 juveniles (under the age of 18) on death row in the US found that nine had major neurological impairments, seven had previous episodes of psychosis, seven showed organic deficits, and only two had IQ scores greater than 90 (Lewis *et al,* 1988).

Working in secure environments

The greatest example of coercive medicine in Britain, and in many other countries, is in forensic psychiatry (Harding, 1986). It is fitting that the last words in this chapter, and indeed the book, should concern the ethics of practising psychiatry in a secure environment. Thousands of patients are detained in secure conditions so that they may receive psychiatric treatment. The scope for abuse is glaring, and detention has been shamelessly exploited throughout the world. The most infamous, and now admitted, examples have been in the former Soviet Union where political dissidents were certified mad and incarcerated under the "care" of psychiatrists in the most appalling conditions.

What Harding (1986) refers to as the "alliance" between state and psychiatry is the very reason why forensic psychiatry is at risk of exploitation. In Britain there is no political abuse of psychiatry; few would suggest it is government policy to manipulate, or intimidate, doctors into detaining healthy citizens on the grounds of their political beliefs. However, the historically institutional approach to forensic psychiatry in Britain has spawned abuse of patients on a large scale. A relentless series of inquiries in English special hospitals has revealed disgraceful standards, dehumanising practices and dismal management (Department of Health and Social Security, 1980; NHS Health Advisory Service and Social Services Inspectorate, 1988; Department of Health, 1992).

Some view with caution the burgeoning growth of the independent sector in providing secure psychiatric facilities. They fear that such units are ethically vulnerable because they accommodate patients who are often isolated hundreds of miles from their families. They have no ties with any particular catchment area and cannot provide the same commitment to aftercare as a regional secure unit. On the other hand, if they did not exist, their patients might well find themselves inappropriately in prisons or special hospitals. That they exist for profit may once have been anathema: in today's business-orientated health service it no longer has quite the same impact.

While the details differ, the breeding ground for abuse in forensic psychiatry is exactly as described in other mental hospital inquiries over the last 30 years (Martin, 1984). Remote institutions (professionally and/

or geographically), uncertainty of function, patients with few outside contacts, low staff morale, poor leadership, interdisciplinary rivalry – these are the elements of a sick institution.

Secure institutions, their patients and staff are all at risk, and the first priority is to achieve and maintain high clinical standards. It is impossible to have regard for ethics if clinical standards are poor. This applies to any hospital setting but the particular ethical responsibilities in secure environments may be summarised as:

(1) awareness of the special implications of treatment in security
(2) the need to review regularly the requirement for secure care
(3) particular regard for the patient's dignity and rights
(4) a duty to remain professionally well-informed
(5) good leadership within the clinical team.

In secure settings these issues must be kept alive. Isolation of a secure unit from colleagues, professionals in different disciplines, other agencies, and the community, is the single most important factor that permits clinical and hence ethical standards to fall. It is a question of whether or not the institution is a part of the wider psychiatric community.

References

Bernadt, M., Gunning, L. & Quenstedt, M. (1991) Patients' access to their own psychiatric records: the patients' view. *Journal of the Royal Society of Medicine*, **81**, 520–522.

Bowden, P. (1976) Medical practice: defendants and prisoners. *Journal of Medical Ethics*, **24**, 163–172.

British Medical Association (1989) *Medicine Betrayed: the Participation of Doctors in Human Rights Abuses*. Report of a working party. London: BMA Zed Books.

—— (1993) *Medical Ethics Today: Its Practice and Philosophy*. London: BMA.

Chiswick, D. (1985) Use and abuse of psychiatric testimony. *British Medical Journal*, **290**, 975–977.

Conference of Medical Royal Colleges and the Faculties in the UK (1992) Interim guidelines on confidentiality and medical audit. *Psychiatric Bulletin*, **16**, 243–245.

Cowley, R. (1994) *Access to Medical Records and Reports. A Practical Guide*. Oxford: Radcliffe Medical Press.

Department of Health (1991) *Local Research Ethics Committees*. London: DoH.

—— (1992) *Report of the Committee of Inquiry into Complaints about Ashworth Hospital*. Cm 2028-1-2. London: HMSO.

Department of Health and Social Security (1980) *Report of the Review of Rampton Hospital* (Boynton report). Cmnd 8073. London: HMSO.

Drife, J. O. (1989) Doctors, lawyers and experts. *British Medical Journal*, **299**, 716.

General Medical Council (1993) *Professional Conduct and Discipline: Fitness to Practise*. London: GMC.

Greene, D. & Cooper, J. (1992) Whistle blowers. *British Medical Journal*, **305**, 1343–1344.

Harding, T. W. (1986) "Treatment under Special Security": a special case of medical coercion. In *Institutions Observed,* pp. 158–164. London: King Edward's Hospital Fund for London.

—— (1989) Prevention of torture and inhuman or degrading treatment: medical implications of a new European convention. *Lancet*, 1191–1193.

Her Majesty's Chief Inspector of Prisons for England and Wales (1990) *Report of a Review of Suicide and Self-harm in Prison Service Establishments in England and Wales.* Cmnd 1383. London: HMSO.

Lancet (1993) Doctors and death row. Editorial. *Lancet*, **341**, 209–210.

Lewis, D. O., Pincus, J. H., Bard, B., *et al* (1988) Neuropsychiatric, psychoeducational, and family characteristics of 14 juveniles condemned to death in the United States. *American Journal of Psychiatry*, **145**, 584–589.

Martin, J. P. (1984) *Hospitals in Trouble.* Oxford: Basil Blackwell.

Medical Research Council (1985) *Responsibility in the Use of Personal Medical Information for Research. Principles and Guide to Practice.* London: MRC.

NHS Health Advisory Service and Social Services Inspectorate (1988) *Report on Services Provided by Broadmoor Hospital.* London: DHSS.

NHS Management Executive (1993) *Guidance for Staff on Relations with the Public and Media.* London: DoH.

Parrott, J., Strathdee, G. & Brown, P. (1988) Patient access to psychiatric records: the patients' view. *Journal of the Royal Society of Medicine*, **81**, 520–522.

Royal College of Psychiatrists (1990) Position statement on confidentiality. *Psychiatric Bulletin*, **14**, 97–109.

—— (1992*a*) Access to Health Records Act 1990. College guidance. *Psychiatric Bulletin*, **16**, 114–123.

—— (1992*b*) Ethical issues concerning psychiatric care in prison. Report from the Special Committee on Unethical Psychiatric Practices. *Psychiatric Bulletin*, **16**, 241–242.

—— (1992*c*) *Resolution Concerning the Participation of Psychiatrists in Executions.* London: Royal College of Psychiatrists

Sadoff, R. L. (1990) The role of the psychiatrist in capital punishment. *Journal of Forensic Psychiatry*, **1**, 73–80.

Showalter, C. R. (1990) Psychiatric participation in capital sentencing procedures: ethical considerations. *International Journal of Law and Psychiatry*, **13**, 261–280.

Stone, A. A. (1984) *Law, Psychiatry and Morality.* Washington: APA.

Tarasoff v Regents of the University of California (1976) 131 Cal Rptr 14.

The Times (1994) Law report. August 16.

World Psychiatric Association (1989) *Declaration on the Participation of Psychiatrists in the Death Penalty (Athens).* Athens: World Psychiatric Association.

W v Egdell (1990) 1 AC 109.

Index

Compiled by Caroline Sheard

Page numbers in italics refer to tables, figures and/or boxes.

347

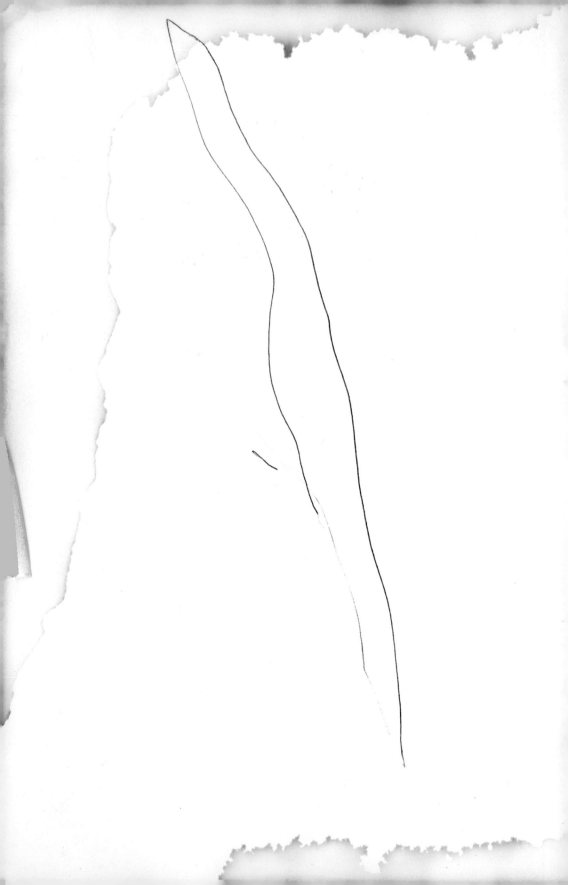